T0321070

IMMUNE SYSTEM DISORDERS

SOURCEBOOK

FIFTH EDITION

Health Reference Series

IMMUNE SYSTEM DISORDERS
SOURCEBOOK

FIFTH EDITION

Basic Consumer Health Information about Disorders of the Immune System, Including Immune System Function and Response, Diagnostic Tests for Immune Disorders, and Information about Primary and Secondary Immunodeficiency Diseases and Autoimmune Diseases, Such as Crohn's Disease, Pernicious Anemia, Antiphospholipid Syndrome, Behçet Disease, Lambert-Eaton Myasthenic Syndrome (LEMS), and Rheumatoid Arthritis (RA)

Along with Treatments for Immune System Disorders, Coping Tips for Immune Diseases, a Glossary of Immunology Terms, and a Directory of Organizations Related to Immune Disorders

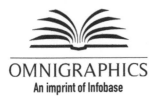

OMNIGRAPHICS
An imprint of Infobase

Bibliographic Note

Because this page cannot legibly accommodate all the copyright notices,
the Bibliographic Note portion of the Preface constitutes an extension
of the copyright notice.

* * *

OMNIGRAPHICS
An imprint of Infobase
132 W. 31st St.
New York, NY 10001
www.infobase.com
James Chambers, *Editorial Director*

* * *

Copyright © 2023 Infobase
ISBN 978-0-7808-2074-6
E-ISBN 978-0-7808-2075-3

Library of Congress Cataloging-in-Publication Data

Names: Chambers, James (Editor), editor.

Title: Immune system disorders sourcebook / edited by James Chambers.

Description: Fifth edition. | New York, NY: Omnigraphics, An imprint of Infobase, [2023] | Series:
Health reference series | Includes index. | Summary: "Provides basic consumer health information
about immune system function, diseases, diagnostic tests, treatments, and management of related
disorders. Includes index, glossary of related terms, and other resources"-- Provided by publisher.

Identifiers: LCCN 2023019335 (print) | LCCN 2023019336 (ebook) | ISBN 9780780820746 (library
binding) | ISBN 9780780820753 (ebook)

Subjects: LCSH: Immunologic diseases--Popular works.

Classification: LCC RC582 .I4626 2023   (print) | LCC RC582 (ebook) | DDC 616.97--dc23/
eng/20230527

LC record available at https://lccn.loc.gov/2023019335

LC ebook record available at https://lccn.loc.gov/2023019336

Table of Contents

Part 4. Autoimmune Diseases

Part 9. Additional Help and Information

Preface

ABOUT THIS BOOK

The body's immune system usually works efficiently to prevent diseases, but things can go wrong. Sometimes, dysfunctions result from inherited conditions. Sometimes, they are caused when bacteria or viruses, such as human immunodeficiency virus (HIV), slip past normal immune system defenses. Sometimes, for reasons poorly understood, the immune system begins to attack normal body cells. This can result in an autoimmune disease. The National Institute of Environmental Health Sciences (NIEHS) estimates that up to 24 million Americans suffer from autoimmune disease and that the prevalence is rising.

Immune System Disorders Sourcebook, Fifth Edition provides information about immune system function and related disorders. It discusses primary and secondary immunodeficiency diseases, hypersensitivity, cancer immunotherapy, and autoimmune diseases, including celiac disease, Behçet disease, systemic lupus erythematosus (SLE), and myasthenia gravis (MG). Moreover, it provides information on symptoms, diagnostic tests, drugs and therapies, coping tips for autoimmune and immune disorders, a glossary of immunology terms, and a directory of additional resources.

HOW TO USE THIS BOOK

This book is divided into parts and chapters. Parts focus on broad areas of interest. Chapters are devoted to single topics within a part.

Part 1: Overview of the Immune System provides a comprehensive understanding of how the immune system functions. It explores the immune response, tolerance, and the role of genetics and epigenetics in immunity. Additionally, it covers different vaccine types and their significance, major disorders of the immune system, including immunodeficiency diseases, allergies, autoimmune diseases, sepsis, and cancer. Furthermore, it discusses the impact of alcohol on immune function.

Part 2: Primary Immunodeficiency Diseases provides an in-depth overview of acquired immune system conditions that develop over time, rather than being present at birth. It covers the symptoms, signs, causes, care, and management of primary immunodeficiency diseases. The included diseases range from Ataxia-telangiectasia and Chédiak-Higashi syndrome to chronic granulomatous disease, common variable immunodeficiency, and severe combined immunodeficiency (SCID), famously known as "bubble boy disease."

Part 3: Secondary Immunodeficiency Diseases offers a comprehensive overview of the associated symptoms, treatments, and prevention measures. It explores conditions such as acquired immunodeficiency syndrome (AIDS), malnutrition and infection, and opportunistic infections including candidiasis, invasive cervical cancer (ICC), coccidioidomycosis, cytomegalovirus (CMV), and toxoplasmosis. Additionally, it delves into topics like chemotherapy-induced neutropenia and infections and cancer in transplant recipients.

Part 4: Autoimmune Diseases covers a wide range of autoimmune disorders affecting various parts of the body, including the intestinal tract, blood, blood vessels, connective tissues, bone, joints, eyes, glands, liver, kidneys, and skin. It explores specific diseases such as Crohn's disease, pernicious anemia, vasculitis, relapsing polychondritis, and primary biliary cholangitis (PBC), along with many others. Additionally, it includes discussions on symptoms, diagnosis, and management of these autoimmune disorders, providing a comprehensive overview of the topic.

Part 5: Hypersensitive Immune Responses delves into the concept of hypersensitivity, covering various types including anaphylaxis (type 1), blood transfusion reaction (type 2), serum sickness (type 3), and transplant rejection (type 4). It explores the causes, symptoms, treatments, and management strategies associated with these hypersensitive immune responses. It also provides insights into understanding and addressing these immune reactions.

Part 6: Diagnostic Tests for Immune Disorders provides information for individuals concerned about the complexities of diagnosing immune disorders. It covers the symptoms and diagnosis methods of immune system disorders, emphasizing how patients can actively contribute to an accurate diagnosis. The section provides information about commonly used tests, including allergy tests, genetic testing, immune assessment tests, and inflammatory markers.

Part 7: Drugs and Therapies for Immune Diseases and Disorders provides comprehensive information about different treatment modalities for immune diseases and disorders. It covers drug therapies, gene therapies, stem cell transplantation, and cancer immunotherapy. It also discusses specific treatments for allergies, autoimmune diseases, immune deficiencies, and cancer.

Part 8: Coping with Immune Diseases provides practical tips for individuals and families dealing with autoimmune or immune system diseases. It offers guidance on immunization recommendations, travel suggestions for those with immune disorders, and support for students with chronic illnesses.

Part 9: Additional Help and Information includes a glossary of immunology terms and a directory of organizations related to immune disorders.

BIBLIOGRAPHIC NOTE

This volume contains documents and excerpts from publications issued by the following U.S. government agencies: Centers for Disease Control and Prevention (CDC); Clinical Center (CC); ClinicalInfo; Genetic and Rare Diseases Information Center (GARD); MedlinePlus; National Cancer Institute (NCI); National Center for Complementary and Integrative Health (NCCIH); National Eye Institute (NEI); National Heart, Lung, and Blood Institute (NHLBI); National Human Genome Research Institute (NHGRI); National Institute of Allergy and Infectious Diseases (NIAID); National Institute of Arthritis and Musculoskeletal and Skin Diseases (NIAMS); National Institute of Diabetes, Digestive, and Kidney Diseases (NIDDK); National Institute of Environmental Health Sciences (NIEHS); National Institute of General Medical Sciences (NIGMS); National Institute of Mental Health (NIMH); National Institute of Neurological Disorders and Stroke (NINDS); National Institutes of Health (NIH); Office on Women's Health (OWH); Small Business Innovation Research (SBIR); Surveillance, Epidemiology, and End Results (SEER) Program; U.S. Department of Health and Human Services (HHS); and U.S. Food and Drug Administration (FDA).

It also contains original material prepared by Infobase and reviewed by medical consultants.

ABOUT THE *HEALTH REFERENCE SERIES*

The *Health Reference Series* is designed to provide basic medical information for patients, families, caregivers, and the general public. Each volume provides comprehensive coverage on a particular topic. This is especially important for people who may be dealing with a newly diagnosed disease or a chronic disorder in themselves or in a family member. People looking for preventive guidance, information about disease warning signs, medical statistics, and risk factors for health problems will also find answers to their questions in the *Health Reference Series*. The *Series*, however, is not intended to serve as a tool for diagnosing illness, in prescribing treatments, or as a substitute for the physician–patient relationship. All people concerned about medical symptoms or the possibility of disease are encouraged to seek professional care from an appropriate health-care provider.

A NOTE ABOUT SPELLING AND STYLE

Health Reference Series editors use *Stedman's Medical Dictionary* as an authority for questions related to the spelling of medical terms and *The Chicago Manual of Style* for questions related to grammatical structures, punctuation, and other editorial concerns. Consistent adherence is not always possible, however, because the individual volumes within the *Series* include many documents from a wide variety of different producers, and the editor's primary goal is to present material from each source as accurately as is possible. This sometimes means that information in different chapters or sections may follow other guidelines and alternate spelling authorities. For example, occasionally a copyright holder may require that eponymous terms be shown in possessive forms (Crohn's disease vs. Crohn disease) or that British spelling norms be retained (leukaemia vs. leukemia).

MEDICAL REVIEW

Infobase contracts with a team of qualified, senior medical professionals who serve as medical consultants for the *Health Reference Series*. As necessary, medical consultants review reprinted and originally written material for currency and accuracy. Medical consultation services are provided to the *Health Reference Series* editors by:

Dr. Vijayalakshmi, MBBS, DGO, MD
Dr. Senthil Selvan, MBBS, DCH, MD
Dr. K. Sivanandham, MBBS, DCH, MS (Research), PhD

HEALTH REFERENCE SERIES UPDATE POLICY

The inaugural book in the *Health Reference Series* was the first edition of *Cancer Sourcebook* published in 1989. Since then, the *Series* has been enthusiastically received by librarians and in the medical community. In order to maintain the standard of providing high-quality health information for the layperson, the editorial staff felt it was necessary to implement a policy of updating volumes when warranted.

Medical researchers have been making tremendous strides, and it is the purpose of the *Health Reference Series* to stay current with the most recent advances. Each decision to update a volume is made on an individual basis. Some of the considerations include how much new information is available and the feedback we receive from people who use the books. If there is a topic you would like to see added to the update list, or an area of medical concern you feel has not been adequately addressed, please write to: custserv@infobaselearning.com.

Part 1 | **An Overview of the Immune System**

Chapter 1 | Understanding the Immune System

WHAT IS THE IMMUNE SYSTEM?

The human immune system is a complex network of specialized cells, tissues, and organs that recognize and defend the body from foreign substances, primarily disease-causing microorganisms such as bacteria, viruses, parasites, and fungi. Granulocytes, macrophages, and T lymphocytes are examples of specialized cells. Organs and tissues of the immune system include the bone marrow, spleen, thymus, tonsils, mucous membranes, and skin. The lymphatic vessels of the immune system carry immune cells, which converge in lymph nodes found throughout the body. A swollen lymph node often indicates an active immune response to a foreign substance (refer to Figure 1.1).[1]

THE FUNCTION OF THE IMMUNE SYSTEM

The overall function of the immune system is to prevent or limit infection. An example of this principle is found in immune-compromised people, including those with genetic immune disorders, those with immune-debilitating infections such as human immunodeficiency virus (HIV), and even pregnant women, who are susceptible to a range of microbes that typically do not cause infection in healthy individuals.

---

[1] ClinicalInfo, "Glossary of HIV/AIDS-Related Terms," U.S. Department of Health and Human Services (HHS), March 29, 2021. Available online. URL: https://clinicalinfo.hiv.gov/sites/default/files/glossary/Glossary-English_HIVinfo.pdf. Accessed April 5, 2023.

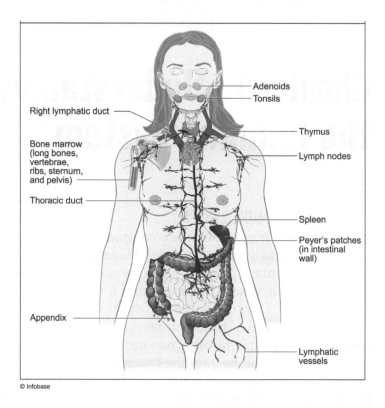

© Infobase

Figure 1.1. The Immune System

Infobase

The immune system can distinguish between normal, healthy cells and unhealthy cells by recognizing a variety of "danger" cues called "danger-associated molecular patterns" (DAMPs). Cells may be unhealthy because of infection or because of cellular damage caused by noninfectious agents such as sunburn or cancer. Infectious microbes such as viruses and bacteria release another set of signals recognized by the immune system called "pathogen-associated molecular patterns" (PAMPs).

When the immune system first recognizes these signals, it responds to address the problem. If an immune response cannot be activated when there is sufficient need, problems arise, such as infection. On the other hand, when an immune response is activated without a real threat or is not turned off once the danger passes, different problems arise, such as allergic reactions and autoimmune diseases.

The immune system is complex and pervasive. There are numerous cell types that either circulate throughout the body or reside in a particular tissue. Each cell type plays a unique role, with different ways of recognizing problems, communicating with other cells, and performing their functions. By understanding all the details behind this network, researchers may optimize immune responses to confront specific issues, ranging from infections to cancer.

CELLS OF THE IMMUNE SYSTEM

- **Granulocytes**. They include basophils, eosinophils, and neutrophils. Basophils and eosinophils are important for host defense against parasites. They are also involved in allergic reactions. Neutrophils, the most numerous innate immune cell, patrol for problems by circulating in the bloodstream. They can phagocytose, or ingest, bacteria, degrading them inside special compartments called "vesicles."
- **Mast cells**. These cells are also important for defense against parasites. Mast cells are found in tissues and can mediate allergic reactions by releasing inflammatory chemicals such as histamine.[2]
- **Monocytes**. A type of immune cell that is made in the bone marrow and travels through the blood to tissues in the body where it becomes a macrophage or a dendritic cell (DC). Macrophages surround and kill microorganisms, ingest foreign material, remove dead cells, and boost immune responses. During inflammation, DCs boost immune responses by showing antigens on their surface to other cells of the immune system.[3]

---

[2] "Overview of the Immune System," National Institute of Allergy and Infectious Diseases (NIAID), December 30, 2013. Available online. URL: www.niaid.nih.gov/research/immune-system-overview. Accessed April 5, 2023.
[3] "Monocyte," National Cancer Institute (NCI), June 30, 2020. Available online. URL: www.cancer.gov/publications/dictionaries/cancer-terms/def/monocyte. Accessed April 5, 2023.

- **DCs**. These cells are important antigen-presenting cells (APCs), and they can also develop from monocytes. Antigens are molecules from pathogens, host cells, and allergens that may be recognized by adaptive immune cells. APCs such as DCs are responsible for processing large molecules into "readable" fragments (antigens) recognized by adaptive B or T cells. However, antigens alone cannot activate T cells. They must be presented with the appropriate major histocompatibility complex (MHC) expressed on the APC. MHC provides a checkpoint and helps immune cells distinguish between host and foreign cells.
- **Natural killer (NK) cells**. These cells have features of both innate and adaptive immunity. They are important for recognizing and killing virus-infected cells or tumor cells. They contain intracellular compartments called "granules," which are filled with proteins that can form holes in the target cell and also cause apoptosis, the process of programmed cell death. It is important to distinguish between apoptosis and other forms of cell-death-like necrosis. Apoptosis, unlike necrosis, does not release danger signals that can lead to greater immune activation and inflammation. Through apoptosis, immune cells can discreetly remove infected cells and limit bystander damage. Nowadays, researchers have shown in mouse models that NK cells, such as adaptive cells, can be retained as memory cells and respond to subsequent infections by the same pathogen.

Adaptive Cells

- **B cells**. These cells have two major functions. They present antigens to T cells, and more importantly, they produce antibodies to neutralize infectious microbes. Antibodies coat the surface of a pathogen and serve three major roles: neutralization, opsonization, and complement activation. Neutralization occurs when the pathogen, because it is covered in antibodies, is unable to bind and infect host cells. In opsonization, an antibody-bound pathogen serves as a red flag to alert immune cells, such as neutrophils and macrophages, to engulf and digest the pathogen. Complement is a process for directly destroying, or lysing, bacteria.

Antibodies are expressed in two ways. The B-cell receptor (BCR), which sits on the surface of a B cell, is actually an antibody. B cells also secrete antibodies to diffuse and bind to pathogens. This dual expression is important because the initial problem—for instance, a bacterium—is recognized by a unique BCR and activates the B cell. The activated B cell responds by secreting antibodies, essentially the BCR but in soluble form. This ensures that the response is specific against the bacterium that started the whole process. Every antibody is unique, but they fall under general categories: IgM, IgD, IgG, IgA, and IgE. (Ig is short for "immunoglobulin," which is another word for antibody.) While they have overlapping roles, IgM generally is important for complement activation; IgD is involved in activating basophils; IgG is important for neutralization, opsonization, and complement activation; IgA is essential for neutralization in the gastrointestinal tract; and IgE is necessary for activating mast cells in parasitic and allergic responses.

- **T cells**. These cells have a variety of roles and are classified by subsets. T cells are divided into two broad categories: cluster of differentiation 8+ (CD8+) T cells or cluster of differentiation 4+ (CD4+) T cells, based on which protein is present on the cell's surface. T cells carry out multiple functions, including killing infected cells and activating or recruiting other immune cells.
  - CD8+ T cells are also called "cytotoxic T cells" or "cytotoxic lymphocytes" (CTLs). They are crucial for recognizing and removing virus-infected cells and cancer cells. CTLs have specialized compartments, or granules, containing cytotoxins that cause apoptosis, which is programmed cell death. Because of its

7

potency, the release of granules is tightly regulated by the immune system.

- The four major CD4$^+$ T-cell subsets are T_H1, T_H2, T_H17, and regulatory T cells (Treg), with "T_H" referring to "T-helper cell." T_H1 cells are critical for coordinating immune responses against intracellular microbes, especially bacteria. They produce and secrete molecules that alert and activate other immune cells, such as bacteria-ingesting macrophages. T_H2 cells are important for coordinating immune responses against extracellular pathogens, such as helminths (parasitic worms), by alerting B cells, granulocytes, and mast cells. T_H17 cells are named for their ability to produce interleukin 17 (IL-17), a signaling molecule that activates immune and nonimmune cells. T_H17 cells are important for recruiting neutrophils.
- As the name suggests, Tregs monitor and inhibit the activity of other T cells. They prevent adverse immune activation and maintain tolerance or the prevention of immune responses against the body's own cells and antigens.[4]

ORGANS OF THE IMMUNE SYSTEM

Lymphoid organs are an essential part of the immune system and are responsible for producing immune cells such as B and T lymphocytes. These organs are dispersed throughout the body and play a vital role in immune function. Injury or dysfunction to these organs can lead to a weakened immune response and increased susceptibility to infection.[5] Lymphoid organs are classified into three categories: primary, secondary, and tertiary. Primary lymphoid organs contain the bone marrow and thymus. Secondary lymphoid organs contain lymph nodes, spleen, mucous-associated

---

[4] See footnote [2].
[5] "Immune Response to Traumatic Injury: Harmony and Discordance of Immune System Homeostasis," National Center for Biotechnology Information (NCBI), January 28, 2014. Available online. URL: www.ncbi.nlm.nih.gov/pmc/articles/PMC5997205. Accessed April 17, 2023.

lymphoid tissue, and tonsils. Tertiary lymphoid organs (TLOs) exhibit structural and functional similarities to secondary lymphoid organs.[6] Lymphoid organs are essential to the body's immune system and important for overall health.[7]

Primary Lymphoid Organs

Primary lymphoid organs are specialized tissues responsible for developing and maturing immune cells, especially lymphocytes, a type of white blood cell (WBC) involved in the immune response. The bone marrow and thymus form the primary lymphoid organs. Immature B and T lymphocytes are produced in the bone marrow. The B lymphocytes attain maturity in the bone marrow and are accountable for producing antibodies. Immature T lymphocytes in the bone marrow migrate to the thymus gland and undergo the process of maturation and differentiation.[8] The mature T lymphocytes help identify and destroy the infected cells. The matured B and T lymphocytes migrate to the secondary lymphoid organs, such as the lymph nodes and spleen, where the invading pathogens are recognized and eliminated. Primary lymphoid organs are necessary for producing active immune cells that help defend the body from diseases and infections.[9]

BONE MARROW

Bone marrow is the spongy tissue inside some of your bones, such as your hip and thigh bones. It contains stem cells. The stem cells can develop into the red blood cells that carry oxygen through your

[6] "Role of Tertiary Lymphoid Organs in the Regulation of Immune Responses in the Periphery," SpringerLink, June 11, 2022. Available online. URL: https://link.springer.com/article/10.1007/s00018-022-04388-x. Accessed June 8, 2023.

[7] "What Are the Organs of the Immune System?" National Center for Biotechnology Information (NCBI), July 30, 2020. Available online. URL: www.ncbi.nlm.nih.gov/books/NBK279395. Accessed April 17, 2023.

[8] "Parts of the Immune System," Children's Hospital of Philadelphia (CHOP), April 22, 2019. Available online. URL: www.chop.edu/centers-programs/vaccine-education-center/human-immune-system/parts-immune-system. Accessed April 17, 2023.

[9] "Lymphocyte," National Human Genome Research Institute (NHGRI), April 14, 2023. Available online. URL: www.genome.gov/genetics-glossary/Lymphocyte. Accessed April 17, 2023.

body, the WBCs that fight infections, and the platelets that help with blood clotting.[10]

THYMUS

The thymus is a soft organ with two lobes that is located anterior to the ascending aorta and posterior to the sternum. It is relatively large in infants and children, but after puberty, it begins to decrease in size so that in older adults it is quite small.

The primary function of the thymus is the processing and maturation of special lymphocytes called "T lymphocytes" or "T cells." While in the thymus, the lymphocytes do not respond to pathogens and foreign agents. After the lymphocytes have matured, they enter the blood and go to other lymphatic organs where they help provide defense against disease. The thymus also produces a hormone, thymosin, which stimulates the maturation of lymphocytes in other lymphatic organs.[11]

Secondary Lymphoid Organs

Secondary lymphoid organs are specialized tissues that activate T and B lymphocytes in response to foreign pathogens. Secondary lymphoid organs are lymph nodes, spleen, mucous-associated lymphoid tissue, and tonsils.[12] The lymph nodes are distributed throughout the body and aid in identifying, trapping, and destroying foreign bodies, such as bacteria and viruses. The spleen in the left hypochondriac region of the abdomen activates immune cells in response to foreign bodies and removes the malformed and old red blood cells from circulation. Tonsils in the throat protect the body against infection and filter out pathogens entering the body

---

[10] MedlinePlus, "Bone Marrow Diseases," National Institutes of Health (NIH), June 2, 2016. Available online. URL: https://medlineplus.gov/bonemarrowdiseases.html. Accessed April 5, 2023.
[11] Surveillance, Epidemiology, and End Results (SEER) Program, "Components of the Lymphatic System," National Cancer Institute (NCI), June 3, 2002. Available online. URL: https://training.seer.cancer.gov/anatomy/lymphatic/components. Accessed April 5, 2023.
[12] See footnote [7].

through the nose and mouth.[13] Mucosa-associated lymphoid tissue protects the body from pathogens that enter through mucosal surfaces, such as the digestive, respiratory, and genitourinary tracts. These organs play a vital role in mounting an effective immune response against foreign invaders and create immunological memory to recognize and respond instantly to previously encountered pathogens.[14]

LYMPH NODE

It is a small bean-shaped structure that is part of the body's immune system. Lymph nodes filter substances that travel through the lymphatic fluid, and they contain lymphocytes (WBCs) that help the body fight infection and disease. There are hundreds of lymph nodes found throughout the body. They are connected to one another by lymph vessels. Clusters of lymph nodes are found in the neck, axilla (underarm), chest, abdomen, and groin. For example, there are about 20–40 lymph nodes in the axilla, also called the "lymph gland."[15]

MUCOUS MEMBRANE

This is the moist, inner lining of some organs and body cavities (such as the nose, mouth, lungs, and stomach). Glands in the mucous membrane make mucus (a thick, slippery fluid), also called "mucosa."[16]

The types of mucous-associated lymphoid tissues are classified based on the mucosal lining of a particular organ, and they are as follows:
- gut-associated lymphoid tissue
- bronchus-associated lymphoid tissue

---

[13] "Lymphatic System," Cleveland Clinic, February 23, 2020. Available online. URL: https://my.clevelandclinic.org/health/articles/21199-lymphatic-system. Accessed April 17, 2023.
[14] "Basic Knowledge of Immunology," ScienceDirect, 2016. Available online. URL: www.sciencedirect.com/science/article/pii/B9780128499030000026. Accessed April 17, 2023.
[15] "Lymph Node," National Cancer Institute (NCI), February 3, 2009. Available online. URL: www.cancer.gov/publications/dictionaries/cancer-terms/def/lymph-node. Accessed April 5, 2023.
[16] "Mucous Membrane," National Cancer Institute (NCI), April 3, 2017. Available online. URL: www.cancer.gov/publications/dictionaries/cancer-terms/def/mucous-membrane. Accessed April 5, 2023.

- nasal-associated lymphoid tissue
- skin-associated lymphoid tissue
- vulvovaginal-associated lymphoid tissue[17]

SPLEEN

The spleen is located in the upper left abdominal cavity, just beneath the diaphragm, and posterior to the stomach. It is similar to a lymph node in shape and structure, but it is much larger. The spleen is the largest lymphatic organ in the body. Surrounded by a connective tissue capsule, which extends inward to divide the organ into lobules, the spleen consists of two types of tissue called "white pulp" and "red pulp." The white pulp is lymphatic tissue consisting mainly of lymphocytes around arteries. The red pulp consists of venous sinuses filled with blood and cords of lymphatic cells, such as lymphocytes and macrophages. Blood enters the spleen through the splenic artery, moves through the sinuses where it is filtered, and then leaves through the splenic vein.

The spleen filters blood in much the way that the lymph nodes filter lymph. Lymphocytes in the spleen react to pathogens in the blood and attempt to destroy them. Macrophages then engulf the resulting debris, the damaged cells, and the other large particles. The spleen, along with the liver, removes old and damaged erythrocytes from the circulating blood. Like other lymphatic tissue, it produces lymphocytes, especially in response to invading pathogens. The sinuses in the spleen are a reservoir for blood. In emergencies such as hemorrhage, smooth muscle in the vessel walls and in the capsule of the spleen contracts. This squeezes the blood out of the spleen into general circulation.

TONSILS

Tonsils are clusters of lymphatic tissue just under the mucous membranes that line the nose, mouth, and throat (pharynx). There are three groups of tonsils. The pharyngeal tonsils are located near the opening of the nasal cavity into the pharynx. The palatine tonsils

[17] "Mucosa-Associated Lymphoid Tissue Lymphomas (MALTomas)," Medscape, January 21, 2022. Available online. URL: https://emedicine.medscape.com/article/207891-overview. Accessed March 29, 2023.

are the ones that are located near the opening of the oral cavity into the pharynx. Lingual tonsils are located on the posterior surface of the tongue, which also places them near the opening of the oral cavity into the pharynx. Lymphocytes and macrophages in the tonsils provide protection against harmful substances and pathogens that may enter the body through the nose or mouth.

Tertiary Lymphoid Organs

TLOs are lymph-node-like structures that form in tissues in the presence of chronic inflammation in response to molecular and pathological damage from exposures (both internal and external). TLOs are found within almost all tumors and may play a critical gatekeeping role in the ability of T cells to access the tumor microenvironment and participate in immune surveillance.[18]

CELL COMMUNICATION

Immune cells communicate in a number of ways, either by cell-to-cell contact or through secreted signaling molecules. Receptors and ligands are fundamental to cellular communication. Receptors are protein structures that may be expressed on the surface of a cell or in intracellular compartments. The molecules that activate receptors are called "ligands," which may be free-floating or membrane-bound.

Ligand–receptor interaction leads to a series of events inside the cell involving networks of intracellular molecules that relay the message. By altering the expression and density of various receptors and ligands, immune cells can dispatch specific instructions tailored to the situation at hand.

Cytokines are small proteins with diverse functions. In immunity, the following are a few categories of cytokines important for immune cell growth, activation, and function:
- Colony-stimulating factors are essential for cell development and differentiation.

---

[18] Small Business Innovation Research (SBIR) and Small Business Technology Transfer (STTR), "Next Generation 3D Tissue Culture Systems with Tertiary Lymphoid Organs," Small Business Administration (SBA), October 19, 2020. Available online. URL: www.sbir.gov/node/1710183. Accessed April 5, 2023.

- Interferons are necessary for immune cell activation. Type I interferons mediate antiviral immune responses, and type II interferons are important for antibacterial responses.
- Interleukins, which come in over 30 varieties, provide context-specific instructions, with activating or inhibitory responses.
- Chemokines are made in specific locations of the body or at a site of infection to attract immune cells. Different chemokines will recruit different immune cells to the site needed.
- The tumor necrosis factor (TNF) family of cytokines stimulates immune cell proliferation and activation. They are critical for activating inflammatory responses, and as such, TNF blockers are used to treat a variety of disorders, including some autoimmune diseases.

Toll-like receptors (TLRs) are expressed on innate immune cells, such as macrophages and DCs. They are located on the cell surface or in intracellular compartments because microbes may be found in the body or inside infected cells. TLRs recognize general microbial patterns, and they are essential for innate immune cell activation and inflammatory responses.

BCRs and T-cell receptors (TCRs) are expressed on adaptive immune cells. They both are found on the cell surface, but BCRs are also secreted as antibodies to neutralize pathogens. The genes for BCRs and TCRs are randomly rearranged at specific cell maturation stages, resulting in unique receptors that may potentially recognize anything. Random generation of receptors allows the immune system to respond to unforeseen problems. They also explain why memory B or T cells are highly specific and, upon reencountering their specific pathogen, can immediately induce a neutralizing immune response.

MHC, or human leukocyte antigen (HLA), proteins serve two general roles. MHC proteins function as carriers to present antigens on cell surfaces. MHC class I proteins are essential for presenting viral antigens and are expressed by nearly all cell types, except red blood cells. Any cell infected by a virus has the ability to signal the problem through MHC class I proteins. In response, CD8$^+$ T cells (also called "CTLs") will recognize and kill infected cells. MHC class II proteins are generally only expressed by APCs such as DCs and macrophages. MHC class II proteins are important for presenting antigens to CD4$^+$ T cells. MHC class II antigens are varied and include both pathogen- and host-derived molecules.

MHC proteins also signal whether a cell is a host cell or a foreign cell. They are very diverse, and every person has a unique set of MHC proteins inherited from his or her parents. As such, there are similarities in MHC proteins between family members. Immune cells use MHC to determine whether a cell is friendly or not. In organ transplantation, the MHC or HLA proteins of donors and recipients are matched to lower the risk of transplant rejection, which occurs when the recipient's immune system attacks the donor tissue or organ. In stem cell or bone marrow transplantation, improper MHC or HLA matching can result in graft versus host disease, which occurs when the donor cells attack the recipient's body.

Complement refers to a unique process that clears away pathogens or dying cells and also activates immune cells. Complement consists of a series of proteins found in the blood that form a membrane attack complex. Complement proteins are only activated by enzymes when a problem, such as an infection, occurs. Activated complement proteins stick to a pathogen, recruiting and activating additional complement proteins, which assemble in a specific order to form a round pore or hole. Complement literally punches small holes into the pathogen, creating leaks that lead to cell death. Complement proteins also serve as signaling molecules that alert immune cells and recruit them to the problem area.[19]

---

[19] See footnote [2].

Chapter 2 | **Immune Response and Tolerance**

An immune response is generally divided into innate and adaptive immunity. Innate immunity occurs immediately when circulating innate cells recognize a problem. Adaptive immunity occurs later, as it relies on the coordination and expansion of specific adaptive immune cells. Immune memory follows the adaptive response when mature adaptive cells, highly specific to the original pathogen, are retained for later use.

INNATE IMMUNITY

Innate immune cells express genetically encoded receptors, called "toll-like receptors" (TLRs), which recognize general danger- or pathogen-associated patterns. Collectively, these receptors can broadly recognize viruses, bacteria, fungi, and even noninfectious problems. However, they cannot distinguish between specific strains of bacteria or viruses.

There are numerous types of innate immune cells with specialized functions. They include neutrophils, eosinophils, basophils, mast cells, monocytes, dendritic cells, and macrophages. Their main feature is the ability to respond quickly and broadly when a problem arises, typically leading to inflammation. Innate immune cells are also important for activating adaptive immunity. Innate cells are critical for host defense, and disorders in innate cell function may cause chronic susceptibility to infection.

ADAPTIVE IMMUNITY

Adaptive immune cells are more specialized, with each adaptive B or T cell bearing unique receptors, B-cell receptors (BCRs) and T-cell receptors (TCRs), that recognize specific signals rather than general patterns. Each receptor recognizes an antigen, which is simply any molecule that may bind to a BCR or TCR. Antigens are derived from a variety of sources including pathogens, host cells, and allergens. Antigens are typically processed by innate immune cells and presented to adaptive cells in the lymph nodes.

The genes for BCRs and TCRs are randomly rearranged at specific cell maturation stages, resulting in unique receptors that may potentially recognize anything. Random generation of receptors allows the immune system to respond to new or unforeseen problems. This concept is especially important because environments may frequently change, for instance, when seasons change or a person relocates, and pathogens are constantly evolving to survive. Because BCRs and TCRs are so specific, adaptive cells may only recognize one strain of a particular pathogen, unlike innate cells, which recognize broad classes of pathogens. In fact, a group of adaptive cells that recognize the same strain will likely recognize different areas of that pathogen.

If a B or T cell has a receptor that recognizes an antigen from a pathogen and also receives cues from innate cells that something is wrong, the B or T cell will activate, divide, and disperse to address the problem. B cells make antibodies, which neutralize pathogens, rendering them harmless. T cells carry out multiple functions, including killing infected cells and activating or recruiting other immune cells. The adaptive response has a system of checks and balances to prevent unnecessary activation that could cause damage to the host. If a B or T cell is autoreactive, meaning its receptor recognizes antigens from the body's own cells, the cell will be deleted. Also, if a B or T cell does not receive signals from innate cells, it will not be optimally activated.

Immune memory is a feature of the adaptive immune response. After B or T cells are activated, they expand rapidly. As the problem resolves, cells stop dividing and are retained in the body as memory cells. The next time this same pathogen enters the body, a memory cell is already poised to react and can clear away the pathogen before it establishes itself.

IMMUNE TOLERANCE

Tolerance is the prevention of an immune response against a particular antigen. For instance, the immune system is generally tolerant of self-antigens, so it does not usually attack the body's own cells, tissues, and organs. However, when tolerance is lost, disorders such as autoimmune disease or food allergy may occur. Tolerance is maintained in a number of ways:

- When adaptive immune cells mature, there are several checkpoints in place to eliminate autoreactive cells. If a B cell produces antibodies that strongly recognize host cells or if a T cell strongly recognizes self-antigen, they are deleted.
- Nevertheless, there are autoreactive immune cells present in healthy individuals. Autoreactive immune cells are kept in a nonreactive, or anergic, state. Even though they recognize the body's own cells, they do not have the ability to react and cannot cause host damage.
- Regulatory immune cells circulate throughout the body to maintain tolerance. Besides limiting autoreactive cells, regulatory cells are important for turning an immune response off after the problem is resolved. They can act as drains, depleting areas of essential nutrients that surrounding immune cells need for activation or survival.
- Some locations in the body are called "immunologically privileged sites." These areas, such as the eye and brain, do not typically elicit strong immune responses. Part of this is because of physical barriers, such as the blood-brain barrier, that limit the degree to which immune cells may enter. These areas may also express higher levels of suppressive cytokines to prevent a robust immune response.

Fetomaternal tolerance is the prevention of a maternal immune response against a developing fetus. Major histocompatibility complex (MHC) proteins help the immune system distinguish between host and foreign cells. MHC is also called "human leukocyte antigen" (HLA). By expressing paternal MHC or HLA proteins and paternal antigens, a fetus can potentially trigger the mother's immune system. However, there are several barriers that may prevent this from occurring: The placenta reduces the exposure of the fetus to maternal immune cells; the proteins expressed on the outer layer of the placenta may limit immune recognition; and regulatory cells and suppressive signals may play a role.[1]

[1] "Immune System Research—Features of an Immune Response," National Institute of Allergy and Infectious Diseases (NIAID), January 16, 2014. Available online. URL: www.niaid.nih.gov/research/immune-response-features. Accessed May 9, 2023.

Chapter 3 | Vaccines and Immunity

Chapter Contents

Section 3.1 | Understanding Vaccines and Immunity

WHAT ARE VACCINES, AND HOW DO THEY WORK?

Vaccines are injections (shots), liquids, pills, or nasal sprays that help your immune system fight infections faster and more effectively. When you get a vaccine, it sparks your immune response, helping your body fight off and remember the germ, so it can attack it if the germ ever invades again. And since vaccines are made of very small amounts of weak or dead germs, they would not make you sick. Vaccines often provide long-lasting immunity to serious diseases without the risk of serious illness.

Before a vaccine is recommended for use in the United States, the Food and Drug Administration (FDA) makes sure that it works—and that it is safe. Since vaccines were invented, the number of babies and adults who get sick or die from vaccine-preventable diseases has gone way down—and some diseases have been wiped out altogether in the United States.

VACCINE INGREDIENTS

Today's vaccines use only the ingredients they need to be safe and effective. Each ingredient in a vaccine serves a specific purpose. For example, vaccine ingredients may:

- help provide immunity (protection) against a specific disease
- help keep the vaccine safe and long-lasting
- be used during the production of the vaccine

Ingredients Provide Immunity

Vaccines include ingredients to help your immune system respond and build immunity to a specific disease. The following are a few examples:

- Antigens are very small amounts of weak or dead germs that can cause diseases. They help your immune system learn how to fight off infections faster and more effectively. The flu virus is an example of an antigen.

23

- Adjuvants, which are in some vaccines, are substances that help your immune system respond more strongly to a vaccine. This increases your immunity against the disease. Aluminum is an example of an adjuvant.

Ingredients Keep Vaccines Safe and Long-Lasting

Some ingredients help make sure a vaccine continues to work like it is supposed to and that it stays free of outside germs and bacteria. The following are a few examples:

- **Preservatives, such as thimerosal**. They protect the vaccine from outside bacteria or fungi. Nowadays, preservatives are usually only used in vials (containers) of vaccines that have more than one dose. That is because, every time an individual dose is taken from the vial, it is possible for harmful germs to get inside. Most vaccines are also available in single-dose vials and do not have preservatives in them.
- **Stabilizers, such as sugar or gelatin**. These ingredients help the active ingredients in vaccines continue to work while the vaccine is made, stored, and moved. Stabilizers keep the active ingredients in vaccines from changing because of something such as a shift in temperature where the vaccine is being stored.

Ingredients Are Used during the Production of Vaccines

Some ingredients that are needed to produce the vaccine are no longer needed for the vaccine to work in a person.

These ingredients are taken out after production, so only tiny amounts are left in the final product. The very small amounts of these ingredients that remain in the final product are not harmful. Examples of ingredients used in some vaccines include the following:

- cell culture (growth) material, such as eggs, to help grow the vaccine antigens
- inactivating (germ-killing) ingredients, such as formaldehyde, to weaken or kill viruses, bacteria, or toxins in the vaccine

- antibiotics, such as neomycin, to help keep outside germs and bacteria from growing in the vaccine[1]

VACCINES ARE SAFE

Before a new vaccine is ever given to people, extensive lab testing is done. Once testing in people begins, it can still take years before clinical studies are complete and the vaccine is licensed.

After a vaccine is licensed, the FDA, the Centers for Disease Control and Prevention (CDC), the National Institutes of Health (NIH), and other federal agencies continue routine monitoring and investigate any potential safety concerns.[2]

VACCINE SIDE EFFECTS

Most people do not have any serious side effects from vaccines. The most common side effects—such as soreness where the shot was given—are usually mild and go away quickly on their own.

What Are the Common Side Effects of Vaccines?

The most common side effects after vaccination are mild. They include:

- pain, swelling, or redness where the shot was given
- mild fever
- chills
- feeling tired
- headache
- muscle and joint aches

Fainting can also happen after any medical procedure, including vaccinations.

Keep in mind that most common side effects are a sign that your body is starting to build immunity (protection) against a disease.

---

[1] "Vaccine Basics," U.S. Department of Health and Human Services (HHS), November 9, 2022. Available online. URL: www.hhs.gov/immunization/basics/index.html. Accessed April 19, 2023.
[2] "Making the Vaccine Decision: Addressing Common Concerns," Centers for Disease Control and Prevention (CDC), March 7, 2023. Available online. URL: www.cdc.gov/vaccines/parents/why-vaccinate/vaccine-decision.html. Accessed April 19, 2023.

What about Serious Side Effects?

Serious side effects from vaccines are extremely rare. For example, if 1 million doses of a vaccine are given, one to two people may have a severe allergic reaction.

Signs of a severe allergic reaction can include:
- difficulty breathing
- swelling of your face and throat
- a fast heartbeat
- a bad rash all over your body
- dizziness and weakness

If you experience a severe allergic reaction, call 911 or go to the nearest hospital. Call your vaccination provider or your health-care provider if you have any side effects that bother you or do not go away. Report any potential side effects experienced from vaccination to the Vaccine Adverse Event Reporting System (VAERS), a program comanaged by the CDC and the FDA to ensure that all recommended vaccines remain safe.

Keep in mind that getting vaccinated is much safer than getting the diseases vaccines prevent.

What If You Feel Sick after Getting Vaccinated?

Talk with your doctor if you are concerned about your health after getting vaccinated. You or your doctor can choose to report the side effect to the VAERS.

In the very rare event that a vaccine causes a serious problem, the National Vaccine Injury Compensation Program (VICP) may offer financial help to individuals who file a petition. The Countermeasure Injury Compensation Program (CICP) may help pay for the costs of medical care and other expenses for people seriously injured from a COVID-19 vaccine.[3]

---

[3] See footnote [1].

WHAT IS A VACCINE SCHEDULE?

A vaccine, or immunization, schedule lists which vaccines are recommended for different groups of people. It includes who should get the vaccines, how many doses they need, and when they should get them. In the United States, the CDC publishes the vaccine schedule. It is important for both children and adults to get their vaccines according to the schedule. Following the schedule allows them to get protection from diseases at exactly the right time.[4]

VACCINES REQUIRE MORE THAN ONE DOSE

The following are four reasons that babies—and even teens or adults—who receive a vaccine for the first time may need more than one dose:

- For some vaccines (primarily nonlive vaccines), the first dose does not provide as much protection as possible. Therefore, more than one dose is needed to build more complete immunity. For example, the *Haemophilus influenzae* type b (Hib) vaccine that protects young children against meningitis requires two or three doses depending on the manufacturer.
- For some vaccines, protection begins to wear off over time. At that point, a "booster" dose is needed to bring protection levels backup. This booster dose usually occurs several years after the initial series of vaccine doses is given. For example, the diphtheria, tetanus, and pertussis (DTaP) vaccine requires the initial series of four shots for an infant to build protection against diphtheria, tetanus, and pertussis. But a booster dose is needed at four to six years old. Another booster against these diseases is needed at 11 or 12 years of age. This booster is called "Tdap."
- For some vaccines (primarily live vaccines), more than one dose is needed for everyone to develop the best protection. For example, after one dose of the measles,

---

[4] MedlinePlus, "Vaccines," National Institutes of Health (NIH), February 22, 2022. Available online. URL: https://medlineplus.gov/vaccines.html. Accessed April 19, 2023.

mumps, and rubella (MMR) vaccine, some people may not develop enough antibodies to fight off infection. The second dose helps make sure that almost everyone is protected.

- Finally, in the case of flu vaccines, everyone six months and older needs to get a dose every year because each year different flu viruses can be circulating and protection from a flu vaccine wears off with time. Children six months to eight years old will need to get two doses the first time they get the flu vaccine, or if they only got one dose in previous years, they should get two doses during the current year.[5]

COMBINATION VACCINES
Fewer Shots but the Same Protection

Combination vaccines reduce the number of shots your child needs while protecting against the same number of serious diseases. Combination vaccines take two or more vaccines that could be given individually and put them into one shot. Therefore, at a doctor's visit, your child may only get two or three shots to protect him or her from five diseases, instead of five individual shots.

Several vaccines are so common that they are generally known by their initials: MMR (measles, mumps, and rubella) and DTaP (diphtheria, tetanus, and pertussis). Each protects your child against three diseases. However, nowadays, these two particular vaccines are not considered true combination vaccines because, in the United States, you cannot get separate vaccines for all of the diseases that MMR and DTaP protect against (refer to Table 3.1).

Benefits of Combination Vaccines

Combining vaccines into fewer shots may mean that more children will get recommended vaccinations on time. And that means fewer delays in disease protection.

---

[5] "Understanding How Vaccines Work," Centers for Disease Control and Prevention (CDC), August 17, 2018. Available online. URL: www.cdc.gov/vaccines/hcp/conversations/understanding-vacc-work.html. Accessed April 19, 2023.

Benefits for children are as follows:
- fewer shots
- less pain and discomfort
- on-time protection

Benefits for parents are as follows:
- fewer visits to the doctor
- less hassle and cost with fewer visits
- less time off from work or family activity

Table 3.1. Common Combination Vaccines for Children

Vaccine Name	Combination	Protection From
Pediarix	DTaP + Hep B + IPV	Five diseases (diphtheria, tetanus, pertussis, hepatitis B, and polio)
Pentacel	DTaP + IPV + Hib	Five diseases (diphtheria, tetanus, pertussis, polio, and Hib)
Kinrix and Quadracel	DTaP + IPV	Four diseases (diphtheria, tetanus, pertussis, and polio)
Vaxelis	DTaP + IPV + Hib + HepB	Six diseases (diphtheria, tetanus, pertussis, polio, hepatitis B, and Hib)
ProQuad Hib – *Haemophilus influenzae* type b HepB – Hepatitis B	MMR + varicella (chickenpox)	Four diseases (measles, mumps, rubella, and varicella)

Safety and Effectiveness

Before a combination vaccine is approved for use, it goes through careful testing to make sure the combination vaccine is as safe and effective as each of the individual vaccines given separately. And, just as with individual vaccines, there are systems in place to watch for any rare reactions to combination vaccines that can be detected only after the vaccine is used widely.

Side Effects

Side effects from combination vaccines are usually mild. They are similar to those of the individual vaccines given separately.

Sometimes, combination vaccines cause slightly more pain or swelling where the shot was given. But, if your child got the shots individually, he or she might have pain or swelling in two or three spots, instead of just one.

If your child has moderate or serious side effects from a combination vaccine, tell your child's doctor. If separate vaccines are available, the doctor may be able to give additional doses of certain vaccines separately.

Growing Future for Combination Vaccines

As scientists develop and test new vaccines to protect children against more diseases, more combination vaccines may become available. This will allow children to get additional protection with fewer shots.[6]

VACCINES DURING AND AFTER PREGNANCY

A pregnant person should get vaccinated against whooping cough and flu during each pregnancy to protect herself and her baby, with immunity for the first few months of life.

Protecting the Mom and Baby with Vaccines

Did you know a baby gets disease immunity (protection) from the mom during pregnancy? This immunity can protect the baby from some diseases during the first few months of life, but immunity decreases over time.

Getting a Whooping Cough Vaccine and a Flu Vaccine during Each Pregnancy

Moms should get a whooping cough vaccine (also called "Tdap") and a flu shot during each pregnancy. Use the CDC's Adult Vaccine

---

[6] See footnote [2].

Self-Assessment Tool (www2.cdc.gov/nip/adultimmsched) to get a customized printout of recommended vaccines to take to the next medical appointment.

WHOOPING COUGH

Whooping cough, known as "pertussis," can be serious for anyone, but for a newborn, it can be life-threatening.

- About 7 in 10 deaths from whooping cough are among babies younger than two months old. These babies are too young to receive a whooping cough vaccine. The younger the baby is when they get whooping cough, the more likely they will need to be treated in a hospital.
- It may be hard to know if a baby has whooping cough because many babies with this disease do not cough at all. Instead, it can cause them to stop breathing and turn blue.

When a pregnant person gets a whooping cough vaccine during pregnancy, her body will create protective antibodies and pass some of them to the baby before birth. These antibodies will provide the baby some short-term, early protection against whooping cough. The CDC recommends getting a whooping cough vaccine during the 27th through 36th week of each pregnancy, preferably during the earlier part of this time period.

FLU

Pregnant people are more likely to have severe illness from flu, possibly due to changes in immune, heart, and lung functions during pregnancy.

Make sure to receive your yearly flu vaccine—it is the best way for a pregnant woman to protect against the flu and protect the baby for several months after birth from flu-related complications.

COVID-19

Pregnant people are more likely to get severely ill with COVID-19 than nonpregnant people. If you are pregnant, you can receive a

COVID-19 vaccine. Getting a COVID-19 vaccine during pregnancy can protect you from severe illness from COVID-19. If you have questions about getting vaccinated, talk to your health-care provider.

OTHER VACCINES

Some women may need other vaccines before, during, or after they become pregnant. For example, if a pregnant woman works in a lab or is traveling to a country where she may be exposed to meningococcal disease, her doctor or health-care professional may recommend meningococcal vaccination.

- **Hepatitis B**. A baby whose mother has hepatitis B is at the highest risk of becoming infected with hepatitis B during delivery. Moms should talk to their health-care professional about getting tested for hepatitis B and whether or not they should get vaccinated.
- **Hepatitis A**. For pregnant women who have a history of chronic liver disease, doctors or health-care professionals may recommend the hepatitis A vaccine.
- **Vaccines for travel**. Pregnant people planning international travel should talk to their doctor or health-care professional at least four to six weeks before their trip to discuss any special precautions or necessary vaccines.

Vaccines after Childbirth

Health-care professionals may recommend some women receive certain vaccines right after giving birth. Postpartum vaccination will help protect moms from getting sick, and they will pass some antibodies to the baby through breastmilk if they are able to breastfeed. Vaccination after pregnancy is especially important if moms did not receive certain vaccines before or during pregnancy.

However, moms will not get protective antibodies immediately if they wait to get vaccinated until after birth. This is because it takes about two weeks after getting vaccinated before the body develops antibodies. The baby will also start to get his or her own vaccines to protect against serious childhood diseases.[7]

VACCINES FOR STRENGTHENING YOUR BABY'S IMMUNE SYSTEM

Immunity is the body's way of preventing disease. Because a baby's immune system is not fully developed at birth, babies face a greater risk of becoming infected and getting seriously ill.

After a few weeks of birth, babies are protected from the germs that cause diseases. This protection is passed before birth from their mother through their placenta. But, after a short period of time, the protection goes away. Vaccines help teach the immune system learn how to defend against germs. Vaccination protects your baby by helping build up their natural defenses.

- Children are exposed to thousands of germs every day. This happens through the food they eat, the air they breathe, and the things they put in their mouth.
- Babies are born with immune systems that can fight most germs, but some germs cause serious or even deadly diseases a baby cannot handle. For those, babies need the help of vaccines.
- Vaccines use very small amounts of antigens to help your child's immune system recognize and learn to fight serious diseases. Antigens are the parts of a germ that cause the body's immune system to go to work.

WHY YOUR CHILD SHOULD GET VACCINATED

Vaccines can prevent common diseases that used to seriously harm or even kill infants, children, and adults. Without vaccines, your child is at risk of becoming seriously ill or even dying from childhood diseases such as measles and whooping cough.

---

[7] "Vaccines during and after Pregnancy," Centers for Disease Control and Prevention (CDC), November 9, 2021. Available online. URL: www.cdc.gov/vaccines/pregnancy/vacc-during-after.html. Accessed April 19, 2023.

It is always better to prevent a disease than to treat one after it occurs.

- Vaccination is a safe, highly effective, and easy way to help keep your family healthy.
- The recommended vaccination schedule balances when a child is likely to be exposed to a disease and when a vaccine will be most effective.
- Vaccines are tested to ensure they can be given safely and effectively at the recommended ages.[8]

VACCINES BY AGE
Birth through Six Years of Age
See which vaccines your child needs from birth through the age of six in the parent-friendly immunization schedule provided in Tables 3.2 and 3.3.

Ages 7–18
See which vaccines your child needs from ages 7 through 18 in the parent-friendly immunization schedule provided in Figures 3.1 and 3.2 and Table 3.4.

Ages 19 or Older
Adults need to keep their vaccinations up-to-date because immunity from childhood vaccines can wear off over time. You are also at risk of different diseases as an adult. Vaccination is one of the most convenient and safest preventive care measures available.

You may need other vaccines based on your age.

---

[8] See footnote [2].

Table 3.2. Recommended Vaccinations for Infants and Children, Birth to Six Years of Age, United States, 2023

Disease	Vaccine	Birth	1 Month	2 Months	4 Months	6 Months	12 Months	15 Months	18 Months	19–23 Months	2–3 Years	4–6 Years
Hepatitis B	HepB vaccine	HepB	HepB			HepB						
Rotavirus	RV* vaccine			RV	RV	RV*						
Diphtheria, pertussis, and tetanus	DTaP vaccine			DTaP	DTaP	DTaP		DTaP				DTaP
Haemophilus influenzae type b	Hib* vaccine			Hib	Hib	Hib*	Hib					
Pneumococcal disease	PCV13 or PCV15 vaccine			PCV	PCV	PCV	PCV					
Polio	Inactivated polio vaccine (IPV)			IPV	IPV	IPV						IPV
Coronavirus disease 2019	COVID-19** vaccine					COVID-19**						

Table 3.2. Continued

Disease	Vaccine	Birth	1 Month	2 Months	4 Months	6 Months	12 Months	15 Months	18 Months	19–23 Months	2–3 Years	4–6 Years
Influenza	Flu† vaccine					Flu (one or two doses yearly)†						
Measles, mumps, and rubella	MMR vaccine						MMR					MMR
Chickenpox	Varicella vaccine						Varicella					Varicella
Hepatitis A	HepA‡ vaccine						HepA‡		HepA‡			

*Administering a third dose at six months depends on the brand of Hib or RV vaccine used for the previous dose.

**Number of doses recommended depends on your child's age and the type of COVID-19 vaccine used.

†Two doses given at least four weeks apart are recommended for children aged six months through eight years who are getting an influenza (flu) vaccine for the first time and for some other children in this age group.

‡Two doses of HepA vaccine are needed for lasting protection. The two doses should be given between the ages of 12 and 23 months. Both doses should be separated by at least six months. Children aged two and older who have not received two doses of HepA should complete the series.

Table 3.3. Vaccine-Preventable Diseases and the Vaccines That Prevent Them (Birth to Six Years)

Disease	Vaccine	Disease Spread By	Disease Symptoms	Disease Complications
Hepatitis B	HepB vaccine protects against hepatitis B.	Contact with blood or body fluids	No symptoms or sometimes, fever, headache, weakness, vomiting, jaundice (yellowing of skin and eyes), joint pain	Chronic liver infection, liver failure, liver cancer, death
Rotavirus	RV vaccine protects against rotavirus.	Through the mouth	Diarrhea, fever, vomiting	Severe diarrhea, dehydration, death
Diphtheria	DTaP* vaccine protects against diphtheria.	Air, direct contact	Sore throat, mild fever, weakness, swollen glands in neck	Swelling of the heart muscle, heart failure, coma, paralysis, death
Pertussis (whooping cough)	DTaP* vaccine protects against pertussis (whooping cough).	Air, direct contact	Severe cough, runny nose, apnea (a pause in breathing in infants)	Pneumonia (infection in the lungs), death
Tetanus	DTaP* vaccine protects against tetanus.	Exposure through cuts in skin	Stiffness in neck and abdominal muscles, difficulty swallowing, muscle spasms, fever	Broken bones, breathing difficulty, death
Haemophilus influenzae type b (Hib)	Hib vaccine protects against *Haemophilus influenzae* type b.	Air, direct contact	No symptoms unless bacteria enter the blood	Meningitis (infection of the covering around the brain and spinal cord), intellectual disability, epiglottitis (life-threatening infection that can block the windpipe and lead to serious breathing problems), pneumonia (infection in the lungs), death

Table 3.3. Continued

Disease	Vaccine	Disease Spread By	Disease Symptoms	Disease Complications
Pneumococcal disease (PCV13, PCV15) polio	PCV vaccine protects against pneumococcal disease.	Air, direct contact	No symptoms or sometimes pneumonia (infection in the lungs)	Bacteremia (blood infection), meningitis (infection of the covering around the brain and spinal cord), death
Polio	IPV vaccine protects against polio.	Air, direct contact, through the mouth	No symptoms or sometimes sore throat, fever, nausea, headache	Paralysis, death
Coronavirus disease 2019 (COVID-19)	COVID-19 vaccine protects against severe complications from COVID-19.	Air, direct contact	No symptoms or sometimes fever, muscle aches, sore throat, cough, runny nose, diarrhea, vomiting, new loss of taste or smell	Pneumonia (infection in the lungs), respiratory failure, blood clots, bleeding disorder, injury to liver, heart or kidney, multisystem inflammatory syndrome, post-COVID syndrome, death
Influenza (flu)	Flu vaccine protects against influenza.	Air, direct contact	Fever, muscle pain, sore throat, cough, extreme fatigue	Pneumonia (infection in the lungs), bronchitis, sinus infections, ear infections, death
Measles	MMR** vaccine protects against measles.	Air, direct contact	Rash, fever, cough, runny nose, pink eye	Encephalitis (brain swelling), pneumonia (infection in the lungs), death

Table 3.3. Continued

Disease	Vaccine	Disease Spread By	Disease Symptoms	Disease Complications
Mumps	MMR** vaccine protects against mumps.	Air, direct contact	Swollen salivary glands (under the jaw), fever, headache, tiredness, muscle pain	Meningitis (infection of the covering around the brain and spinal cord), encephalitis (brain swelling), inflammation of testicles or ovaries, deafness, death
Rubella	MMR** vaccine protects against rubella.	Air, direct contact, through the mouth	Sometimes rash, fever, swollen lymph nodes	Very serious in pregnant women—can lead to miscarriage, stillbirth, premature delivery, birth defects
Chickenpox	Varicella vaccine protects against chickenpox.	Air, direct contact	Rash, tiredness, headache, fever	Infected blisters, bleeding disorders, encephalitis (brain swelling), pneumonia (infection in the lungs), death
Hepatitis A	HepA vaccine protects against hepatitis A.	Direct contact, contaminated food or water	No symptoms or sometimes fever, stomach pain, loss of appetite, fatigue, vomiting, jaundice (yellowing of skin and eyes), dark urine	Liver failure, arthralgia (joint pain), kidney, pancreatic and blood disorders, death

*DTaP provides combined protection against diphtheria, tetanus, and pertussis.
**MMR provides combined protection against measles, mumps, and rubella.

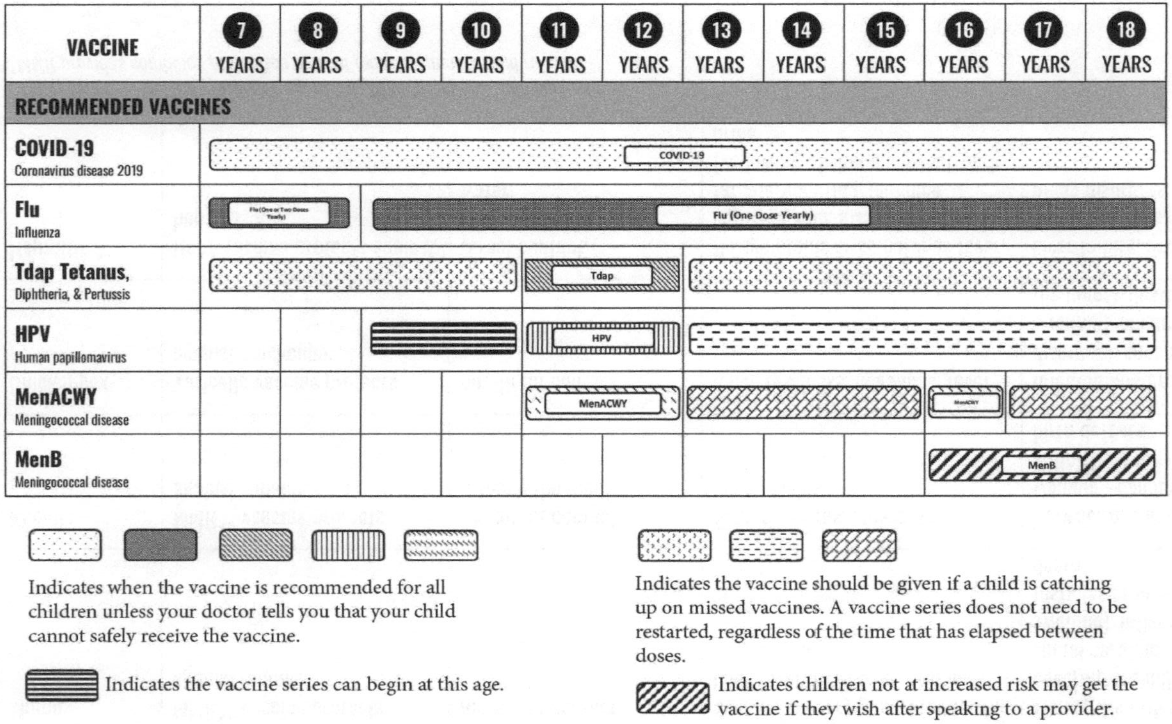

Figure 3.1. Recommended Vaccinations for Children Aged 7–18, United States, 2023

Centers for Disease Control and Prevention (CDC)

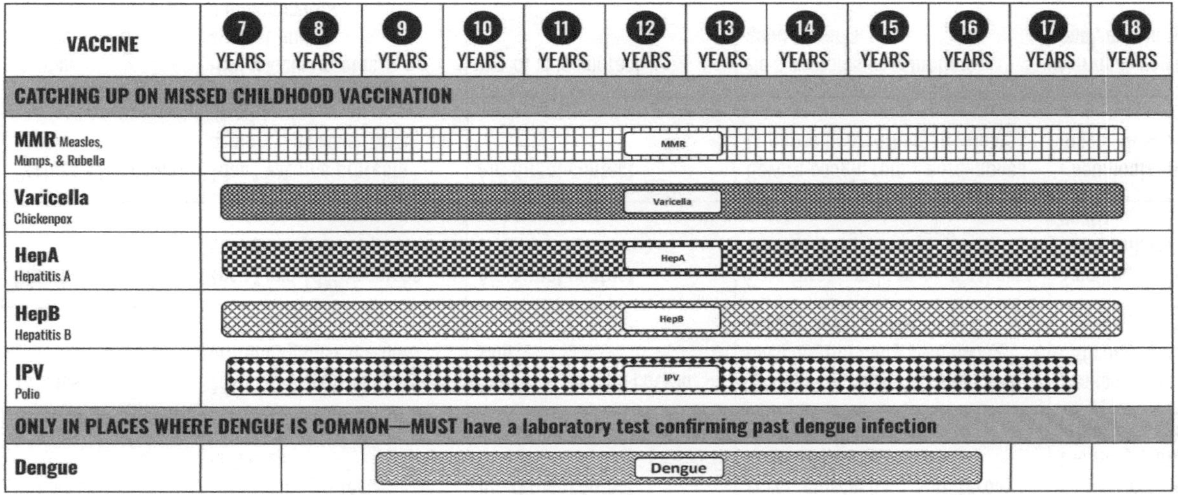

Indicates when the vaccine is recommended for all children unless your doctor tells you that your child cannot safely receive the vaccine.

Indicates the vaccine should be given if a child is catching up on missed vaccines. A vaccine series does not need to be restarted, regardless of the time that has elapsed between doses.

Figure 3.2. Missed Childhood and Dengue Vaccination for Children Aged 7–18

Centers for Disease Control and Prevention (CDC)

Table 3.4. Vaccine-Preventable Diseases and the Vaccines That Prevent Them (7–18 Years)

Disease	Vaccine	Disease Spread By	Disease Symptoms	Disease Complications
Coronavirus disease 2019 (COVID-19)	COVID-19 vaccine protects against severe complications from COVID-19.	Air, direct contact	No symptoms or sometimes fever, muscle aches, sore throat, cough, runny nose, diarrhea, vomiting, new loss of taste or smell	Pneumonia (infection in the lungs), respiratory failure, blood clots, bleeding disorder, injury to liver, heart or kidney, multisystem inflammatory syndrome, post-COVID syndrome, death
Influenza (flu)	Flu vaccine protects against influenza.	Air, direct contact	Fever, muscle pain, sore throat, cough, extreme fatigue	Pneumonia (infection in the lungs), bronchitis, sinus infections, ear infections, death
Tetanus	Tdap* and Td** vaccines protect against tetanus.	Exposure through cuts in skin	Stiffness in neck and abdominal muscles, difficulty swallowing, muscle spasms, fever	Broken bones, breathing difficulty, death
Diphtheria	Tdap* and Td** vaccines protects against diphtheria.	Air, direct contact	Sore throat, mild fever, weakness, swollen glands in neck	Swelling of the heart muscle, heart failure, coma, paralysis, death
Pertussis (whooping cough)	Tdap* vaccine protects against pertussis (whooping cough).	Air, direct contact	Severe cough, runny nose, apnea (a pause in breathing in infants)	Pneumonia (infection in the lungs), death
Human papillomavirus	HPV vaccine protects against human papillomavirus.	Direct skin contact	No symptoms or sometimes genital warts	Cervical, vaginal, vulvar, penile, anal, oropharyngeal cancers

Table 3.4. Continued

Disease	Vaccine	Disease Spread By	Disease Symptoms	Disease Complications
Meningococcal disease	MenACWY and MenB vaccines protect against meningococcal disease.	Air, direct contact	Sudden onset of fever, headache, and stiff neck, dark purple rash	Loss of limb, deafness, nervous system disorders, developmental disabilities, seizure disorder, stroke, death
Measles	MMR† vaccine protects against measles.	Air, direct contact	Rash, fever, cough, runny nose, pink eye	Encephalitis (brain swelling), pneumonia (infection in the lungs), death
Mumps	MMR† vaccine protects against mumps.	Air, direct contact	Swollen salivary glands (under the jaw), fever, headache, tiredness, muscle pain	Meningitis (infection of the covering around the brain and spinal cord), encephalitis (brain swelling), inflammation of testicles or ovaries, deafness, death
Rubella	MMR† vaccine protects against rubella.	Air, direct contact	Sometimes rash, fever, swollen lymph nodes	Very serious in pregnant women—can lead to miscarriage, stillbirth, premature delivery, birth defects
Chickenpox	Varicella vaccine protects against chickenpox.	Air, direct contact	Rash, tiredness, headache, fever	Infected blisters, bleeding disorders, encephalitis (brain swelling), pneumonia (infection in the lungs), death

Table 3.4. Continued

Disease	Vaccine	Disease Spread By	Disease Symptoms	Disease Complications
Hepatitis A	HepA vaccine protects against hepatitis A.	Direct contact, contaminated food or water	No symptoms or sometimes fever, stomach pain, loss of appetite, fatigue, vomiting, jaundice (yellowing of skin and eyes), dark urine	Liver failure, arthralgia (joint pain), kidney, pancreatic and blood disorders, death
Hepatitis B	HepB vaccine protects against hepatitis B.	Contact with blood or body fluids	No symptoms or sometimes fever, headache, weakness, vomiting, jaundice (yellowing of skin and eyes), joint pain	Chronic liver infection, liver failure, liver cancer, death
Polio	IPV vaccine protects against polio.	Air, direct contact, through the mouth	No symptoms or sometimes sore throat, fever, nausea, headache	Paralysis, death
Dengue	Dengue vaccine† protects against dengue.	Bite from infected mosquito	No symptoms or sometimes fever, headache, pain behind the eyes, rash, joint pain, body ache, nausea, loss of appetite, feeling tired, abdominal pain	Severe bleeding; seizures; shock; damage to the liver, heart, and lungs; death

*Tdap provides combined protection against diphtheria, tetanus, and pertussis.
**Td provides combined protection against diphtheria and tetanus.
†MMR provides combined protection against measles, mumps, and rubella.
†This vaccine is recommended where dengue is common.

ADULTS AGED 19–26
All adults aged 19–26 should make sure they are up-to-date on the following vaccines:
- chickenpox vaccine (varicella)
- COVID-19 vaccine
- flu vaccine (influenza)
- hepatitis B vaccine
- HPV vaccine (human papillomavirus)
- MMR vaccine (measles, mumps, and rubella)
- Tdap vaccine (tetanus, diphtheria, and whooping cough) or Td (tetanus and diphtheria)

You may need other vaccines, too:
- MenB vaccine (meningococcal disease)—for adults up to 23 years of age

ADULTS AGED 27–49
All adults aged 27–49 years should make sure they are up-to-date on the following vaccines:
- COVID-19 vaccine
- flu vaccine (influenza)
- hepatitis B vaccine
- MMR vaccine (measles, mumps, and rubella)
- Tdap vaccine (tetanus, diphtheria, and whooping cough) or Td (tetanus and diphtheria)

You may need other vaccines, too:
- chickenpox vaccine (varicella)—if born in 1980 or later
- HPV vaccine (human papillomavirus)

ADULTS AGED 50–64
All adults aged 50–64 years should make sure they are up-to-date on these vaccines:
- COVID-19 vaccine
- flu vaccine (influenza)
- shingles vaccine (zoster)

- Tdap (tetanus, diphtheria, and whooping cough) or Td (tetanus and diphtheria)

You may need other vaccines, too:
- hepatitis B vaccine—recommended for all adults up to 59 years of age
- MMR vaccine (measles, mumps, and rubella) if born in 1957 or later

ADULTS AGED 65 AND OLDER

As we get older, our immune systems tend to weaken over time, putting us at a higher risk for certain diseases. All adults aged 65 and older should make sure they are up-to-date on the following vaccines:
- COVID-19 vaccine
- flu vaccine (influenza)
- pneumococcal vaccine
- shingles vaccine (zoster)
- Tdap (tetanus, diphtheria, and whooping cough) or Td (tetanus and diphtheria)[9]

Section 3.2 | Vaccine Types

There are several different types of vaccines. Each type is designed to teach your immune system how to fight off certain kinds of germs—and the serious diseases they cause.

When scientists create vaccines, they consider:
- how your immune system responds to the germ
- who needs to be vaccinated against the germ
- the best technology or approach to create the vaccine

---

[9] "Immunization Schedules," Centers for Disease Control and Prevention (CDC), February 10, 2023. Available online. URL: www.cdc.gov/vaccines/schedules/easy-to-read/child-easyread.html. Accessed April 19, 2023.

Based on these factors, scientists decide which type of vaccine they will make. There are several types of vaccines, including:
- inactivated vaccines
- live-attenuated vaccines
- messenger ribonucleic acid (mRNA) vaccines
- subunit, recombinant, polysaccharide, and conjugate vaccines
- toxoid vaccines
- viral vector vaccines

INACTIVATED VACCINES
Inactivated vaccines use the killed version of the germ that causes a disease.

Inactivated vaccines usually do not provide immunity (protection) that is as strong as live vaccines. So you may need several doses over time (booster shots) in order to get ongoing immunity against diseases.

Inactivated vaccines are used to protect against:
- hepatitis A
- flu (shot only)
- polio (shot only)
- rabies

LIVE-ATTENUATED VACCINES
Live vaccines use a weakened (or attenuated) form of the germ that causes a disease.

Because these vaccines are so similar to the natural infection that they help prevent, they create a strong and long-lasting immune response. Just one or two doses of most live vaccines can give you a lifetime of protection against a germ and the disease it causes.

But live vaccines also have some limitations:
- Because they contain a small amount of the weakened live virus, some people should talk to their health-care provider before receiving them, such as people with weakened immune systems, people with long-term

health problems, or people who have had an organ transplant.
- They need to be kept cool, so they do not travel well. That means they cannot be used in countries with limited access to refrigerators.

Live vaccines are used to protect against:
- measles, mumps, rubella (MMR combined vaccine)
- rotavirus
- smallpox
- chickenpox
- yellow fever

MESSENGER RIBONUCLEIC ACID VACCINES

Researchers have been studying and working with mRNA vaccines for decades, and this technology was used to make some of the COVID-19 vaccines. mRNA vaccines make proteins in order to trigger an immune response. mRNA vaccines have several benefits compared to other types of vaccines, including shorter manufacturing times and, because they do not contain a live virus, no risk of causing disease in the person getting vaccinated. COVID-19 mRNA vaccines are used to protect against COVID-19.

SUBUNIT, RECOMBINANT, POLYSACCHARIDE, AND CONJUGATE VACCINES

Subunit, recombinant, polysaccharide, and conjugate vaccines use specific pieces of the germ—such as its protein, sugar, or capsid (a casing around the germ).

Because these vaccines use only specific pieces of the germ, they give a very strong immune response that is targeted to key parts of the germ. They can also be used on almost everyone who needs them, including people with weakened immune systems and long-term health problems. One limitation of these vaccines is that you may need booster shots to get ongoing protection against diseases.

These vaccines are used to protect against:
- *Haemophilus influenzae* type b (Hib) disease
- hepatitis B
- human papillomavirus (HPV)
- whooping cough (part of the DTaP combined vaccine)
- pneumococcal disease
- meningococcal disease
- shingles

TOXOID VACCINES

Toxoid vaccines use a toxin (harmful product) made by the germ that causes a disease. They create immunity to the parts of the germ that cause a disease instead of the germ itself. That means the immune response is targeted to the toxin instead of the whole germ. Like some other types of vaccines, you may need booster shots to get ongoing protection against diseases.

Toxoid vaccines are used to protect against:
- diphtheria
- tetanus

VIRAL VECTOR VACCINES

For decades, scientists studied viral vector vaccines. Some vaccines recently used for Ebola outbreaks have used viral vector technology, and a number of studies have focused on viral vector vaccines against other infectious diseases such as Zika, flu, and human immunodeficiency virus (HIV). Scientists used this technology to make COVID-19 vaccines as well.

Viral vector vaccines use a modified version of a different virus as a vector to deliver protection. Several different viruses have been used as vectors, including influenza, vesicular stomatitis virus (VSV), measles virus, and adenovirus, which causes the common cold. Adenovirus is one of the viral vectors used in some COVID-19 vaccines being studied in clinical trials. Viral vector vaccines are used to protect against COVID-19.

THE FUTURE OF VACCINES

New types of vaccines are in research and development, and the following are the examples of future vaccines:

- Deoxyribonucleic acid (DNA) vaccines are easy and inexpensive to make and they produce strong, long-term immunity.
- Recombinant vector vaccines (platform-based vaccines) act like a natural infection, so they are especially good at teaching the immune system how to fight germs.[10]

Section 3.3 | Infant Immunization: An Overview

Most parents choose to vaccinate their children according to the recommended schedule, but many parents may still have questions about the vaccines recommended for their child.

VACCINE SAFETY
Are Vaccines Safe for Children?

Yes. Vaccines are very safe. The United States' long-standing vaccine safety system ensures that vaccines are as safe as possible. Currently, the United States has the safest vaccine supply in its history. Millions of children safely receive vaccines each year. The most common side effects are very mild, such as pain or swelling at the injection site.

What Are the Risks and Benefits of Vaccines?

Vaccines can prevent infectious diseases that once killed or harmed many infants, children, and adults. Without vaccines, your child is at risk of getting seriously ill and suffering pain, disability, and even death from diseases such as measles and whooping cough. The

---

[10] "Vaccine Types," U.S. Department of Health and Human Services (HHS), December 22, 2022. Available online. URL: www.hhs.gov/immunization/basics/types/index.html. Accessed April 24, 2023.

main risks associated with getting vaccines are side effects, which are almost always mild (redness and swelling at the injection site) and go away within a few days. Serious side effects after vaccination, such as a severe allergic reaction, are very rare, and doctors and clinic staff are trained to deal with them. The disease prevention benefits of getting vaccines are much greater than the possible side effects for almost all children. The only exceptions to this are cases in which a child has a serious chronic medical condition, such as cancer or a disease that weakens the immune system, or has had a severe allergic reaction to a previous vaccine dose.

Is There a Link between Vaccines and Autism?

No. Scientific studies and reviews continue to show no relationship between vaccines and autism.

SIDE EFFECTS
What Are the Common Side Effects of Vaccines?

Vaccines, such as any medication, may cause some side effects. Most of these side effects are very minor, such as soreness where the shot was given, fussiness, or a low-grade fever. These side effects typically only last a couple of days and are treatable. For example, you can apply a cool, wet washcloth on the sore area to ease discomfort.

Can Vaccines Overload Your Baby's Immune System?

Vaccines do not overload the immune system. Every day, a healthy baby's immune system successfully fights off thousands of germs. Antigens are parts of germs that cause the body's immune system to go to work to build antibodies, which fight off diseases.

The antigens in vaccines come from the germs themselves, but the germs are weakened or killed so that they cannot cause serious illness. Even if babies receive several vaccinations in one day, vaccines contain only a tiny fraction of the antigens they encounter every day in their environment. Vaccines give your child the antibodies they need to fight off serious vaccine-preventable diseases.

SCHEDULE FOR VACCINES
Why Do Vaccines Start So Early?

The recommended schedule protects infants and children by providing protection early in life, before they come into contact with life-threatening diseases. Children receive vaccinations early because they are susceptible to diseases at a young age.

Should Your Child Get Shots If Your Child Is Sick?

Talk with your child's doctor, but children can usually get vaccinated even if they have a mild illness such as a cold, earache, mild fever, or diarrhea. If the doctor says it is okay, your child can still get vaccinated.

Should You Delay Some Vaccines or Follow a Nonstandard Schedule?

Children do not receive any known benefits from following schedules that delay vaccines. Infants and young children who follow immunization schedules that spread out or leave out shots are at risk of developing diseases during the time you delay their shots.

Why Can You Not Delay Some Vaccines If You Are Planning for Your Baby to Get Them All Eventually?

Young children have the highest risk of having a serious case of disease that could cause hospitalization or death. Delaying or spreading out vaccine doses leaves your child unprotected during the time when they need vaccine protection the most. For example, diseases such as *Haemophilus influenzae* type b (Hib) or pneumococcus almost always occur in the first two years of a baby's life. And some diseases, such as hepatitis B and whooping cough (pertussis), are more serious when babies get them.

If You Are Breastfeeding, Do You Vaccinate Your Baby on Schedule?

Yes, even breastfed babies need to be protected with vaccines at the recommended ages. The immune system is not fully developed at birth, which puts newborns at greater risk of infections.

Breastmilk provides important protection from some infections as your baby's immune system is developing. For example, babies who are breastfed have a lower risk of ear infections, respiratory tract infections, and diarrhea. However, breastmilk does not protect children against all diseases. Even in breastfed infants, vaccines are the most effective way to prevent many diseases. Your baby needs the long-term protection that can only come from following the schedule recommended by the Center for Disease Control and Prevention (CDC).

Can You Wait to Vaccinate Your Baby since Your Baby Is Not in Childcare?

No, even young children who are cared for at home can be exposed to vaccine-preventable diseases, so it is important for them to get all their vaccines at the recommended ages. Children can catch these illnesses from any number of people or places, including from parents, from brothers or sisters, from visitors to their home, on playgrounds, or even at the grocery store. Regardless of whether your baby is cared for outside the home, your baby comes in contact with people throughout the day, some of whom may have a vaccine-preventable disease.

Many of these diseases can be especially dangerous to young children, so it is safest to vaccinate your child at the recommended ages.

Can You Wait until Your Child Goes to School to Catch Up on Immunizations?

No. Before entering school, young children can be exposed to vaccine-preventable diseases. Children under the age of five are especially susceptible to diseases because their immune systems have not built up the necessary defenses to fight infection.

Why Do Adolescents Need Vaccines?

Vaccines are recommended throughout your lives to protect against serious diseases. As protection from childhood vaccines wears off, adolescents need vaccines that will extend protection. Adolescents need protection from additional infections as well, before the risk of exposure increases.

Why Are Multiple Doses Needed for Each Vaccine?

Getting every recommended dose of each vaccine provides your child with the best protection possible. Depending on the vaccine, your child will need more than one dose to build high enough immunity to help prevent disease or to boost immunity that fades over time. Your child may also receive more than one dose to make sure they are protected if they did not get immunity from a first dose or to protect them against germs that change over time, such as flu. Every dose is important because each protects against an infectious disease that can be especially serious for infants and very young children.

PROTECTION FROM DISEASES
Do Infants Have Natural Immunity?

Babies may get some temporary protection from the mom during the last few weeks of pregnancy but only for diseases to which the mom is immune. Breastfeeding may also protect your baby temporarily from minor infections, such as colds. These antibodies do not last long, leaving your baby vulnerable to disease.

Vaccines Control Now Uncommon Diseases

Some vaccine-preventable diseases, such as pertussis (whooping cough) and chickenpox, remain common in the United States. On the other hand, other diseases vaccines prevent are no longer common in this country because of vaccines. If you stopped vaccinating, the few cases you have in the United States could very quickly become tens or hundreds of thousands of cases. Even though many serious vaccine-preventable diseases are uncommon in the United States, some are common in other parts of the world. Even if your family does not travel internationally, you could come into contact with international travelers anywhere in your community. Children who do not receive all vaccinations and are exposed to a disease can become seriously sick and spread it throughout a community.[11]

---

[11] "Common Questions about Vaccines," Center for Disease Control and Prevention (CDC), July 7, 2022. Available online. URL: www.cdc.gov/vaccines/parents/parent-questions.html. Accessed April 28, 2023.

Chapter 4 | Major Disorders of the Immune System

Chapter Contents

Section 4.1 | An Overview of the Disorders of the Immune System

Complications arise when the immune system does not function properly. Some issues are less pervasive, such as pollen allergy, while others are extensive, such as genetic disorders that wipe out the presence or function of an entire set of immune cells.

IMMUNE DEFICIENCIES

Immune deficiencies may be temporary or permanent. Temporary immune deficiency can be caused by a variety of sources that weaken the immune system. Common infections, including influenza and mononucleosis, can suppress the immune system.

When immune cells are the target of infection, severe immune suppression can occur. For example, human immunodeficiency virus (HIV) specifically infects T cells, and their elimination allows for secondary infections by other pathogens. Patients receiving chemotherapy, bone marrow transplants, or immunosuppressive drugs experience weakened immune systems until immune cell levels are restored. Pregnancy also suppresses the maternal immune system, increasing susceptibility to infections by common microbes.

Primary immune deficiency diseases (PIDDs) are inherited genetic disorders and tend to cause chronic susceptibility to infection. There are over 150 PIDDs, and almost all are considered rare (affecting fewer than 200,000 people in the United States). They may result from altered immune signaling molecules or the complete absence of mature immune cells. For instance, X-linked severe combined immunodeficiency (SCID) is caused by a mutation in a signaling receptor gene, rendering immune cells insensitive to multiple cytokines. Without the growth and activation signals delivered by cytokines, immune cell subsets, particularly T and natural killer cells, fail to develop normally.

ALLERGIES

Allergies are a form of hypersensitivity reaction, typically in response to harmless environmental allergens, such as pollen or food. Hypersensitivity reactions are divided into four classes. Classes I, II, and III are caused by antibodies, immunoglobulin E (IgE) or immunoglobulin G (IgG), which are produced by B cells in response to an allergen. The overproduction of these antibodies activates immune cells such as basophils and mast cells, which respond by releasing inflammatory chemicals such as histamine. Class IV reactions are caused by T cells, which may either directly cause damage themselves or activate macrophages and eosinophils that damage host cells.

AUTOIMMUNE DISEASES

Autoimmune diseases occur when self-tolerance is broken. Self-tolerance breaks when adaptive immune cells that recognize host cells persist unchecked. B cells may produce antibodies targeting host cells, and active T cells may recognize self-antigens. This amplifies when they recruit and activate other immune cells.

Autoimmunity is either organ-specific or systemic, meaning it affects the whole body. For instance, type I diabetes is organ-specific and caused by immune cells erroneously recognizing insulin-producing pancreatic beta cells as foreign. However, systemic lupus erythematosus, commonly called "lupus," can result from antibodies that recognize antigens expressed by nearly all healthy cells. Autoimmune diseases have a strong genetic component, and with advances in gene sequencing tools, researchers have a better understanding of what may contribute to specific diseases.

SEPSIS

Sepsis may refer to an infection of the bloodstream, or it can refer to a systemic inflammatory state caused by the uncontrolled, broad release of cytokines that quickly activate immune cells throughout the body. Sepsis is an extremely serious condition and is typically triggered by an infection. However, the damage itself is caused by cytokines (the adverse response is sometimes referred to as a "cytokine storm"). The systemic release of cytokines may lead to loss of blood pressure, resulting in septic shock and possible multiorgan failure.

CANCER

Some forms of cancer are directly caused by the uncontrolled growth of immune cells. Leukemia is cancer caused by white blood cells (WBCs), which is another term for immune cells. Lymphoma is cancer caused by lymphocytes, which is another term for adaptive B or T cells. Myeloma is cancer caused by plasma cells, which are mature B cells. Unrestricted growth of any of these cell types causes cancer.

In addition, an emerging concept is that cancer progression may partially result from the ability of cancer cells to avoid immune detection. The immune system is capable of removing infectious pathogens and dangerous host cells such as tumors. Cancer researchers are studying how the tumor microenvironment may allow cancer cells to evade immune cells. Immune evasion may result from the abundance of suppressive, regulatory immune cells, excessive inhibitory cytokines, and other features that are not well understood.[1]

Section 4.2 | Immunodeficiency Diseases

Immunodeficiency is when your body's defense system (immune system), which fights against harmful invaders such as germs and cancer cells, does not function properly or is disrupted. This means that you are more vulnerable to getting sick from things that your body would normally be able to fight off.

TYPES OF IMMUNODEFICIENCY DISEASES

The following are the two main types of diseases that affect your immune system:

- **Primary immunodeficiency (PI).** This is inherited immunity, which with you are born.
- **Secondary immunodeficiency (SI).** When a condition or disease attacks or weakens your immune system,

---

[1] "Disorders of the Immune System," National Institute of Allergy and Infectious Diseases (NIAID), January 17, 2014. Available online. URL: www.niaid.nih.gov/research/immune-system-disorders. Accessed May 12, 2023.

your immune system develops defenses against it (acquired).

Primary Immunodeficiency

PI disorder is usually present from birth and is hereditary. Most PIs manifest during childhood and infancy. There are many types of PIs, and all are relatively rare.

PI disorders are conditions where the body's immune system does not work properly. This can happen because of changes in a person's genes or because of things in the environment that make it hard for the immune system to do its job. These disorders are classified based on which part of the immune system is affected and is not working as it should.

Secondary Immunodeficiency

SI is more common than PI and is acquired and not inherited. It is commonly acquired from primary illnesses or other treatment and environmental factors such as malnutrition, chemotherapy, immunosuppressive drugs, or human immunodeficiency virus (HIV).

SYMPTOMS OF IMMUNODEFICIENCY DISEASES

If someone frequently gets sick and their infections take longer to go away or are difficult to cure, it could be a classical sign that they have an immunodeficiency disorder. This means that the body has a harder time fighting off germs, and they might get sick more often than people who are healthy. The signs and symptoms of immunodeficiency diseases include the following:

- infection and inflammation of internal organs
- blood disorders (anemia or low platelet counts)
- delayed growth and development
- autoimmune disorders (type 1 diabetes, lupus, or rheumatoid arthritis)
- problems in the digestive system (cramping, loss of appetite, nausea, and diarrhea)

- frequent and recurrent infections in the sinuses, ears, or skin
- bacterial infections that may cause pus-filled sores
- chronic gum disease (gingivitis)
- frequent fever and chillness
- infections in the ears, nose, and digestive tract

These symptoms vary based on the duration and severity of the infection.

DIAGNOSIS OF IMMUNODEFICIENCY DISEASES

The diagnosis of immunodeficiency disease is as follows:
- physical examination
- blood tests
- biopsy

Physical Examination

The doctor may conduct a physical examination to find the presence of immunodeficiency diseases by examining the following:
- enlargement in the spleen
- problems with lymph nodes and tonsils

The doctor may ask questions about your history, such as drug usage for any previous illness, exposure to toxic substances, the possibility of family members with an immunodeficiency disorder, use of intravenous drugs, and previous blood transfusions.

Blood Tests

The doctor will order blood tests, including a complete blood count (CBC). A CBC test can detect abnormalities in blood cells, which can help your doctor determine the presence of immunodeficiency disease. A blood sample is taken and tested to determine your white blood cell (WBC) count. The sample is observed under a microscope to check for abnormalities. The immunoglobulin levels are also checked after vaccination.

Biopsy

A biopsy is performed to identify the type of immunodeficiency disease. The doctor takes a sample from bone marrow and/or lymph nodes. These samples are used to determine whether the immune cells are present.

TREATMENT FOR IMMUNODEFICIENCY DISEASES

The treatment for immunodeficiency diseases is based on specific conditions and involves immunoglobulin therapy and antibiotics. Antiviral drugs, such as acyclovir and amantadine or a drug called "interferon," are used to treat viral infections caused by immunodeficiency disorders.

Your doctor may suggest an immunoglobulin injection to replace the missing antibodies in your body. If the severity of the immunodeficiency disease is high, the doctor may perform a stem cell transplant.

The risk of contagious diseases is high if you have immunodeficiency diseases such as HIV or cancer. If the disorder is identified and treated early, people with immunodeficiency disorders can have full productive lives.

References

Carey, Elea. "Immunodeficiency Disorders," Healthline, December 9, 2021. Available online. URL: www.healthline.com/health/immunodeficiency-disorders. Accessed April 20, 2023.

"CVID Community Center," Immune Deficiency Foundation, June 25, 2013. Available online. URL: https://primaryimmune.org/about-primary-immunodeficiencies/specific-disease-types/common-variable-immune-deficiency. Accessed April 20, 2023.

Fernandez, James. "Overview of Immunodeficiency Disorders," MSD and the MSD Manuals, January 25, 2023. Available online. URL: www.msdmanuals.com/en-in/home/immune-disorders/immunodeficiency-disorders/overview-of-immunodeficiency-disorders. Accessed April 20, 2023.

"Immunodeficiency," British Society for Immunology, March 27, 2017. Available online. URL: www.immunology. org/policy-and-public-affairs/briefings-and-position-statements/immunodeficiency. Accessed April 20, 2023.

"Primary Immunodeficiency," Mayo Foundation for Medical Education and Research (MFMER), March 12, 2022. Available online. URL: www.mayoclinic.org/diseases-conditions/primary-immunodeficiency/symptoms-causes/syc-20376905. Accessed April 20, 2023.

"Primary Immunodeficiency Disease," American Academy of Allergy, Asthma & Immunology (AAAAI), July 29, 2011. Available online. URL: www.aaaai.org/conditions-and-treatments/primary-immunodeficiency-disease. Accessed April 20, 2023.

Section 4.3 | Allergies

An allergy is a reaction by the immune system to something that does not bother most other people. People who have allergies often are sensitive to more than one thing. Substances that often cause reactions are as follows:

- pollen
- dust mites
- mold spores
- pet dander
- food
- insect stings
- medicines

Normally, the immune system fights germs. It is the body's defense system. In most allergic reactions, however, it is responding to a false alarm. Genes and the environment probably both play a role.

Allergies can cause a variety of symptoms such as runny nose, sneezing, itching, rashes, swelling, or asthma. Allergies can range from minor to severe. Anaphylaxis is a severe reaction that can be life-threatening. Doctors use skin and blood tests to diagnose allergies. Treatments include medicines, allergy shots, and avoiding the substances that cause the reactions.[2]

TYPES OF ALLERGIES
Asthma

Asthma is a chronic lung disease characterized by episodes of airway narrowing and obstruction, causing wheezing, coughing, chest tightness, and shortness of breath.

UNDERSTANDING ASTHMA TRIGGERS

Asthma is a chronic disease in which the airways in the lungs become inflamed. The inflammation causes swelling and increases the tendency of the airways to tighten in response to irritants or other triggers. The airways become narrower, causing difficulty breathing and symptoms such as wheezing, coughing, and chest tightness. Airway inflammation can be caused by allergens, such as those from dust mites, mold, and cockroaches; viral infections; and air pollution, such as diesel exhaust and environmental tobacco smoke.

The research supported by the National Institute of Allergy and Infectious Diseases (NIAID) has enhanced understanding of the factors that contribute to asthma severity. Studies have shown that reducing allergens in the home can lessen asthma symptoms. Results from the Asthma Phenotypes in the Inner City (APIC) study, reported in 2016, pinpointed sensitivity to multiple allergens, poor lung function, allergic rhinitis, and exposure to secondhand smoke as major factors associated with asthma severity in children.

The other NIAID-supported research studies have shown that bacterial and viral infections are linked to asthma symptoms. In 2014, researchers at the University of Wisconsin–Madison reported that combined viral and bacterial infections are associated with the increase in asthma symptoms that many children experience

---

[2] MedlinePlus, "Allergy," National Institutes of Health (NIH), May 16, 2018. Available online. URL: https://medlineplus.gov/allergy.html. Accessed May 2, 2023.

during the fall. The same researchers in 2015 identified a cellular receptor for rhinovirus C—a cold-causing virus that is strongly associated with severe asthma attacks—pointing to a novel target for the development of prevention and treatment strategies against rhinovirus C–induced colds and asthma attacks.

Eczema (Atopic Dermatitis)

Atopic dermatitis, also known as "eczema," is a noncontagious inflammatory skin condition. It is a chronic disease characterized by dry and itchy skin that can weep clear fluid when scratched. People with eczema may also be particularly susceptible to bacterial, viral, and fungal skin infections.

CAUSES OF ECZEMA (ATOPIC DERMATITIS) AND STRATEGIES FOR PREVENTION

A combination of genetic and environmental factors appears to be involved in the development of eczema. The condition is often associated with other allergic diseases such as asthma, hay fever, and food allergy. Children whose parents have asthma and allergies are more likely to develop atopic dermatitis than children of parents without allergic diseases. Approximately 30 percent of children with atopic dermatitis have food allergies, and many develop asthma or respiratory allergies. People who live in cities or drier climates also appear more likely to develop the disease. The condition tends to worsen when a person is exposed to certain triggers, such as:

- pollen, mold, dust mites, animals, and certain foods (for allergic individuals)
- cold and dry air
- colds or the flu
- skin contact with irritating chemicals
- skin contact with rough materials such as wool
- emotional factors such as stress
- fragrances or dyes added to skin lotions or soaps

Taking too many baths or showers and not moisturizing the skin properly afterward may also make eczema worse.

ECZEMA (ATOPIC DERMATITIS) COMPLICATIONS

The skin of people with atopic dermatitis lacks infection-fighting proteins, making them susceptible to skin infections caused by bacteria and viruses. Fungal infections are also common in people with atopic dermatitis.

- **Bacterial infections**. A major health risk associated with atopic dermatitis is skin colonization or infection by bacteria such as *Staphylococcus aureus*. Around 60–90 percent of people with atopic dermatitis are likely to have staph bacteria on their skin. Many eventually develop infection, which worsens the atopic dermatitis.
- **Viral infections**. People with atopic dermatitis are highly vulnerable to certain viral infections of the skin. For example, if infected with the herpes simplex virus, they can develop a severe skin condition called "atopic dermatitis" with eczema herpeticum.

Those with atopic dermatitis should not receive the currently licensed smallpox vaccine, even if their disease is in remission, because they are at risk of developing a severe infection called "eczema vaccinatum." This infection is caused when the live vaccinia virus in the smallpox vaccine reproduces and spreads throughout the body. Furthermore, those in close contact with people who have atopic dermatitis or a history of the disease should not receive the smallpox vaccine because of the risk of transmitting the live vaccine virus to the person with atopic dermatitis.

Food Allergy

In a person with a food allergy, the immune system reacts abnormally to a component of a food, sometimes producing a severe and life-threatening response. A food allergy is a condition that affects approximately 8 percent of children and nearly 11 percent of adults in the United States.

The NIAID support for food allergy research encompasses basic research in allergy and immunology, epidemiological and observational studies to identify risk factors, and clinical trials of new strategies for prevention and treatment.

IDENTIFYING CAUSES OF THE FOOD ALLERGY AND ASSESSING STRATEGIES FOR PREVENTION

Food allergies develop when a person consumes or comes in contact with their allergen, and the immune system makes an antibody called "immunoglobulin E" (IgE). IgE then circulates through the blood and attaches to immune cells called "mast cells" and "basophils." This initial exposure does not cause an allergic reaction; however, subsequent contact with the same allergen may allow previously created IgE antibodies to recognize it. This recognition then launches an immune response that can result in a severe allergic reaction. However, some people make IgE against a certain food without developing an allergy, and others still may develop only a mild allergy compared to those who experience severe reactions. Researchers are investigating why severe allergies develop in some people and whether this process can be avoided.

Investigators, including the NIAID-funded researchers, have discovered several factors that can increase a person's risk of developing food allergies. Those who already have a food allergy or another allergic disease are more likely to develop food allergies than those who do not. Young children are also more likely to develop food allergies than older children or adults. In 2014, the NIAID-funded researchers discovered that the presence of some naturally occurring gut bacteria may influence a person's chance of developing food allergies.

Genetics are also likely to play a role. People who come from a family in which allergic diseases—such as food allergies, eczema, hay fever, or asthma—are common are more likely to develop food allergies. Likewise, a person with two allergic parents is even more likely to develop a food allergy than someone with one allergic parent. Specifically, researchers working within the NIAID-sponsored Consortium for Food Allergy Research discovered genes that increase the risk of peanut allergy among European Americans.[3]

Food allergic reactions vary in severity from mild symptoms involving hives and lip swelling to severe, life-threatening

---

[3] "Diseases & Conditions," National Institute of Allergy and Infectious Diseases (NIAID), April 29, 2019. Available online. URL: www.niaid.nih.gov/diseases-conditions/allergic-diseases. Accessed May 2, 2023.

symptoms, often called "anaphylaxis," that may involve fatal respiratory problems and shock. While promising prevention and therapeutic strategies are being developed, food allergies currently cannot be cured. Early recognition and learning how to manage food allergies, including which foods to avoid, are important measures to prevent serious health consequences.

To protect those with food allergies and other food hypersensitivities, the U.S. Food and Drug Administration (FDA) enforces regulations requiring companies to list ingredients on packaged foods and beverages. For certain foods or substances that cause allergies or other hypersensitivity reactions, there are more specific labeling requirements.

The FDA provides guidance to the food industry, consumers, and other stakeholders on the best ways to assess and manage allergen hazards in food. The FDA also conducts inspections and sampling to check that major food allergens are properly labeled on products and to determine whether food facilities implement controls to prevent allergen cross-contact (the inadvertent introduction of a major food allergen into a product) and labeling controls to prevent undeclared allergens during manufacturing and packaging. When problems are found, the FDA works with firms to recall products and provide public notification to immediately alert consumers. In addition, the FDA has the authority to seize and remove violative products from the marketplace or refuse entry of imported products.[4]

CHILDREN AND ALLERGIES

The immune system responds to the invading allergen by releasing histamine and other chemicals that typically trigger symptoms in the nose, lungs, throat, sinuses, ears, eyes, skin, or stomach lining.

In some children, allergies can also trigger symptoms of asthma—a disease that causes wheezing or difficulty breathing. If a child has allergies and asthma, "not controlling the allergies can make asthma worse," says Anthony Durmowicz, M.D., a pediatric pulmonary doctor at the FDA.

---

[4] "Food Allergies," U.S. Food and Drug Administration (FDA), January 10, 2023. Available online. URL: www.fda.gov/food/food-labeling-nutrition/food-allergies. Accessed May 2, 2023.

AVOID POLLEN, MOLD, AND OTHER ALLERGY TRIGGERS

If the child has seasonal allergies, pay attention to pollen counts and try to keep the child inside when the levels are high.

- In the late summer and early fall, during the ragweed pollen season, pollen levels are highest in the morning.
- In the spring and summer, during the grass pollen season, pollen levels are highest in the evening.
- Some molds, another allergy trigger, may also be seasonal. For example, leaf mold is more common in the fall.
- Sunny, windy days can be especially troublesome for pollen allergy sufferers.

It may also help to keep windows closed in the house and car and run the air conditioner.

ALLERGY MEDICINES FOR CHILDREN

For most children, symptoms may be controlled by avoiding the allergen, if known, and using over-the-counter (OTC) medicines. But, if a child's symptoms are persistent and not relieved by OTC medicines, see a health-care professional. Although some allergy medicines are approved for use in children as young as six months, the FDA cautions that simply because a product's box says that it is intended for children does not mean it is intended for children of all ages. Always read the label to make sure the product is right for the child's age.

When the child is taking more than one medication, read the label to be sure that the active ingredients are not the same. Although the big print may say the product is to treat a certain symptom, different products may have the same medicine (active ingredient). It might seem that you are buying different products to treat different symptoms, but in fact, the same medicine could be in all the products. The result is that you might accidentally be giving too much of one type of medicine to the child. Children are more sensitive to many drugs than adults. For example, some antihistamines can have adverse effects at lower doses on young patients, causing excitability or excessive drowsiness.

ALLERGY SHOTS AND CHILDREN

Jay E. Slater, M.D., a pediatric allergist at the FDA, says that children who do not respond to either OTC or prescription medications or who suffer from frequent complications of allergic rhinitis may be candidates for allergen immunotherapy—commonly known as "allergy shots."

After allergy testing, typically by skin testing to detect what allergens the child may react to, a health-care professional injects the child with "extracts"—small amounts of the allergens that trigger a reaction. The doses are gradually increased so that the body builds up immunity to these allergens. Allergen extracts are manufactured from natural substances, such as pollens, insect venoms, animal hair, and foods. More than 1,200 extracts are licensed by the FDA.

In 2014, the FDA approved three new immunotherapy products that are taken under the tongue for the treatment of hay fever caused by certain pollens, two of them for use in children. All of them are intended for daily use, before and during the pollen season. They are not meant for immediate symptom relief. Although they are intended for at-home use, these are prescription medications, and the first doses are taken in the presence of a health-care provider. The products are Oralair, Grastek, and Ragwitek (which are approved for use in adults only).

In 2017, the FDA approved Odactra, the first immunotherapy product administered under the tongue for the treatment of house dust mite–induced allergic rhinitis (nasal inflammation) with or without conjunctivitis (eye inflammation). Odactra is approved for use only in adults. "Allergy shots are never appropriate for food allergies," adds Dr. Slater, "but it is common to use extracts to test for food allergies, so the child can avoid those foods."

"In the last 20 years, there has been a remarkable transformation in allergy treatments," says Dr. Slater. "Kids used to be miserable for months out of the year, and drugs made them incredibly sleepy. But today's products offer proven approaches for relief of seasonal allergy symptoms."[5]

---

[5] "Allergy Relief for Your Child," U.S. Food and Drug Administration (FDA), June 1, 2017. Available online. URL: www.fda.gov/consumers/consumer-updates/allergy-relief-your-child. Accessed May 2, 2023.

Section 4.4 | Autoimmune Diseases

WHAT ARE AUTOIMMUNE DISEASES?

The human body has an immune system, which is a complex network of special cells and organs, that defends the body from germs and other foreign invaders. At the core of the immune system is the ability to tell the difference between self and nonself: recognizing what is "you" and what is "foreign." A flaw can make the body unable to tell the difference between self and nonself. When this happens, the body makes autoantibodies that attack normal cells by mistake. At the same time, special cells called "regulatory T cells" fail to do their job of keeping the immune system in line. The result is a misguided attack on your own body. This causes the damage known as "autoimmune disease." The body parts that are affected depend on the type of autoimmune disease. There are more than 80 known types.

HOW COMMON ARE AUTOIMMUNE DISEASES?

Overall, autoimmune diseases are common, affecting more than 23.5 million Americans. They are a leading cause of death and disability. Some autoimmune diseases are rare, while others, such as Hashimoto disease, affect many people.

WHO GETS AUTOIMMUNE DISEASES?

Autoimmune diseases can affect anyone. Yet certain people are at greater risk, including the following:

- **Women of childbearing age**. More women have autoimmune diseases than men, which often start during their childbearing years.
- **People with a family history**. Some autoimmune diseases, such as lupus and multiple sclerosis (MS) run in families. It is also common for different types of autoimmune diseases to affect different members of a single family. Inheriting certain genes can make it more likely to get an autoimmune disease. But a combination of genes and other factors may trigger the disease to start.

- **People who are around certain things in the environment.** Certain events or environmental exposures may cause some autoimmune diseases or make them worse. Sunlight, chemicals called "solvents," and viral and bacterial infections are linked to many autoimmune diseases.
- **People of certain races or ethnic backgrounds.** Some autoimmune diseases are more common or affect certain groups of people more severely. For instance, type 1 diabetes is more common in White people. Lupus is most severe for African American and Hispanic people.

WHAT AUTOIMMUNE DISEASES AFFECT WOMEN, AND WHAT ARE THEIR SYMPTOMS?

The diseases listed in Table 4.1 either are more common in women than men or affect many women and men.

Although each disease is unique, many share hallmark symptoms, such as fatigue, dizziness, and low-grade fever. For many autoimmune diseases, symptoms come and go or can be mild sometimes and severe at others. When symptoms go away for a while, it is called "remission." Flares are the sudden and severe onset of symptoms.

Table 4.1. Types of Autoimmune Diseases and Their Symptoms

Disease	Symptoms
Alopecia areata. The immune system attacks hair follicles (the structures from which hair grows). It usually does not threaten health, but it can greatly affect the way a person looks.	• patchy hair loss on the scalp, face, or other areas of your body
Antiphospholipid antibody syndrome (aPL). A disease that causes problems in the inner lining of blood vessels resulting in blood clots in arteries or veins.	• blood clots in veins or arteries • multiple miscarriages • lacy, netlike red rash on the wrists and knees

Table 4.1. Continued

Disease	Symptoms
Autoimmune hepatitis. A disease in which the immune system attacks and destroys the liver cells. This can lead to scarring and hardening of the liver and possibly liver failure.	• fatigue • enlarged liver • yellowing of the skin or whites of the eyes • itchy skin • joint pain • stomach pain or upset
Celiac disease. A disease in which people cannot tolerate gluten, a substance found in wheat, rye, and barley, and also some medicines. When people with celiac disease eat foods or use products that have gluten, the immune system responds by damaging the lining of the small intestines.	• abdominal bloating and pain • diarrhea or constipation • weight loss or weight gain • fatigue • missed menstrual periods • itchy skin rash • infertility or miscarriages
Diabetes type 1. A disease in which your immune system attacks the cells that make insulin, a hormone needed to control blood sugar levels. As a result, your body cannot make insulin. Without insulin, too much sugar stays in your blood. High blood sugar can hurt the eyes, kidneys, nerves, and gums and teeth. But the most serious problem caused by diabetes is heart disease.	• being very thirsty • urinating often • feeling very hungry or tired • losing weight without trying • having sores that heal slowly • dry, itchy skin • losing the feeling in your feet or having tingling in your feet • having blurry eyesight
Graves disease (overactive thyroid). A disease that causes the thyroid to make too much thyroid hormone.	• insomnia • irritability • weight loss • heat sensitivity • sweating • fine, brittle hair • muscle weakness • light menstrual periods • bulging eyes • shaky hands • sometimes no symptoms

Table 4.1. Continued

Disease	Symptoms
Guillain-Barré syndrome. A disease in which your immune system attacks the nerves that connect your brain and spinal cord with the rest of your body. Damage to the nerves makes it hard for them to transmit signals. As a result, the muscles have trouble responding to the brain.	• weakness or tingling feeling in the legs that might spread to the upper body • paralysis in severe cases Symptoms often progress relatively quickly, over a period of days or weeks, and often occur on both sides of the body.
Hashimoto. A disease that causes the thyroid not to make enough thyroid hormone.	• fatigue • weakness • weight gain • sensitivity to cold • muscle aches and stiff joints • facial swelling • constipation
Hemolytic anemia. A disease in which your immune system destroys red blood cells (RBCs). Yet the body cannot make new RBCs fast enough to meet the body's needs. As a result, your body does not get the oxygen it needs to function well, and your heart must work harder to move oxygen-rich blood throughout the body.	• fatigue • shortness of breath • dizziness • headache • cold hands or feet • paleness • yellowish skin or whites of eyes • heart problems, including heart failure
Idiopathic thrombocytopenic purpura (ITP). A disease in which the immune system destroys blood platelets, which are needed for blood to clot.	• very heavy menstrual period • tiny purple or red dots on the skin that might look like a rash • easy bruising • nosebleed or bleeding in the mouth
Inflammatory bowel disease (IBD). A disease that causes chronic inflammation of the digestive tract. Crohn's disease and ulcerative colitis are the most common forms of IBD.	• abdominal pain • diarrhea, which may be bloody Some people also have: • rectal bleeding • fever • weight loss • fatigue • mouth ulcers (in Crohn's disease) • painful or difficult bowel movements (in ulcerative colitis)

Table 4.1. Continued

Disease	Symptoms
Inflammatory myopathies. A group of diseases that involve muscle inflammation and muscle weakness. Polymyositis and dermatomyositis are two types more common in women than men.	• slow but progressive muscle weakness beginning in the muscles closest to the trunk of the body (Polymyositis affects muscles involved with making movement on both sides of the body. With dermatomyositis, a skin rash comes before or at the same time as muscle weakness.) Some may also have: • fatigue after walking or standing • tripping or falling • difficulty swallowing or breathing
Multiple sclerosis (MS). A disease in which the immune system attacks the protective coating around the nerves. The damage affects the brain and spinal cord.	• weakness and trouble with coordination, balance, speaking, and walking • paralysis • tremors • numbness and tingling feeling in arms, legs, hands, and feet • varied symptoms because the location and extent of each attack vary
Myasthenia gravis (MG). A disease in which the immune system attacks the nerves and muscles throughout the body.	• double vision, trouble keeping a steady gaze, and drooping eyelids • trouble swallowing, with frequent gagging or choking • weakness or paralysis • muscles that work better after rest • drooping head • trouble climbing stairs or lifting things • trouble talking
Primary biliary cholangitis. A disease in which the immune system slowly destroys the liver's bile ducts. Bile is a substance made in the liver. It travels through the bile ducts to help with digestion. When the ducts are destroyed, the bile builds up in the liver and hurts it. The damage causes the liver to harden and scar and eventually stop working.	• fatigue • itchy skin • dry eyes and mouth • yellowing of skin and whites of eyes

Table 4.1. Continued

Disease	Symptoms
Psoriasis. A disease that causes new skin cells that grow deep in your skin to rise too fast and pile up on the skin surface.	• thick red patches covered with scales, usually appearing on the head, elbows, and knees • itching and pain, which can make it hard to sleep, walk, and care for yourself Some people may also have: • a form of arthritis that often affects the joints and the ends of the fingers and toes • back pain that can occur if the spine is involved
Rheumatoid arthritis (RA). A disease in which the immune system attacks the lining of the joints throughout the body.	• painful, stiff, swollen, and deformed joints • reduced movement and function Some people may also have: • fatigue • fever • weight loss • eye inflammation • lung disease • lumps of tissue under the skin, often the elbows • anemia
Scleroderma. A disease-causing abnormal growth of connective tissue in the skin and blood vessels.	• fingers and toes that turn white, red, or blue in response to heat and cold • pain, stiffness, and swelling of fingers and joints • thickening of the skin • skin that looks shiny on the hands and forearm • tight and mask-like facial skin • sores on the fingers or toes • trouble swallowing • weight loss • diarrhea or constipation • shortness of breath

Table 4.1. Continued

Disease	Symptoms
Sjögren syndrome. A disease in which the immune system targets the glands that make moisture, such as tears and saliva.	• dry eyes or eyes that itch • dryness of the mouth, which can cause sores • trouble swallowing • loss of sense of taste • severe dental cavities • hoarse voice • fatigue • joint swelling or pain • swollen glands • cloudy eyes
Systemic lupus erythematosus. A disease that can damage the joints, skin, kidneys, heart, lungs, and other parts of the body. It is also called "SLE" or "lupus."	• fever • weight loss • hair loss • mouth sores • fatigue • "butterfly" rash across the nose and cheeks • rashes on other parts of the body • painful or swollen joints and muscle pain • sensitivity to the sun • chest pain • headache, dizziness, seizure, memory problems, or change in behavior
Vitiligo. The immune system destroys the cells that give your skin its color. It can also affect the tissue inside your mouth and nose.	• white patches on areas exposed to the sun or on armpits, genitals, and rectum • hair turns gray early • loss of color inside your mouth

HOW DO YOU FIND OUT IF YOU HAVE AN AUTOIMMUNE DISEASE?

Getting a diagnosis can be a long and stressful process. Although each autoimmune disease is unique, many share some of the same symptoms. And many symptoms of autoimmune diseases are the same for other types of health problems too. This makes it hard for doctors to find out if you really have an autoimmune disease and which one it might be.

But, if you are having symptoms that bother you, it is important to find the cause. Do not give up if you are not getting any answers. You can take the following steps to find out the cause of your symptoms:

- Write down a complete family health history that includes extended family and share it with your doctor.
- Record any symptoms you have, even if they seem unrelated, and share them with your doctor.
- See a specialist who has experience dealing with your most major symptom. For instance, if you have symptoms of IBD, start with a gastroenterologist. Ask your regular doctor, friends, and others for suggestions.
- Get a second, third, or fourth opinion if need be. If your doctor does not take your symptoms seriously or tells you they are stress related or in your head, see another doctor.

WHAT TYPES OF DOCTORS TREAT AUTOIMMUNE DISEASES?

Juggling your health-care needs among many doctors and specialists can be hard. But specialists, along with your primary doctor, may be helpful in managing some symptoms of your autoimmune disease. If you see a specialist, make sure you have a supportive primary doctor to help you. Often, your family doctor may help you coordinate care if you need to see one or more specialists. Here are some specialists who treat autoimmune diseases:

- **Nephrologist**. A doctor who treats kidney problems, such as inflamed kidneys caused by lupus.
- **Rheumatologist**. A doctor who treats arthritis and other rheumatic diseases, such as scleroderma and lupus.
- **Endocrinologist**. A doctor who treats gland and hormone problems, such as diabetes and thyroid disease.
- **Neurologist**. A doctor who treats nerve problems, such as MS and MG.
- **Hematologist**. A doctor who treats diseases that affect the blood, such as some forms of anemia.
- **Gastroenterologist**. A doctor who treats problems with the digestive system, such as IBD.

- **Dermatologist**. A doctor who treats diseases that affect the skin, hair, and nails, such as psoriasis and lupus.
- **Physical therapist**. A health-care worker who uses proper types of physical activity to help patients with stiffness, weakness, and restricted body movement.
- **Occupational therapist**. A health-care worker who can find ways to make activities of daily living easier for you despite your pain and other health problems. This could be teaching you new ways of doing things or how to use special devices or suggesting changes to make in your home or workplace.
- **Speech therapist**. A health-care worker who can help people with speech problems from illnesses such as MS.
- **Audiologist**. A health-care worker who can help people with hearing problems, including inner ear damage from autoimmune diseases.
- **Vocational therapist**. A health-care worker who offers job training for people who cannot do their current jobs because of their illness or other health problems. You can find this type of person through both public and private agencies.
- **Counselor for emotional support**. A health-care worker who is specially trained to help you find ways to cope with your illness. You can work through your feelings of anger, fear, denial, and frustration.

ARE THERE MEDICINES TO TREAT AUTOIMMUNE DISEASES?

There are many types of medicines used to treat autoimmune diseases. The type of medicine you need depends on which disease you have, how severe it is, and your symptoms. Treatment can do the following:

- **Relieve symptoms**. Some people can use over-the-counter (OTC) drugs such as aspirin and ibuprofen for mild pain or mild symptoms. Others with more severe symptoms may need prescription drugs to help relieve symptoms such as pain, swelling, depression, anxiety, sleep problems, fatigue, or rashes. For others, treatment may be as involved as having surgery.

- **Replace vital substances the body can no longer make on its own**. Some autoimmune diseases, such as diabetes and thyroid disease, can affect the body's ability to make substances it needs to function. With diabetes, insulin injections are needed to regulate blood sugar. Thyroid hormone replacement restores thyroid hormone levels in people with an underactive thyroid.
- **Suppress the immune system**. Some drugs can suppress immune system activity. These drugs can help control the disease process and preserve organ function. For instance, these drugs are used to control inflammation in affected kidneys in people with lupus to keep the kidneys working. Medicines used to suppress inflammation include chemotherapy given at lower doses than for cancer treatment and drugs used in patients who have had an organ transplant to protect against rejection. A class of drugs called "anti-TNF medications" blocks inflammation in some forms of autoimmune arthritis and psoriasis.

New treatments for autoimmune diseases are being studied all the time.

ARE THERE ALTERNATIVE TREATMENTS THAT CAN HELP?

Many people try some form of complementary and alternative medicine (CAM) at some point in their lives. Some examples of CAM are herbal products, chiropractic care, acupuncture, and hypnosis. If you have an autoimmune disease, you might wonder if CAM therapies can help some of your symptoms. This is hard to know. Studies on CAM therapies are limited. Also, some CAM products can cause health problems or interfere with how the medicines you might need work. If you want to try a CAM treatment, be sure to discuss it with your doctor. Your doctor can tell you about the possible benefits and risks of trying CAM.

YOU WANT TO HAVE A BABY. DOES HAVING AN AUTOIMMUNE DISEASE AFFECT PREGNANCY?

Women with autoimmune diseases can safely have children. But there could be some risks for the mother or baby, depending on the disease and how severe it is. For instance, pregnant women with lupus have a higher risk of preterm birth and stillbirth. Pregnant women with MG might have symptoms that lead to trouble breathing during pregnancy. For some women, symptoms tend to improve during pregnancy, while others find their symptoms tend to flare up. Also, some medicines used to treat autoimmune diseases might not be safe to use during pregnancy.

If you want to have a baby, talk to your doctor before you start trying to get pregnant. Your doctor might suggest that you wait until your disease is in remission or suggest a change in medicines before you start trying. You might also need to see a doctor who cares for women with high-risk pregnancies.

Some women with autoimmune diseases may have problems getting pregnant. This can happen for many reasons. Tests can tell if fertility problems are caused by an autoimmune disease or an unrelated reason. Fertility treatments are able to help some women with autoimmune diseases become pregnant.

HOW CAN YOU MANAGE YOUR LIFE NOW THAT YOU HAVE AN AUTOIMMUNE DISEASE?

Although most autoimmune diseases do not go away, you can treat your symptoms and learn to manage your disease, so you can enjoy life! Your life goals should not have to change. It is important, though, to see a doctor who specializes in these types of diseases, follow your treatment plan, and adopt a healthy lifestyle.[6]

---

[6] Office on Women's Health (OWH), "Autoimmune Diseases," U.S. Department of Health and Human Services (HHS), February 22, 2021. Available online. URL: www.womenshealth.gov/a-z-topics/autoimmune-diseases. Accessed May 23, 2023.

WHAT IS SEPSIS?

Sepsis is a person's overwhelming or impaired whole-body immune response to an insult—an infection or an injury to the body or something else that provokes such a response. It is a serious condition and a leading cause of death in hospitals. It is also the main reason why people are readmitted to the hospital.

Sepsis occurs unpredictably and can progress rapidly. In severe cases, one or more organ systems fail. In the worst cases, blood pressure drops; the heart weakens; and the patient spirals toward septic shock. Once this happens, multiple organs—lungs, kidneys, and liver—may quickly fail, and the patient can die.

WHAT CAUSES SEPSIS?

Most sepsis is caused by bacterial infections, but it can also be caused by viral infections, such as coronavirus disease 2019 (COVID-19) or influenza; fungal infections; or noninfectious insults, such as traumatic injury. Normally, the body releases chemical or protein immune mediators into the blood to combat the infection or insult. If unchecked, those immune mediators trigger widespread inflammation, blood clots, and leaky blood vessels. As a result, blood flow is impaired, depriving organs of nutrients and oxygen and leading to organ damage. Noninfectious insults can lead to sepsis because they can activate the body's immune responses just like infections do. In some cases, the cause can no longer be determined, particularly when a patient is given antibiotics, which can make infectious agents no longer detectable.

WHO GETS SEPSIS?

Anyone can develop sepsis. The people at the highest risk are infants, children, older adults, and people who have underlying medical problems such as diabetes, acquired immunodeficiency syndrome (AIDS), cancer, or liver disease; have concurrent injuries or surgeries; or are taking certain medications. There are also unknown biological characteristics in the body that may increase or decrease a person's susceptibility to sepsis and cause some people to decline more rapidly while others recover quickly. Scientists are conducting studies to identify these individual factors.

PREVALENCE OF SEPSIS

Each year, according to the Centers for Disease Control and Prevention (CDC), at least 1.7 million adults in the United States develop sepsis, and nearly 270,000 die as a result. The number of sepsis cases per year in the United States has been on the rise, likely due to several factors:

- There is increased awareness and tracking of sepsis, so more cases may be recognized than they were previously.
- People with chronic diseases are living longer. Sepsis is more common and more dangerous in those with other illnesses and in older adults.
- Some infections can no longer be eliminated with antibiotic drugs. Antibiotic-resistant infections can lead to sepsis.
- Organ transplants are more common. People are at a higher risk for sepsis if they have undergone any procedure that requires the use of medications to suppress the immune system, including organ transplantation.

WHAT ARE THE SYMPTOMS OF SEPSIS?

Common symptoms of sepsis are fever, chills, rapid breathing and heart rate, rash, confusion, and disorientation. Many of these symptoms are also common in other conditions, making sepsis challenging to recognize, especially in its early stages.

HOW IS SEPSIS DIAGNOSED?

Doctors start by checking for the symptoms mentioned above. They may also test a person's blood for the presence of bacteria or an abnormal number of white blood cells (WBCs) or use a chest x-ray or a computed tomography (CT) scan to locate an infection. In addition, they can use a scoring system to determine if the function of a particular organ is declining and note the number of organ systems affected.

HOW IS SEPSIS TREATED?

Doctors typically treat people with sepsis in hospital intensive care units (ICUs). They try to stop an infection, protect vital organs, and prevent a drop in blood pressure. This almost always includes the use of antibiotic medications and fluids.[7]

Antibiotics are critical tools for treating life-threatening infections, such as those that can lead to sepsis. However, as antibiotic resistance grows, infections are becoming more difficult to treat. Antibiotic side effects range from minor, such as rash, dizziness, nausea, diarrhea, and yeast infections, to very severe health problems, such as life-threatening allergic reactions.[8]

More seriously affected patients might need a breathing tube, kidney dialysis, or surgery to remove an infection. Despite years of research, scientists have not yet been successful in developing an approved medicine that specifically targets the aggressive or impaired immune response seen with sepsis. Sepsis patients vary in their immune responses and in their responses to treatment due to individual differences. Scientists are trying to find new therapies and to determine which patients are likely to benefit most from a certain approach.

ARE THERE ANY LONG-TERM EFFECTS OF SEPSIS?

Many patients who survive severe sepsis recover completely, and their lives return to normal. But some people can have permanent organ damage. For example, in someone who already has impaired kidneys, sepsis can lead to kidney failure that requires lifelong

---

[7] "Sepsis," National Institute of General Medical Sciences (NIGMS), September 10, 2021. Available online. URL: www.nigms.nih.gov/education/fact-sheets/Pages/sepsis.aspx. Accessed May 5, 2023.
[8] "How Is Sepsis Diagnosed and Treated?" Centers for Disease Control and Prevention (CDC), August 9, 2022. Available online. URL: www.cdc.gov/sepsis/diagnosis/index.html. Accessed May 5, 2023.

dialysis. If sepsis affects the brain, a person may have problems with thinking, memory, or concentration.

There is also some evidence that severe sepsis permanently disrupts a person's immune system, placing them at greater risk of future infections. Studies have shown that people who have experienced sepsis may have higher risk of various medical conditions or death, even several years after the episode.[9]

YOU SURVIVED SEPSIS. WHAT IS NEXT?
What Are the First Steps in Recovery?

After you have had sepsis, rehabilitation usually starts in the hospital by slowly helping you to move around and look after yourself: bathing, sitting up, standing, walking, taking yourself to the restroom, and so on. The purpose of rehabilitation is to restore you back to your previous level of health or as close to it as possible. Work with your health-care professional to determine the most appropriate rehabilitation plan and what activities are safe for you. Begin your rehabilitation by building up your activities slowly and rest when you are tired.

How Will You Feel When You Get Home?

You have been seriously ill, and your body and mind need time to get better. You may experience the following physical symptoms upon returning home:

- general to extreme weakness and fatigue
- breathlessness
- general body pains or aches
- difficulty moving around
- difficulty sleeping
- weight loss, lack of appetite, food not tasting normal
- dry and itchy skin that may peel
- brittle nails
- hair loss

---

[9] See footnote [7].

You may also experience the following feelings once you are at home:
- unsure of yourself
- not caring about your appearance
- wanting to be alone, avoiding friends and family
- flashbacks, bad memories
- confusing reality (e.g., not sure what is real and what is not)
- feeling anxious, more worried than usual
- poor concentration
- depressed, angry, unmotivated
- frustration at not being able to do everyday tasks

Talk with your health-care professional if you or your caregivers are concerned about any physical symptoms or feelings you are experiencing.

What Can You Do to Recover at Home?

Work with your health-care professional to determine the most appropriate rehabilitation plan and what activities are safe for you. The following are a few examples:
- Set small, achievable goals for yourself each week, such as taking a bath, dressing yourself, or walking up the stairs.
- Rest and rebuild your strength.
- Talk about what you are feeling to family and friends.
- Record your thoughts, struggles, and milestones in a journal.
- Learn about sepsis to understand what happened.
- Ask your family to fill in any gaps you may have in your memory about what happened to you.
- Eat a balanced diet.
- Exercise if you feel up to it.
- Make a list of questions to ask your health-care professional when you go for a checkup.

Are There Any Long-Term Effects of Sepsis?

Many people who survive sepsis recover completely, and their lives return to normal. However, as with some other illnesses requiring intensive medical care, some patients have long-term effects. These problems may not become apparent until several weeks after your hospital stay and may include consequences such as:

- insomnia and difficulty getting to or staying asleep
- nightmares, vivid hallucinations, and panic attacks
- disabling muscle and joint pains
- decreased mental (cognitive) function
- loss of self-esteem and self-belief
- organ dysfunction (kidney failure, lung problems, etc.)
- amputations (loss of limb(s))

Talk with your health-care professional if you have concerns about what you might experience in the weeks and months after getting home from the hospital.

Do the Effects of Sepsis Get Better? Are You at Risk of Sepsis Again? What Should You Do If You Think You Have Sepsis Again?

Generally, the effects of sepsis do improve with time. Some hospitals have follow-up clinics or staff to help patients and families once they have been discharged. Find out if yours does or if there are local resources available to help you while you get better. However, if you feel you are not getting better or finding it difficult to cope, call your health-care professional.

Keep in mind that people who survived sepsis are at a higher risk of getting sepsis again. If you or your loved one has an infection that is not getting better or is getting worse, act fast. Get medical care immediately. Ask your health-care professional, "Could this infection be leading to sepsis?" and if you should go to the emergency room. With fast recognition and treatment, most people survive.[10]

---

[10] See footnote [8].

Section 4.6 | **Cancer**

Cancer is a disease in which some of the body's cells grow uncontrollably and spread to other parts of the body. Cancer can start almost anywhere in the human body, which is made up of trillions of cells. Normally, human cells grow and multiply (through a process called "cell division") to form new cells as the body needs them. When cells grow old or become damaged, they die, and new cells take their place.

Sometimes, this orderly process breaks down, and abnormal or damaged cells grow and multiply when they should not. These cells may form tumors, which are lumps of tissue. Tumors can be cancerous or noncancerous (benign). Cancerous tumors spread into, or invade, nearby tissues and can travel to distant places in the body to form new tumors (a process called "metastasis"). Cancerous tumors may also be called "malignant tumors." Many cancers form solid tumors, but cancers of the blood, such as leukemias, generally do not.

Benign tumors do not spread into, or invade, nearby tissues. When removed, benign tumors usually do not grow back, whereas cancerous tumors sometimes do. Benign tumors can sometimes be quite large, however. Some can cause serious symptoms or be life-threatening, such as benign tumors in the brain.

TYPES OF CANCER

There are more than 100 types of cancer. Types of cancer are usually named for the organs or tissues where the cancers form. For example, lung cancer starts in the lung, and brain cancer starts in the brain. Cancers may also be described by the type of cell that formed them, such as an epithelial cell or a squamous cell.

Carcinoma

Carcinomas are the most common type of cancer. They are formed by epithelial cells, which are the cells that cover the inside and outside surfaces of the body. There are many types of epithelial cells, which often have a column-like shape when viewed under a microscope. Carcinomas that begin in different epithelial cell types have specific names:

- **Adenocarcinoma**. This cancer forms in epithelial cells that produce fluids or mucus. Tissues with this type of epithelial cells are sometimes called "glandular tissues." Most cancers of the breast, colon, and prostate are adenocarcinomas.
- **Basal cell carcinoma**. This cancer begins in the lower or basal (base) layer of the epidermis, which is a person's outer layer of skin.
- **Squamous cell carcinoma**. This cancer forms in squamous cells, which are epithelial cells that lie just beneath the outer surface of the skin. Squamous cells also line many other organs, including the stomach, intestines, lungs, bladder, and kidneys. Squamous cells look flat, like fish scales, when viewed under a microscope. Squamous cell carcinomas are sometimes called "epidermoid carcinomas."
- **Transitional cell carcinoma**. This cancer forms in a type of epithelial tissue called "transitional epithelium" or "urothelium." This tissue, which is made up of many layers of epithelial cells that can get bigger and smaller, is found in the linings of the bladder, ureters, part of the kidneys (renal pelvis), and a few other organs. Some cancers of the bladder, ureters, and kidneys are transitional cell carcinomas.

Sarcoma

Sarcomas are cancers that form in bone and soft tissues, including muscle, fat, blood vessels, lymph vessels, and fibrous tissue (such as tendons and ligaments). Osteosarcoma is the most common cancer of bone. The most common types of soft tissue sarcoma are leiomyosarcoma, Kaposi sarcoma, malignant fibrous histiocytoma, liposarcoma, and dermatofibrosarcoma protuberans.

Leukemia

Cancers that begin in the blood-forming tissue of the bone marrow are called "leukemias." These cancers do not form solid tumors. Instead, large numbers of abnormal white blood cells (WBCs; leukemia cells and leukemic blast cells) build up in the blood and bone marrow, crowding out normal blood cells. The low level of normal blood cells can make it harder for the body to get oxygen to its tissues, control bleeding, or fight infections.

There are four common types of leukemia, which are grouped based on how quickly the disease gets worse (acute or chronic) and on the type of blood cell the cancer starts in (lymphoblastic or myeloid). Acute forms of leukemia grow quickly, and chronic forms grow more slowly.

Lymphoma

Lymphoma is a cancer that begins in lymphocytes (T cells or B cells). These are disease-fighting WBCs that are part of the immune system. In lymphoma, abnormal lymphocytes build up in lymph nodes and lymph vessels, as well as in other organs of the body.

The following are the two main types of lymphoma:
- **Hodgkin lymphoma**. People with this disease have abnormal lymphocytes that are called "Reed-Sternberg cells." These cells usually form from B cells.
- **Non-Hodgkin lymphoma**. This is a large group of cancers that start in lymphocytes. The cancers can grow quickly or slowly and can form from B cells or T cells.

Multiple Myeloma

Multiple myeloma is a cancer that begins in plasma cells, another type of immune cell. The abnormal plasma cells, called "myeloma cells," build up in the bone marrow and form tumors in bones all through the body. Multiple myeloma is also called "plasma cell myeloma" and "Kahler disease."

Melanoma

Melanoma is a cancer that begins in cells that become melanocytes, which are specialized cells that make melanin (the pigment that gives skin its color). Most melanomas form on the skin, but melanomas can also form in other pigmented tissues, such as the eye.

Brain and Spinal Cord Tumors

There are different types of brain and spinal cord tumors. These tumors are named based on the type of cell in which they formed and where the tumor first formed in the central nervous system. For example, an astrocytic tumor begins in star-shaped brain cells called "astrocytes," which help keep nerve cells healthy. Brain tumors can be benign (not cancer) or malignant (cancer).

Other Types of Tumors

GERM CELL TUMORS

Germ cell tumors are a type of tumor that begins in the cells that give rise to sperm or eggs. These tumors can occur almost anywhere in the body and can be either benign or malignant.

NEUROENDOCRINE TUMORS

Neuroendocrine tumors form from cells that release hormones into the blood in response to a signal from the nervous system. These tumors, which may make higher-than-normal amounts of hormones, can cause many different symptoms. Neuroendocrine tumors may be benign or malignant.

CARCINOID TUMORS

Carcinoid tumors are a type of neuroendocrine tumor. They are slow-growing tumors that are usually found in the gastrointestinal system (most often in the rectum and small intestine). Carcinoid tumors may spread to the liver or other sites in the body, and they may secrete substances such as serotonin or prostaglandins, causing carcinoid syndrome.[11]

IMMUNOTHERAPY TO TREAT CANCER

Immunotherapy is a type of cancer treatment that helps your immune system fight cancer. The immune system helps your body fight infections and other diseases. It is made up of WBCs and organs and tissues of the lymph system.

Immunotherapy is a type of biological therapy. Biological therapy is a type of treatment that uses substances made from living organisms to treat cancer.

HOW DOES IMMUNOTHERAPY WORK AGAINST CANCER?

As part of its normal function, the immune system detects and destroys abnormal cells and most likely prevents or curbs the growth of many cancers. For instance, immune cells are sometimes found in and around tumors. These cells, called "tumor-infiltrating lymphocytes" (TILs), are a sign that the immune system is responding to the tumor. People whose tumors contain TILs often do better than people whose tumors do not contain them.

Even though the immune system can prevent or slow cancer growth, cancer cells have ways to avoid destruction by the immune system. For example, cancer cells may:

- have genetic changes that make them less visible to the immune system
- have proteins on their surface that turn off immune cells
- change the normal cells around the tumor, so they interfere with how the immune system responds to the cancer cells

Immunotherapy helps the immune system better act against cancer.

---

[11] "What Is Cancer?" National Cancer Institute (NCI), October 11, 2021. Available online. URL: www.cancer.gov/about-cancer/understanding/what-is-cancer. Accessed May 8, 2023.

WHAT ARE THE TYPES OF IMMUNOTHERAPY?

Several types of immunotherapy are used to treat cancer. These include the following:

- **Immune checkpoint inhibitors**. These are drugs that block immune checkpoints. These checkpoints are a normal part of the immune system and keep immune responses from being too strong. By blocking them, these drugs allow immune cells to respond more strongly to cancer.
- **T-cell transfer therapy**. This is a treatment that boosts the natural ability of your T cells to fight cancer. In this treatment, immune cells are taken from your tumor. Those that are most active against your cancer are selected or changed in the lab to better attack your cancer cells, grown in large batches, and put back into your body through a needle in a vein. T-cell transfer therapy may also be called "adoptive cell therapy," "adoptive immunotherapy," or "immune cell therapy."
- **Monoclonal antibodies**. These are immune system proteins created in the lab that are designed to bind to specific targets on cancer cells. Some monoclonal antibodies mark cancer cells so that they will be better seen and destroyed by the immune system. Such monoclonal antibodies are a type of immunotherapy. Monoclonal antibodies may also be called "therapeutic antibodies."
- **Treatment vaccines**. They work against cancer by boosting your immune system's response to cancer cells. Treatment vaccines are different from the ones that help prevent disease.
- **Immune system modulators**. They enhance the body's immune response against cancer. Some of these agents affect specific parts of the immune system, whereas others affect the immune system in a more general way.

WHICH CANCERS ARE TREATED WITH IMMUNOTHERAPY?

Immunotherapy drugs have been approved to treat many types of cancer. However, immunotherapy is not yet as widely used as surgery, chemotherapy, or radiation therapy.

What Are the Side Effects of Immunotherapy?

Immunotherapy can cause side effects, many of which happen when the immune system that has been revved up to act against the cancer also acts against healthy cells and tissues in your body.

Different people have different side effects. The ones you have and how they make you feel will depend on:

- how healthy you are before treatment
- your type of cancer
- how advanced your cancer is
- the type and dose of immunotherapy you are getting

You might be on immunotherapy for a long time. And side effects can occur at any point during and after treatment. Doctors and nurses cannot know for certain when or if side effects will occur or how serious they will be. Therefore, it is important to talk with your doctors and nurses about what signs to look for and what to do if you start to have problems.

Some side effects are common with all types of immunotherapy. For instance, you might have skin reactions at the needle site, which include:

- pain
- swelling
- soreness
- redness
- itchiness
- rash

You may have flu-like symptoms, and other side effects might include:

- swelling and weight gain from retaining fluid
- heart palpitations
- sinus congestion

- diarrhea
- infection
- organ inflammation

Some types of immunotherapy may cause severe or fatal allergic and inflammation-related reactions. But these reactions are rare.

HOW IS IMMUNOTHERAPY GIVEN?

Different forms of immunotherapy may be given in different ways. These include the following:

- **Intravenous (IV)**. The immunotherapy goes directly into a vein.
- **Oral**. The immunotherapy comes in pills or capsules that you swallow.
- **Topical**. The immunotherapy comes in a cream that you rub onto your skin. This type of immunotherapy can be used for very early skin cancer.
- **Intravesical**. The immunotherapy goes directly into the bladder.

WHERE DO YOU GO FOR IMMUNOTHERAPY?

You may receive immunotherapy in a doctor's office, clinic, or out-patient unit in a hospital. Outpatient means you do not spend the night in the hospital.

HOW OFTEN DO YOU RECEIVE IMMUNOTHERAPY?

How often and how long you receive immunotherapy depend on:

- your type of cancer and how advanced it is
- the type of immunotherapy you get
- how your body reacts to treatment

You may have treatment every day, week, or month. Some types of immunotherapy are given in cycles. A cycle is a period of treatment followed by a period of rest. The rest period gives your body a chance to recover, respond to immunotherapy, and build new healthy cells.

HOW CAN YOU TELL IF IMMUNOTHERAPY IS WORKING?

You will see your doctor often. He or she will give you physical exams and ask you how you feel. You will have medical tests, such as blood tests and different types of scans. These tests will measure the size of your tumor and look for changes in your blood work.

WHAT IS THE CURRENT RESEARCH IN IMMUNOTHERAPY?

Researchers are focusing on several major areas to improve immunotherapy, including the following:

- **Finding solutions for resistance**. Researchers are testing combinations of immune checkpoint inhibitors and other types of immunotherapy, targeted therapy, and radiation therapy to overcome resistance to immunotherapy.
- **Finding ways to predict responses to immunotherapy**. Only a small portion of people who receive immunotherapy will respond to the treatment. Finding ways to predict which people will respond to treatment is a major area of research.
- **Learning more about cancer cells**. It is important to learn how cancer cells evade or suppress immune responses against them. A better understanding of how cancer cells get around the immune system could lead to the development of new drugs that block those processes.
- **Reducing the side effects of treatment**. Know how to reduce the side effects of treatment with immunotherapy.[12]

---

[12] "Immunotherapy to Treat Cancer," National Cancer Institute (NCI), September 24, 2019. Available online. URL: www.cancer.gov/about-cancer/treatment/types/immunotherapy. Accessed May 8, 2023.

Chapter 5 | **Genetics and Epigenetics of Immunity**

GENETICS

Numerous studies have reported that certain diseases are inherited. But genetics also plays a role in immune response, affecting our ability to stave off disease, according to a team of international researchers. Understanding the genes affecting immune system cells and the risk for autoimmune disease is the first step in developing therapies that are personalized according to an individual's needs although more research is needed to further characterize the role genetics plays in the complex dynamics of the immune system, the researchers pointed out.

The human immune system is a complex network of cells, tissues, and organs working together to fight disease and keep us in optimal health and function. Our first line of defense, the innate immune system, includes barriers, such as skin and mucus, as well as specific cells and molecules providing a prompt but nonspecific response to harmful germs—pathogens—preventing them from entering the body or eliminating them rapidly after infection. The second line of defense, the adaptive immune system, engages the body to produce, store, and transport cells and molecules providing more specific responses to combat pathogens. The immune system has evolved to reject pathogens and even some cancers, but high levels of immune function can also make the body prone to autoimmune disease. Autoimmune diseases occur when the body uses the immune system against itself, attacking normal, healthy cells.

The number of adaptive immune system cells available to attack a pathogen or, in the case of autoimmune disease, attack healthy cells is what appears to be regulated by genetics. Small, single-letter variations in genes naturally occur throughout the deoxyribonucleic acid (DNA) code and are generally without effect on any specific trait. However, in some instances, scientists find that a particular variant is more common among people with a trait or disease.[1]

THE LINK BETWEEN POWERFUL GENE REGULATORY ELEMENTS AND AUTOIMMUNE DISEASES

Investigators with the National Institutes of Health (NIH) have discovered the genomic switches of a blood cell key to regulating the human immune system. Autoimmune diseases occur when the immune system mistakenly attacks its own cells, causing inflammation. Different tissues are affected in different diseases: For example, the joints become swollen and inflamed in rheumatoid arthritis (RA), and the brain and spinal cord are damaged in multiple sclerosis. The causes of these diseases are not well understood, but scientists believe that they have a genetic component because they often run in families.

Identifying autoimmune disease susceptibility genes can be a challenge because, in most cases, a complex mix of genetic and environmental factors is involved. Genetic studies have shown that people with autoimmune diseases possess unique genetic variants, but most of the alterations are found in regions of the DNA that do not carry genes. Scientists have suspected that the variants are in DNA elements called "enhancers," which act like switches to control gene activities.[2]

WHAT IS EPIGENETICS?

Your genes play an important role in your health, but so do your behaviors and environment, such as what you eat and how

[1] "Gene Variants Found Associated with Human Immune System, Autoimmune Disease," National Institutes of Health (NIH), September 26, 2013. Available online. URL: www.nih.gov/news-events/news-releases/gene-variants-found-associated-human-immune-system-autoimmune-disease. Accessed May 4, 2023.
[2] "NIH Researchers Reveal Link between Powerful Gene Regulatory Elements and Autoimmune Diseases," National Institutes of Health (NIH), February 17, 2015. Available online. URL: www.nih.gov/news-events/news-releases/nih-researchers-reveal-link-between-powerful-gene-regulatory-elements-autoimmune-diseases. Accessed May 4, 2023.

physically active you are. Epigenetics is the study of how your behaviors and environment can cause changes that affect the way your genes work. Unlike genetic changes, epigenetic changes are reversible and do not change your DNA sequence, but they can change how your body reads a DNA sequence.

Gene expression refers to how often or when proteins are created from the instructions within your genes. While genetic changes can alter which protein is made, epigenetic changes affect gene expression to turn genes "on" and "off." Since your environment and behaviors, such as diet and exercise, can result in epigenetic changes, it is easy to see the connection between your genes and your behaviors and environment.

HOW DOES EPIGENETICS WORK?

Epigenetic changes affect gene expression in different ways. The types of epigenetic changes include the following:

- **DNA methylation**. DNA methylation works by adding a chemical group to DNA. Typically, this group is added to specific places on the DNA, where it blocks the proteins that attach to DNA to "read" the gene. This chemical group can be removed through a process called "demethylation." Typically, methylation turns genes "off," and demethylation turns genes "on."
- **Histone modification**. DNA wraps around proteins called "histones." When histones are tightly packed together, proteins that "read" the gene cannot access the DNA as easily, so the gene is turned "off." When histones are loosely packed, more DNA is exposed or not wrapped around a histone and can be accessed by proteins that "read" the gene, so the gene is turned "on." Chemical groups can be added or removed from histones to make the histones more tightly or loosely packed, turning genes "off" or "on."
- **Noncoding ribonucleic acid (RNA)**. Your DNA is used as instructions for making coding and noncoding RNA. Coding RNA is used to make proteins. Noncoding RNA helps control gene expression by attaching to coding

RNA, along with certain proteins, to break down the coding RNA so that it cannot be used to make proteins. Noncoding RNA may also recruit proteins to modify histones to turn genes "on" or "off."

HOW CAN YOUR EPIGENETICS CHANGE?

Your epigenetics changes as you age, both as part of normal development and aging and in response to your behaviors and environment.

Epigenetics and Development

Epigenetic changes begin before you are born. All your cells have the same genes but look and act differently. As you grow and develop, epigenetics helps determine which function a cell will have, for example, whether it will become a heart cell, nerve cell, or skin cell. For example—nerve cells versus muscle cells—your muscle cells and nerve cells have the same DNA but work differently. A nerve cell transports information to other cells in your body. A muscle cell has a structure that aids in your body's ability to move. Epigenetics allows the muscle cell to turn "on" genes to make proteins important for its job and turn "off" genes important for a nerve cell's job.

Epigenetics and Age

Your epigenetics changes throughout your life. Your epigenetics at birth is not the same as your epigenetics during childhood or adulthood. For example, in the study of newborn versus 26-year-old versus 103-year-old, DNA methylation at millions of sites was measured in a newborn, 26-year-old, and 103-year-old. The level of DNA methylation decreases with age. A newborn had the highest DNA methylation; the 103-year-old had the lowest DNA methylation; and the 26-year-old had a DNA methylation level between the newborn and the 103-year-old.

Epigenetics and Reversibility

Not all epigenetic changes are permanent. Some epigenetic changes can be added or removed in response to changes in behavior or environment. For example—smokers versus nonsmokers versus former smokers—smoking can result in epigenetic changes. At certain parts of the AHRR gene, smokers tend to have less DNA methylation than nonsmokers. The difference is greater for heavy smokers and long-term smokers. After quitting smoking, former smokers can begin to have increased DNA methylation at this gene. Eventually, they can reach levels similar to those of nonsmokers. In some cases, this can happen in under a year, but the length of time depends on how long and how much someone smoked before quitting.

EPIGENETICS AND HEALTH

Epigenetic changes can affect your health in different ways:

- **Infections**. Germs can change your epigenetics to weaken your immune system. This helps the germ survive.
- **Cancer**. Certain mutations make you more likely to develop cancer. Likewise, some epigenetic changes increase your cancer risk. For example, having a mutation in the BRCA1 gene that prevents it from working properly makes you more likely to get breast and other cancers. Similarly, increased DNA methylation that results in decreased BRCA1 gene expression raises your risk for breast and other cancers. While cancer cells have increased DNA methylation at certain genes, overall DNA methylation levels are lower in cancer cells than those in normal cells. Different types of cancer that look alike can have different DNA methylation patterns. Epigenetics can be used to help determine which type of cancer a person has or can help find hard-to-detect cancers earlier. Epigenetics alone cannot diagnose cancer, and cancers would need to be confirmed with further screening tests. For example, colorectal cancers have abnormal methylation at DNA regions near certain genes, which affects the expression of these genes. Some commercial colorectal cancer screening tests use stool samples to look for

abnormal DNA methylation levels at one or more of these DNA regions. It is important to know that if the test result is positive or abnormal, a colonoscopy test is needed to complete the screening process.

- **Nutrition during pregnancy.** A pregnant woman's environment and behavior during pregnancy, such as whether she eats healthy food, can change the baby's epigenetics. Some of these changes can remain for decades and might make the child more likely to get certain diseases.[3]

ENVIRONMENTAL EPIGENETICS

Epigenetic processes are particularly important in early life when cells are first receiving the instructions that will dictate their future development and specialization. These processes can also be initiated or disrupted by environmental factors, such as diet, stress, aging, and pollutants.

In 2005, a team of Italian researchers provided the first concrete evidence for the role of environmental epigenetics in explaining why twins with the same genetic background can have vastly different disease susceptibilities. The researchers showed that at birth, pairs of identical twins have similar epigenetic patterns, including DNA methylation and histone modifications.

However, over time, the epigenetic patterns of individuals become different, even in twins. Since identical twins are the same genetically, the differences are thought to result from a combination of different environmental influences that each individual experiences over a lifetime.[4]

[3] "What Is Epigenetics?" Centers for Disease Control and Prevention (CDC), August 15, 2022. Available online. URL: www.cdc.gov/genomics/disease/epigenetics.htm. Accessed May 4, 2023.
[4] "Epigenetics," National Institute of Environmental Health Sciences (NIEHS), November 16, 2021. Available online. URL: www.niehs.nih.gov/health/topics/science/epigenetics/index.cfm. Accessed May 4, 2023.

Chapter 6 | **Alcohol Impairment of Immune Function**

Alcohol use disorders (AUDs) were estimated to be the third most common nongenetic cause of mortality in the United States in the year 2000. Epidemiological and clinical studies have established that alcohol abuse predisposes individuals to opportunistic infections and to organ damage, the two most prominent alcohol-related medical complications. Important alcohol-related infections include bacterial pneumonia and viral hepatitis. Significant alcohol-related illnesses involving organ damage or tissue injury include chronic liver diseases, respiratory distress syndrome, pancreatitis, renal disease, and cancer (in particular cancer of the upper aerodigestive tract, liver, and breast). Other organ systems adversely affected by excessive alcohol consumption include the cardiovascular system, muscle, and bone. In addition, alcohol abuse exacerbates tissue injury caused by various comorbid conditions such as viral hepatitis, trauma, surgical challenge, obesity, diabetes, smoking (in the case of cancer), and human immunodeficiency virus/acquired immunodeficiency syndrome (HIV/AIDS).

SYSTEMIC AND ORGAN-SPECIFIC IMMUNE DYSFUNCTION DUE TO ALCOHOL EXPOSURE

Innate immune cells are the first line of response against pathogens and tissue injury, sensing, killing, and removing pathogens and damaged cells. Among these cells, monocytes and monocyte-derived tissue macrophages are critical for initiating inflammation, producing cytokines, and eliminating pathogens and damaged cells by phagocytosis. Acute alcohol feeding in animal models inhibits both the phagocytic activity of monocytes and macrophages and their cytokine production in response to inducers of inflammation such as lipopolysaccharides (LPSs).

Chronic alcohol feeding also inhibits the phagocytic activity of these cells, especially monocytes and liver macrophages (Kupffer cells), in response to inflammation inducers yet potentiates excessive cytokine expression. Excessive alcohol use has been shown to adversely affect the function of important innate immune cells including neutrophils, natural killer (NK) and NK T cells, and dendritic cells. Changes in cytokine production, together with the effects on immune cells, foster a pro-inflammatory environment that has been causally linked to tissue injury. The integrity of barrier function is also an essential part of innate host defense. Epithelial tissues at mucosal surfaces in the gut and the lung and at the blood-brain barrier are increasingly recognized for their roles in restricting infections and shaping host immune systems. Impairment of barrier function of these cells due to alcohol use has been extensively reported.

Adaptive immune cells, in contrast, provide a more specific and long-lasting defense against infection, and their activation is achieved with the help of innate immune cells, especially dendritic cells. T cells and B cells, respectively, represent the cell and antibody-based adaptive immune responses. Chronic alcohol consumption has a generally immunosuppressive effect on the adaptive immune response, especially cell-mediated immunity. In addition, a chronic alcohol-induced shift from a naïve CD8$^+$ T cell phenotype to a memory cell CD8$^+$ phenotype has been observed in both humans and mouse models.

Different lineages of helper CD4$^+$ T cells play critical roles in directing pathogen-specific adaptive immune responses. For example, CD4$^+$ T-helper 1 (T$_h$1) cells are essential for combating intracellular bacterial infections, whereas T$_h$2 cells are critical for combating extracellular parasites. T$_h$1 cell-produced cytokines help to sustain an inflammatory response by stimulating macrophages, with feed-forward stimulation by macrophage-produced cytokines. In alcohol-fed animal models with primary infection and human alcoholics undergoing surgery, a significant shift of the T_h1/T_h2 balance has been observed and suggested to be critical in the susceptibility to infection. The current understanding of the polarization of immune function has expanded beyond T-helper cells to a somewhat analogous diversity of function in macrophages. While classically activated macrophages stimulate and maintain inflammation by releasing pro-inflammatory cytokines that influence T_h1 development, alternatively activated macrophages are anti-inflammatory and serve different homeostatic functions, including tissue repair.

Chronic and systemic inflammation, evident in the rise of circulating pro-inflammatory cytokines, is a common feature in alcoholics, especially those with liver diseases. Along with long-term exposure to alcohol, a confluence of factors induce and sustain the inflammatory environment, causing tissue injury in the liver and gut, increasing circulating LPSs, and exerting an impact on the host immune system and neuroendocrine function.

IMMUNE DYSFUNCTION AND ORGAN INJURY
Lung
Impairment of pulmonary defense by alcohol is a major contributor to the medical burden of alcohol consumption. Chronic alcoholics account for 50 percent of all cases of acute respiratory distress syndrome (ARDS). The high incidence of this often-fatal condition and of other respiratory infections in chronic alcoholics reflects the fact that alcohol has multiple effects on lung homeostasis. Alveolar integrity and pulmonary immune function are compromised by alcohol exposure; mucociliary clearance in the upper airway is disrupted; and alcohol is known to contribute to oxidative stress in the lung. Antioxidant therapy has shown some promise in restoring pulmonary immune function in preclinical models.

Alcoholic Liver Diseases
A number of immune alterations are associated with alcoholic liver diseases (ALDs). Early research has shown that alcoholics with cirrhosis have elevated pro-inflammatory cytokines in circulation in addition to clinical symptoms of systemic inflammation

that are closely linked to an increased leakage of gut microbial products such as LPSs. Polymorphisms of cytokine genes have been found to be associated with ALDs. Consistently, studies of mouse models have shown that LPS and its host cell sensor TLR4, liver-resident macrophages (Kupffer cells), and pro-inflammatory cytokine tumor necrosis factor-alpha (TNF-α) all play a causal role in the early stages of alcohol-induced liver pathology. Consistently, probiotics use in alcoholics has shown promise as an effective preventive treatment. Other immune alterations are associated with ALD, including:

- autoimmune activity, including liver deposition of IgG and IgA against liver proteins that form adducts with the alcohol metabolite acetaldehyde
- enrichment of a pro-inflammatory effector T cell, T_h17 cells, in the liver of alcoholics with liver diseases
- activation of hepatic stellate cells by cytokines made by Kupffer cells, an event critical for the progression of fibrosis to cirrhosis
- enrichment of neutrophils in the liver as a characteristic of ALD

The relative importance of these immune alterations in the pathogenesis of human ALD remains to be determined.

Neuropathy

Alcohol-induced brain inflammation is now believed to be an underlying cause for impairment of cognitive function and structural changes to the brain, common in alcoholics. Alcohol administration induces the pro-inflammatory cytokine TNF-α in the brains of mice and potentially contributes to neural damage. In addition, alcohol alters the permeability of the blood-brain barrier by oxidative stress and by damaging basement membranes and modifying tight junction proteins. The disruption of the blood-brain barrier allows the accumulation of neutrophils and T cells in the brain, leading to an inflammatory state that is harmful to neurons.

IMMUNE DYSFUNCTION IN SIGNIFICANT COMORBID CONDITIONS
Trauma

In patients who sustain trauma, alcohol exposure occurring either prior to or at the time of injury contributes to enhanced morbidity and mortality due to sepsis and shock. Tissue injury at remote sites not only leads to a systemic inflammatory response but also affects the immune homeostasis of important organs—in particular, the lung and the gut. Consequently, trauma victims are more susceptible to infections after acute or chronic alcohol exposure. Alcohol's contribution to a poorer outcome has been observed with fractures, burns, blood loss, and other forms of trauma. In addition, the incidence of postsurgical complications is greater in chronic alcoholics than that in the general population. Insight into the mechanism by which alcohol exposure increases the progression of the systemic inflammatory response leading to sepsis and ultimately multiple organ failure would be of clinical benefit.

Pathogenesis of Viral Hepatitis

Four million Americans and 120 million people worldwide are infected with the hepatitis C virus (HCV), and up to 70–80 percent of patients with primary infection fail to clear the virus. Alcohol abuse further reduces viral clearance and accelerates the progression of fibrosis and hepatocellular carcinoma (HCC). Chronic HCV infection, like alcohol abuse, is a major cause of chronic liver disease and HCC. Alcohol affects anti-HCV immunity through the impairment of the dendritic cell activation of T_h1 CD4$^+$ cells, an adaptive immune cell type critical for HCV clearance, and through oxidative stress, reducing the proteasomal activity in hepatocytes necessary for viral antigen presentation, further attenuating the adaptive immune response.

HIV/AIDS

An estimated 1.1 million Americans and more than 30 million people worldwide are living with HIV/AIDS. The prevalence of alcohol use in this population is associated with increased mortality.

In animal models with HIV/simian immunodeficiency virus (SIV) infection, alcohol feeding increases viral replication and accelerates mortality and morbidity. These medical consequences coincide with alcohol-induced alteration of T cells in the mucosa. The impact of alcohol on the mucosal immune system is still largely unknown.

As an increasing number of HIV-infected patients live longer with antiretroviral medications, non-AIDS-defining conditions have become the major causes of mortality and multiple morbidities. For example, a significant percentage of HIV patients have HCV or hepatitis B virus (HBV) coinfections and are at a greater risk to develop end-stage liver diseases. These coinfected patients are particularly vulnerable to the adverse impact of alcohol abuse. Other alcohol-affected conditions include neuropathological problems.

Alcohol, Immune Function, and Cancer

Alcohol consumption is associated with cancers originating in the upper aerodigestive tract, liver, colon, and breast. Chronic alcohol consumption leads to chronic inflammation, and a causative link between inflammation and cancer has been postulated. In addition, disruption of immune function, specifically immune surveillance, by alcohol may contribute to the incidence of cancer at these sites. Alterations in NK cells and myeloid-derived suppressor cells (MDSCs) in alcohol-fed animals have been reported in the context of cancer models. However, immune surveillance is a complex physiological process likely involving all immune cell types. The effects of alcohol on antitumor immunity remain an underexplored area of research.[1]

---

[1] "Alcohol Impairment of Immune Function, Host Defense and Tissue Homeostasis (R01 Clinical Trial Optional)," National Institutes of Health (NIH), November 1, 2017. Available online. URL: https://grants.nih.gov/grants/guide/pa-files/PA-18-191.html. Accessed May 9, 2023.

Part 2 | Primary Immunodeficiency Diseases

Chapter 7 | **Understanding Primary Immune Deficiency Diseases**

PRIMARY IMMUNODEFICIENCY

Your immune system helps your body fight infections. People with primary immunodeficiency (PI) have an immune system that does not work correctly. This means that people with PI are more likely to get and become very sick from infections.

There are more than 400 types of PI that vary in severity, which affects how early they are detected. In some cases, a person with a mild form may not find out that they have PI until adulthood. In other cases, the disorder causes problems in infancy and is found soon after birth. All states include testing for one type of PI called "severe combined immunodeficiency" (SCID) as part of newborn screening. Treatments can help the immune system work better. Which treatment works best depends on the type of PI a person has.

SIGNS AND SYMPTOMS OF PRIMARY IMMUNODEFICIENCY

People with PI are more likely to have the following:
- more frequent or repeated infections, such as:
  - ear infections
  - sinus infections
  - pneumonia
  - bronchitis
  - meningitis
  - skin infections

- thrush (a fungal infection of the mouth or skin, also called "candidiasis")
- infections that last longer than in most people
- infections that are hard to treat and do not respond to antibiotics or require intravenous (IV) antibiotics
- infections that are more severe and require hospitalization, such as sepsis or abscesses (pus-filled infections) of internal organs
- infections that most people do not get (sometimes called "opportunistic infections")
- lack of weight gain or growth in an infant (failure to thrive)
- digestive problems, such as chronic diarrhea

People with PI are more likely to have autoimmune disorders and certain blood disorders. Because your immune system protects your body against cancer, people with PI are more likely to have certain cancers. In some cases, PI is due to a genetic disorder that involves other health problems, such as 22q11.2 deletion syndrome (also called "DiGeorge syndrome").

Talk to your doctor if you think that you or your child has signs of PI. Your doctor might refer you or your child to a clinical immunologist, a doctor who specializes in the immune system. You can use the American Academy of Allergy, Asthma, and Immunology's Find an Allergist/Immunologist tool (https://allergist.aaaai.org/find) to find a doctor near you.

PI often has an underlying genetic cause and can run in families. Sharing your family history of PI with your doctor can be important for your and your children's health or if you are pregnant or planning a pregnancy. If you or your child has been diagnosed with PI, be sure to share this information with your family members. Your doctor might refer you for genetic counseling and testing if you have been diagnosed with PI or have a family health history of PI.

PREVENTION OF PRIMARY IMMUNODEFICIENCY

Early diagnosis can help prevent or delay some of the health problems caused by PI. Left untreated, some types of PI can result in serious health problems, including organ damage, and even death. Even with treatment, most PIs do not have a cure. Taking steps to prevent infection is very important if you have PI. These steps include the following:

- washing your hands the right way
- taking good care of your teeth
- maintaining healthy habits, including being physically active, eating healthy, and getting enough sleep
- avoiding exposure to people who are sick and crowds
- asking your doctor which vaccinations are safe for you (In some cases, people with PI cannot have live vaccines such as rotavirus, chickenpox, oral polio, measles, mumps, and rubella. Newborn screening for SCID can find babies with this PI early, before they receive these vaccines.)

TREATMENT FOR PEOPLE WITH PRIMARY IMMUNODEFICIENCY

Treatments vary, depending on the type of PI, and can include the following:

- antibiotics to prevent certain infections
- treatments that help your immune system work better (including immunoglobulin replacement therapy and interferon gamma therapy)
- growth factors to help increase the number of white blood cells (WBCs), which are part of the immune system
- stem cell transplant to provide your body with working immune cells from another person (donor)
- gene therapy to replace the gene that does not work correctly with the one that does[1]

---

[1] "Primary Immunodeficiency (PI)," Centers for Disease Control and Prevention (CDC), May 20, 2022. Available online. URL: www.cdc.gov/genomics/disease/primary_immunodeficiency.htm. Accessed April 18, 2023.

Chapter 8 | **Ataxia-Telangiectasia**

WHAT IS ATAXIA-TELANGIECTASIA?

Ataxia-telangiectasia (AT) is a rare inherited disorder that affects the nervous system, immune system, and other body systems. This disorder is characterized by progressive difficulty with coordinating movements (ataxia) beginning in early childhood, usually before the age of five. Affected children typically develop difficulty walking, problems with balance and hand coordination, involuntary jerking movements (chorea), muscle twitches (myoclonus), and disturbances in nerve function (neuropathy). The movement problems typically cause people to require wheelchair assistance by adolescence. People with this disorder also have slurred speech and trouble moving their eyes to look side-to-side (oculomotor apraxia). Small clusters of enlarged blood vessels called "telangiectases," which occur in the eyes and on the surface of the skin, are also characteristic of this condition.

Affected individuals tend to have high amounts of a protein called "alpha-fetoprotein" (AFP) in their blood. The level of this protein is normally increased in the bloodstream of pregnant women, but it is unknown why individuals with AT have elevated AFP or what effects it has in these individuals.

People with AT often have a weakened immune system, and many develop chronic lung infections. They also have an increased risk of developing cancer, particularly cancer of blood-forming cells (leukemia) and cancer of immune system cells (lymphoma). Affected individuals are very sensitive to the effects of radiation exposure, including medical x-rays. AT has no cure though treatments might improve some symptoms. These treatments include physical and speech therapy and improving deficits in the immune system and nutrition. The life expectancy of people with AT varies greatly, but affected individuals typically live into early adulthood.

Other Names of This Condition
- A-T
- ataxia-telangiectasia syndrome
- ataxia-telangiectasia mutated (ATM)
- Louis-Bar syndrome
- cerebello-oculocutaneous telangiectasia

FREQUENCY OF ATAXIA-TELANGIECTASIA
Ataxia-telangiectasia occurs in 1 in 40,000–100,000 people worldwide.

CAUSES OF ATAXIA-TELANGIECTASIA
Variants, also called "mutations," in the *ATM* gene cause AT. The *ATM* gene provides instructions for making a protein that helps control cell division and is involved in deoxyribonucleic acid (DNA) repair. This protein plays an important role in the normal development and activity of several body systems, including the nervous system and immune system. The ATM protein assists cells in recognizing damaged or broken DNA strands and coordinates DNA repairs by activating enzymes that fix the broken strands. Efficient repair of damaged DNA strands helps maintain the stability of the cell's genetic information.

Variants in the *ATM* gene reduce or eliminate the function of the ATM protein. Without this protein, cells become unstable and die. Cells in the part of the brain involved in coordinating movements (the cerebellum) are particularly affected by the loss of the ATM protein. The loss of these brain cells causes some of the movement problems characteristic of AT. Variants in the *ATM* gene also prevent cells from responding correctly to DNA damage, which allows breaks in DNA strands to accumulate and can lead to the formation of cancerous tumors.

INHERITANCE OF ATAXIA-TELANGIECTASIA

Ataxia-telangiectasia is inherited in an autosomal recessive pattern, which means both copies of the *ATM* gene in each cell have variants. Most often, the parents of an individual with an autosomal recessive condition each carry one copy of the altered gene but do not show signs and symptoms of the condition.

About 1 percent of the U.S. population carry one altered copy and one normal copy of the *ATM* gene in each cell. These individuals are called "carriers." Although *ATM* gene variant carriers do not have AT, they are more likely than people without an *ATM* gene variant to develop cancer; female carriers are particularly at risk for developing breast cancer. Carriers of a variant in the *ATM* gene may also have an increased risk of heart disease.[1]

HOW CAN YOU OR YOUR LOVED ONE HELP IMPROVE CARE FOR PEOPLE WITH ATAXIA-TELANGIECTASIS?

Consider participating in a clinical trial, so clinicians and scientists can learn more about AT and related disorders. Clinical research uses human volunteers to help researchers learn more about a disorder and perhaps find better ways to safely detect, treat, or prevent disease. All types of volunteers are needed—those who are healthy or may have an illness or disease—of all different ages, sexes, races, and ethnicities to ensure that study results apply to as many people as possible and that treatments will be safe and effective for everyone who will use them.

For information about participating in clinical research, visit the National Institutes of Health (NIH) Clinical Research Trials and You web page (www.nih.gov/health/clinicaltrials). Learn about clinical trials currently looking for people with AT at http://clinicaltrials.gov.[2]

---

[1] MedlinePlus, "Ataxia-Telangiectasia," National Institutes of Health (NIH), September 19, 2022. Available online. URL: https://medlineplus.gov/genetics/condition/ataxia-telangiectasia. Accessed April 18, 2023.

[2] "Ataxia Telangiectasia," National Institute of Neurological Disorders and Stroke (NINDS), February 7, 2023. Available online. URL: www.ninds.nih.gov/health-information/disorders/ataxia-telangiectasia. Accessed April 18, 2023.

Chapter 9 | **Autoimmune Lymphoproliferative Syndrome**

Autoimmune lymphoproliferative syndrome (ALPS) is an inherited disorder in which the body cannot properly regulate the number of immune system cells (lymphocytes). ALPS is characterized by the production of an abnormally large number of lymphocytes (lymphoproliferation). Accumulation of excess lymphocytes results in enlargement of the lymph nodes (lymphadenopathy), the liver (hepatomegaly), and the spleen (splenomegaly).

Autoimmune disorders are also common in ALPS. Autoimmune disorders occur when the immune system malfunctions and attacks the body's own tissues and organs. Most of the autoimmune disorders associated with ALPS target and damage blood cells. For example, the immune system may attack red blood cells (RBCs; autoimmune hemolytic anemia), white blood cells (WBCs; autoimmune neutropenia), or platelets (autoimmune thrombocytopenia). Less commonly, autoimmune disorders that affect other organs and tissues occur in people with ALPS. These disorders can damage the kidneys (glomerulonephritis), liver (autoimmune hepatitis), eyes (uveitis), or nerves (Guillain-Barré syndrome). Skin problems, usually rashes or hives (urticaria), can also occur in ALPS.

ALPS can have varying patterns of signs and symptoms. Most commonly, lymphoproliferation becomes apparent during childhood. Enlargement of the lymph nodes and spleen frequently occurs in affected individuals. Autoimmune disorders typically

119

develop several years later, most frequently as a combination of hemolytic anemia and thrombocytopenia, also called "Evans syndrome." People with this classic form of ALPS generally have a near-normal life span but have a greatly increased risk of developing cancer of the immune system cells (lymphoma) compared with the general population.

Some people have signs and symptoms that resemble those of ALPS, including lymphoproliferation, lymphadenopathy, splenomegaly, and low blood counts, but the specific pattern of these signs and symptoms or the genetic cause may be different. Researchers disagree on whether individuals with these nonclassic forms should be considered to have ALPS or a separate condition.

Other Names of This Condition
- ALPS
- Canale-Smith syndrome

CAUSES OF AUTOIMMUNE LYMPHOPROLIFERATIVE SYNDROME
Mutations in the *FAS* gene cause ALPS in approximately 75 percent of affected individuals; these mutations are associated with the classic form of the disorder. The *FAS* gene provides instructions for making a protein involved in cell signaling that results in the self-destruction of cells (apoptosis).

When the immune system is turned on (activated) to fight an infection, large numbers of lymphocytes are produced. Normally, these lymphocytes undergo apoptosis when they are no longer required.

FAS gene mutations lead to an abnormal protein that interferes with apoptosis. As a result, excess lymphocytes accumulate in the body's tissues and organs and often begin attacking them, leading to autoimmune disorders. Interference with apoptosis allows cells to multiply without control, leading to the lymphomas that often occur in people with this disorder.

Nonclassic forms of ALPS may be caused by mutations in additional genes, some of which have not been identified.

FREQUENCY OF AUTOIMMUNE LYMPHOPROLIFERATIVE SYNDROME

Autoimmune lymphoproliferative syndrome is a rare disorder; its prevalence is unknown.

INHERITANCE OF AUTOIMMUNE LYMPHOPROLIFERATIVE SYNDROME

In most people with ALPS, including the majority of those with *FAS* gene mutations, this condition is inherited in an autosomal dominant pattern, which means one copy of an altered gene in each cell is sufficient to cause the disorder. In these cases, an affected person usually inherits the mutation from one affected parent. Other cases with an autosomal dominant pattern result from new (de novo) gene mutations that occur early in embryonic development in people with no history of the disorder in their family.

In a small number of cases, including some cases caused by *FAS* gene mutations, ALPS is inherited in an autosomal recessive pattern, which means both copies of a gene in each cell have mutations. The parents of an individual with an autosomal recessive condition each carry one copy of the mutated gene, but they typically do not show signs and symptoms of the condition.

ALPS can also arise from a mutation in lymphocytes that is not inherited but instead occurs during an individual's lifetime. This alteration is called a "somatic mutation."[1]

[1] MedlinePlus, "Autoimmune Lymphoproliferative Syndrome," National Institutes of Health (NIH), December 1, 2018. Available online. URL: https://medlineplus.gov/genetics/condition/autoimmune-lymphoproliferative-syndrome. Accessed June 12, 2023.

Chapter 10 | **Autoimmune Polyglandular Syndrome Type 1**

Autoimmune polyglandular syndrome type 1 (APS-1), also called "autoimmune polyendocrinopathy-candidiasis-ectodermal dystrophy" (APECED), is a genetic immune disorder. This disorder has a diverse range of symptoms, including autoimmunity against different organs and an increased susceptibility to candidiasis, a fungal infection caused by *Candida* yeast. The syndrome is caused by mutations in the *autoimmune regulator* (*AIRE*) gene. The National Institute of Allergy and Infectious Diseases (NIAID) researchers are exploring how AIRE mutations impact the function of cells by studying people with APS-1 (APECED), as well as using mouse models of AIRE deficiency. With a better understanding of how these mutations affect the immune system and other cells in the body, researchers hope to uncover promising therapeutic targets to prevent and treat persistent candidiasis and autoimmune disorders.[1]

SYMPTOMS OF AUTOIMMUNE POLYGLANDULAR SYNDROME TYPE 1

Autoimmune polyendocrinopathy-candidiasis-ectodermal dystrophy is a disorder with striking variability, even within the same family. This implies that complex interactions among genetic, epigenetic (influences on gene expression not explained by the

---

[1] "APS-1 (APECED)," National Institute of Allergy and Infectious Diseases (NIAID), April 22, 2019. Available online. URL: www.niaid.nih.gov/diseases-conditions/aps-1-apeced. Accessed April 18, 2023.

deoxyribonucleic acid (DNA) sequence), and environmental factors contribute to the disease.

Chronic Mucocutaneous Candidiasis

Chronic mucocutaneous candidiasis—persistent *Candida* infection of the skin, nails, or mucosal membranes—is typically the first symptom to appear, usually in the form of oral candidiasis, commonly known as "oral thrush." Thrush can range in severity from redness and soreness at the corners of the mouth to whole-mouth involvement, which can interfere with eating spicy or acidic foods. Chronic inflammation of the mouth and throat makes some APECED patients (5–10%) susceptible to oral squamous cell carcinoma, a type of cancer. Candidiasis can also affect the esophagus, intestines, or vagina.

Autoimmunity

Autoimmunity can affect virtually any tissue or organ. Doctors have identified autoantibodies—immune system proteins that recognize and counteract numerous tissues and organs in the body—in people with APECED. In addition, autoreactive T cells, which are normally removed in the thymus in the presence of functional AIRE, attack different organs in people with APECED. Most commonly, autoantibodies and autoreactive T cells attack the parathyroid glands, adrenal glands, thyroid gland, and ovaries or testes. This can result in hypoparathyroidism, adrenal insufficiency, hypothyroidism, and ovarian or testicular failure. Autoimmunity affecting the gastrointestinal tract, ectodermal structures (skin, teeth, nails, and parts of the eyes), spleen, blood, lungs, and other organs and tissues has also been reported in APECED patients (refer to Figure 10.1).

Ectodermal Symptoms

APECED can affect structures of the ectoderm, resulting in a wide variety of symptoms. These include keratitis of the eye, rashes with fever, alopecia, vitiligo, nail dystrophy, tooth enamel hypoplasia, and calcification of the inner ear's tympanic membrane. Some, but not all, of these symptoms may be caused by underlying autoimmune problems. The National Institutes of Health (NIH) researchers are working to better understand the constellation of symptoms that people with APECED experience and the immune and non-immune mechanisms that contribute to the syndrome.

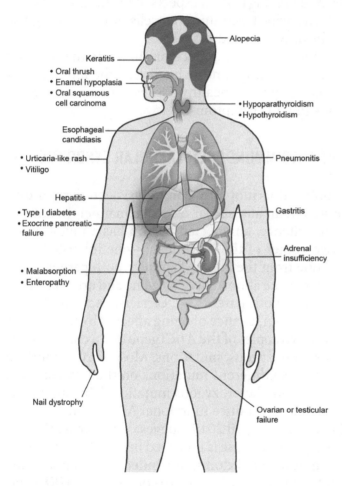

Figure 10.1. Autoimmune Polyglandular Syndrome Type 1 Symptoms and the Organs They Affect

National Institute of Allergy and Infectious Diseases (NIAID)

CAUSES OF AUTOIMMUNE POLYGLANDULAR SYNDROME TYPE 1

Autoimmune polyendocrinopathy-candidiasis-ectodermal dystrophy syndrome is caused by mutations in the gene *AIRE*. *AIRE* provides instructions for making a protein called the "AIRE," which helps control when other genes get "turned on," or expressed. The AIRE protein is expressed in the thymus, a key immune organ located behind the breastbone. As its name suggests, AIRE plays an important role in regulating certain aspects of the immune system. In particular, AIRE helps teach immune cells how to distinguish the body's own healthy cells and tissues.

Mutations in the *AIRE* gene reduce or eliminate the function of the AIRE protein, making it more likely that the immune system will attack the body's own healthy tissues. This autoimmunity underlies many APECED symptoms.

INHERITANCE OF AUTOIMMUNE POLYGLANDULAR SYNDROME TYPE 1 PATTERN

Autoimmune polyendocrinopathy-candidiasis-ectodermal dystrophy is inherited in an autosomal recessive manner. In autosomal recessive inheritance, an affected person has a mutation on each of their two copies of the *AIRE* gene—one inherited from the mother and one from the father. Typically, both parents of an affected person carry one abnormal *AIRE* gene and are unaffected by the disease. When both parents are carriers, each child has a 25 percent, or one in four, chance of being affected by the disease.

Sometimes, the two copies of the *AIRE* gene that a child inherits have identical, or homozygous, mutations. Most North American APECED patients have different mutations on the two copies of AIRE, called "compound heterozygous mutations." In either case, the patient is not able to produce functional AIRE protein.

Recent evidence (as of April 2019) suggested that in a minority of APECED patients, the disease is inherited in an autosomal dominant manner. In autosomal dominant inheritance, an affected person has a mutation on one of their two copies of the *AIRE* gene. The mutation is inherited from a parent who is also affected by the syndrome. The other parent does not carry a mutation in the *AIRE* gene and is healthy. In this situation, each child has a 50 percent, or one in two, chance of being affected by the disease. Such mutations have been reported in European APECED patients but so far have not been observed in North American APECED patients.

About 15–20 percent of North American patients with APECED symptoms do not have detectable mutations in both copies of the *AIRE* gene, suggesting that other undiscovered genetic factors are also involved in the syndrome. Understanding the genetic factors that contribute to APECED in families without *AIRE* gene mutations is an area of active research at the NIH.

DIAGNOSIS OF AUTOIMMUNE POLYGLANDULAR SYNDROME TYPE 1

Doctors may diagnose APECED based on genetic testing and the presence of at least two of the three classic components of the syndrome: chronic mucocutaneous candidiasis, hypoparathyroidism, and adrenal insufficiency. However, these criteria are imperfect. Some patients have other symptoms for decades before the classic APECED symptoms become apparent or their doctor performs a targeted evaluation for APECED. The rarity of APECED and the variation in disease symptoms and severity among people with the disease contribute to the likely underdiagnosis of this condition. As researchers work toward a better characterization of APECED, the diagnostic criteria will likely evolve.

TREATMENT FOR AUTOIMMUNE POLYGLANDULAR SYNDROME TYPE 1

Treatment is based on a person's clinical condition and may include medications and other strategies to manage *Candida*, autoimmunity, and endocrine problems. Some treatments may be specific for APECED, while others are standard treatments for conditions experienced by APECED patients, such as hypoparathyroidism. Because APECED affects many of the body's organs and tissues, optimal care requires a team of specialists working closely with the patient. The goal of treatment is to preserve the patient's quality of life (QOL) and recognize and address early signs of new disease symptoms, which may appear throughout life.

COPING STRATEGIES FOR FAMILIES AFFECTED BY AUTOIMMUNE POLYGLANDULAR SYNDROME TYPE 1

Living with APECED can be difficult not only for the person who has it but also for their family members. It is important for families to talk openly about APECED and about how the family is dealing with it so that misconceptions can be corrected and everyone can learn to cope to the best of their ability. Some people with APECED have to work hard to develop their self-confidence and sense of security. Everyone benefits from being reminded that they have many positive characteristics, but this is especially important when a person's appearance attracts attention (e.g., due to candidiasis, alopecia, or vitiligo) or affects their QOL (e.g., because of malabsorption).

Some children who have siblings with APECED feel anxious about their brother or sister being in pain or even dying from the disease. Some think that they may develop symptoms because they look or act like a sibling who has the disease or that the disease is contagious. Some children struggle with how much time their parents spend with their sick siblings. Many families benefit from meeting or talking to other families affected by the same rare disease. Patient organizations such as the Immune Deficiency Foundation (www.primaryimmune.org) or an APECED support group (www.apstype1.org) are great resources for providing useful information and connecting families. Counseling can also help families cope with the challenges of APECED.[2]

---

[2] "APECED," National Institute of Allergy and Infectious Diseases (NIAID), August 2016. Available online. URL: www.niaid.nih.gov/sites/default/files/APECED-Factsheet.pdf. Accessed April 18, 2023.

Chapter 11 | Chédiak-Higashi Syndrome

WHAT IS CHÉDIAK-HIGASHI SYNDROME?

Chédiak-Higashi syndrome (CHS) is a condition that affects many parts of the body, particularly the immune system. This disease damages immune system cells, leaving them less able to fight off invaders such as viruses and bacteria. As a result, most people with CHS have repeated and persistent infections starting in infancy or early childhood. These infections tend to be very serious or life-threatening.

CHS is also characterized by a condition called "oculocutaneous albinism," which causes abnormally light coloring (pigmentation) of the skin, hair, and eyes. Affected individuals typically have fair skin and light-colored hair, often with a metallic sheen. Oculocutaneous albinism also causes vision problems such as reduced sharpness, rapid involuntary eye movements (nystagmus), and increased sensitivity to light (photophobia).

Many people with CHS have problems with blood clotting (coagulation) that lead to easy bruising and abnormal bleeding. In adulthood, CHS can also affect the nervous system, causing weakness, clumsiness, difficulty with walking, and seizures.

CAUSES OF CHÉDIAK-HIGASHI SYNDROME

Chédiak-Higashi syndrome is caused by mutations in the *lysosomal trafficking regulator* (*LYST*) gene. This gene provides instructions for making a protein known as a "lysosomal trafficking regulator." Researchers believe that this protein plays a role in the transport (trafficking) of materials into structures called "lysosomes" and similar cell structures. Lysosomes act as recycling centers within cells. They use digestive enzymes to break down toxic substances, digest bacteria that invade the cell, and recycle worn-out cell components.

Mutations in the *LYST* gene impair the normal function of the lysosomal trafficking regulator protein, which disrupts the size, structure, and function of lysosomes and related structures in cells throughout the body. In many cells, the lysosomes are abnormally large and interfere with normal cell functions. For example, enlarged lysosomes in certain immune system cells prevent these cells from responding appropriately to bacteria and other foreign invaders. As a result, the malfunctioning immune system cannot protect the body from infections.

In pigment cells called "melanocytes," cellular structures called "melanosomes" (which are related to lysosomes) are abnormally large. Melanosomes produce and distribute a pigment called "melanin," which is the substance that gives skin, hair, and eyes their color. People with CHS have oculocutaneous albinism because melanin is trapped within the giant melanosomes and is unable to contribute to skin, hair, and eye pigmentation.

Researchers believe that abnormal lysosome-like structures inside blood cell fragments called "platelets" underlie the abnormal bruising and bleeding seen in people with CHS. Similarly, abnormal lysosomes in nerve cells probably cause neurological problems associated with this disease.

INHERITANCE PATTERN OF CHÉDIAK-HIGASHI SYNDROME

This condition is inherited in an autosomal recessive pattern, which means both copies of the gene in each cell have mutations. The parents of an individual with an autosomal recessive condition each carry one copy of the mutated gene, but they typically do not show signs and symptoms of the condition.[1]

---

[1] MedlinePlus, "Chediak-Higashi Syndrome," National Institutes of Health (NIH), January 1, 2014. Available online. URL: https://medlineplus.gov/genetics/condition/chediak-higashi-syndrome. Accessed April 18, 2023.

Chapter 12 | **Chronic Granulomatous Disease**

Chronic granulomatous disease (CGD) is a genetic disorder in which white blood cells (WBCs) called "phagocytes" are unable to kill certain types of bacteria and fungi. People with CGD are highly susceptible to frequent and sometimes life-threatening bacterial and fungal infections (refer to Figure 12.1).

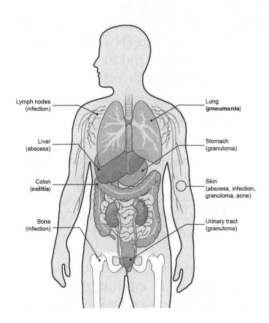

Figure 12.1. Locations of Chronic Granulomatous Disease Infections and Inflammation

National Institute of Allergy and Infectious Diseases (NIAID)

SYMPTOMS AND DIAGNOSIS OF CHRONIC GRANULOMATOUS DISEASE

People with CGD are highly susceptible to infections caused by certain bacteria and fungi, such as *Staphylococcus aureus*, *Serratia marcescens*, *Burkholderia cepacia*, *Nocardia* species, and *Aspergillus* species. These people may develop abscesses (boils) in their lungs, liver, spleen, bones, or skin and masses of cells called "granulomas" that can obstruct the bowel or urinary tract. In some people, granulomas can cause an inflammatory bowel disease (IBD) similar to Crohn's disease. In addition, heart or kidney problems, diabetes, and autoimmune disease may occur in people with CGD, but this varies depending on which gene is mutated.

CGD is diagnosed by special blood tests that show how well phagocytes produce hydrogen peroxide, an indicator that they are functioning properly.

CAUSES OF CHRONIC GRANULOMATOUS DISEASE

Chronic granulomatous disease is caused by defects in an enzyme, nicotinamide adenine dinucleotide phosphate (NADPH) oxidase, that phagocytes need to kill certain bacteria and fungi. Mutations in one of five different genes can cause these defects.

TREATMENT FOR CHRONIC GRANULOMATOUS DISEASE

People with CGD take lifelong regimens of antibiotics and anti-fungals to prevent infections. Injections with interferon gamma, a protein that improves the activity of phagocytes, may also help reduce the number of severe infections. Abscesses need aggressive care that may include surgery. Granulomas may require steroid therapy. Some people with CGD have been treated successfully with bone marrow transplantation.

The National Institute of Allergy and Infectious Diseases (NIAID) also supports the development of antifungal drugs and other therapies to curb infections and improve outcomes for people with CGD.[1]

---

[1] "Chronic Granulomatous Disease (CGD)," National Institute of Allergy and Infectious Diseases (NIAID), May 22, 2020. Available online. URL: www.niaid.nih.gov/diseases-conditions/chronic-granulomatous-disease-cgd. Accessed April 19, 2023.

Chapter 13 | **Congenital Neutropenia Syndromes**

Congenital neutropenia syndromes are a group of rare disorders present from birth that are characterized by low levels of neutrophils, a type of white blood cell (WBC) necessary for fighting infections. Congenital neutropenia syndromes may also be referred to as congenital agranulocytosis, severe congenital neutropenia, severe infantile genetic neutropenia, infantile genetic agranulocytosis, or Kostmann disease.

Researchers have identified numerous genetic mutations that cause congenital neutropenia syndromes. Generally, mutations that result in congenital neutropenia affect the development, life span, or function of neutrophils. Congenital neutropenia syndromes are inherited through autosomal recessive, autosomal dominant, and X-linked inheritance patterns. The genes linked to these syndromes include the following:

- *ELANE*
- *HAX1*
- *G6PC3*
- *GFI1*
- *CSF3R*
- X-linked *WAS*
- *CXCR4*
- *VPS45A*
- *JAGN1*

In some people with congenital neutropenia, however, the disease-causing mutation is unknown.

People with congenital neutropenia experience bacterial infections early in life. These may cause inflammation of the umbilical cord stump, abscesses (or boils) on the skin, oral infections, and pneumonia.

Congenital neutropenia also increases one's risk for developing myelodysplastic syndromes (MDS), blood disorders that are distinguished by low levels of various blood cells. MDS may progress to a type of blood cell cancer called "acute myeloid leukemia" (AML).

Bone marrow and blood tests can measure the levels of various WBCs to test for deficiencies. A person suspected of having congenital neutropenia may also undergo genetic testing.

Standard therapy for congenital neutropenia includes injections of granulocyte colony-stimulating factor (G-CSF), which can help restore immune system function. People on G-CSF therapy may have a lower incidence and severity of infections, improving their quality of life (QOL), but the effects vary. For some individuals, a bone marrow transplant may be recommended to replace defective immune cells with healthy ones from a donor.[1]

---

[1] "Congenital Neutropenia Syndromes," National Institute of Allergy and Infectious Diseases (NIAID), April 1, 2019. Available online. URL: www.niaid.nih.gov/diseases-conditions/congenital-neutropenia-syndromes. Accessed April 20, 2023.

Chapter 14 |
Common Variable Immunodeficiency

Common variable immunodeficiency (CVID) is a primary immune deficiency disease characterized by low levels of protective antibodies and an increased risk of infections. Although the disease is usually diagnosed in adults, it can also occur in children. CVID is also known as "hypogammaglobulinemia," "adult-onset agammaglobulinemia," "late-onset hypogammaglobulinemia," and "acquired agammaglobulinemia."

CAUSES OF COMMON VARIABLE IMMUNODEFICIENCY

Common variable immunodeficiency is caused by a variety of different genetic abnormalities that result in a defect in the capability of immune cells to produce normal amounts of all types of antibodies. Only a few of these defects have been identified, and the cause of most cases of CVID is unknown. Many people with CVID carry a deoxyribonucleic acid (DNA) variation called a "polymorphism" in a gene known as "*TACI.*" However, while this genetic abnormality confers an increased risk of developing CVID, it alone is not capable of causing CVID.

CVID is also linked to immunoglobulin A (IgA) deficiency, a related condition in which only the level of the antibody IgA is low, while levels of other antibody types are usually normal or near normal. IgA deficiency typically occurs alone, but in some cases, it may precede the development of CVID or occur in family members of CVID patients.

SYMPTOMS AND DIAGNOSIS OF COMMON VARIABLE IMMUNODEFICIENCY

People with CVID may experience frequent bacterial and viral infections of the upper airway, sinuses, and lungs. Acute lung infections can cause pneumonia, and long-term lung infections may cause a chronic form of bronchitis known as "bronchiectasis," which is characterized by thickened airway walls colonized by bacteria.

People with CVID may also have diarrhea, problems absorbing food nutrients, reduced liver function, and impaired blood flow to the liver. Autoimmune problems that cause reduced levels of blood cells or platelets may also occur. People with CVID may develop an enlarged spleen and swollen glands or lymph nodes, as well as painful swollen joints in the knee, ankle, elbow, or wrist. In addition, people with CVID may have an increased risk of developing some cancers.

Doctors can diagnose CVID by weighing factors including infection history, digestive symptoms, lab tests showing very low immunoglobulin levels, and low antibody responses to immunization.

TREATMENT FOR COMMON VARIABLE IMMUNODEFICIENCY

Common variable immunodeficiency is treated with intravenous immunoglobulin infusions or subcutaneous (under the skin) immunoglobulin injections to partially restore immunoglobulin levels. The immunoglobulin given by either method provides antibodies from the blood of healthy donors. The frequent bacterial infections experienced by people with CVID are treated with antibiotics. Other problems caused by CVID may require additional, tailored treatments.[1]

---

[1] "Common Variable Immunodeficiency (CVID)," National Institute of Allergy and Infectious Diseases (NIAID), April 23, 2019. Available online. URL: www.niaid.nih.gov/diseases-conditions/common-variable-immunodeficiency-cvid. Accessed April 19, 2023.

Chapter 15 | **CTLA4 Deficiency**

Cytotoxic T-lymphocyte-associated protein 4 (CTLA4) deficiency is a rare disorder that severely impairs the normal regulation of the immune system, resulting in conditions such as intestinal disease, respiratory infections, autoimmune problems, and enlarged lymph nodes, liver, and spleen.

CTLA4 deficiency is a primary immune deficiency disease (PIDD) and is caused by mutations in a gene called "*CTLA4*," which gives cells instructions for making the CTLA4 protein. This protein functions as a brake to slow down and control the action of the immune system.

Each person has two copies of the *CTLA4* gene, one from each parent. In 2014, National Institute of Allergy and Infectious Diseases (NIAID) scientists found that people with only one functional copy of *CTLA4* experience abnormal T-cell activity; lower levels of healthy, antibody-producing B cells; higher levels of autoimmune B cells; and the disruption of organs by infiltrating immune cells. The researchers determined that having a single working copy of *CTLA4* is not sufficient to produce enough CTLA4 protein for a normal immune system.

CTLA4 deficiency is characterized by infiltration of immune cells into the gut, lungs, bone marrow, central nervous system (CNS), kidneys, and possibly other organs. Most people with CTLA4 deficiency experience diarrhea or intestinal disease. Enlarged lymph nodes, liver, and spleen are also common, as are respiratory infections. People with CTLA4 deficiency often experience autoimmune problems that can affect various organs and tissues, including the blood, thyroid, skin, and joints. The disease may also slightly increase the risk of lymphoma, a type of immune cell cancer.

CTLA4 deficiency is diagnosed based on clinical symptoms, laboratory findings, and genetic testing. Treatment for CTLA4 deficiency may include standard therapies for autoimmune problems and immunoglobulin deficiencies. A potential new therapy is a drug called "CTLA-4-Ig," also known as "abatacept," which mimics the action of the CTLA4 protein and reduces immune activity. Abatacept is used to treat autoimmune diseases such as rheumatoid arthritis (RA), but its effectiveness for treating CTLA4 deficiency requires further study. In 2019, NIAID investigators launched a small clinical trial to test the safety and efficacy of intravenous infusions of abatacept for correcting or improving the numbers of blood cells in people with CTLA4 deficiency.[1]

[1] "CTLA4 Deficiency," National Institute of Allergy and Infectious Diseases (NIAID), April 11, 2019. Available online. URL: www.niaid.nih.gov/diseases-conditions/ctla4-deficiency. Accessed April 19, 2023.

Chapter 16 | **DiGeorge Syndrome**

WHAT IS DIGEORGE SYNDROME?

DiGeorge syndrome is a disorder caused by the deletion of a small piece of chromosome 22. The deletion occurs near the middle of the chromosome at a location designated q11.2.

DiGeorge syndrome has many possible signs and symptoms that can affect almost any part of the body. The features of this syndrome vary widely, even among affected members of the same family. Common signs and symptoms include heart abnormalities that are often present from birth, an opening in the roof of the mouth (a cleft palate), and distinctive facial features. People with DiGeorge syndrome often experience recurrent infections caused by problems with the immune system, and some develop auto-immune disorders such as rheumatoid arthritis (RA) and Graves disease in which the immune system attacks the body's own tissues and organs. Affected individuals may also have breathing problems, kidney abnormalities, low levels of calcium in the blood (which can result in seizures), a decrease in blood platelets (thrombocytopenia), significant feeding difficulties, gastrointestinal problems, and hearing loss. Skeletal differences are possible, including mild short stature and, less frequently, abnormalities of the spinal bones.

Many children with DiGeorge syndrome have developmental delays, including delayed growth and speech development, and learning disabilities. Later in life, they are at an increased risk of developing mental illnesses such as schizophrenia, depression, anxiety, and bipolar disorder. Additionally, affected children are more likely than children without DiGeorge syndrome to have attention deficit hyperactivity disorder (ADHD) and developmental conditions such as autism spectrum disorder (ASD) that affect communication and social interaction.

Because the signs and symptoms of DiGeorge syndrome are so varied, different groupings of features were once described as separate conditions. In addition, some children with the 22q11.2 deletion were diagnosed with the autosomal dominant form of Opitz G/BBB syndrome and Cayler cardiofacial syndrome. Once the genetic basis for these disorders was identified, doctors determined that they were all part of a single syndrome with many possible signs and symptoms. To avoid confusion, this condition is usually called "DiGeorge syndrome," a description based on its underlying genetic cause.

CAUSES OF DIGEORGE SYNDROME

Most people with DiGeorge syndrome are missing a sequence of about 3 million deoxyribonucleic acid (DNA) building blocks (base pairs) on one copy of chromosome 22 in each cell. This region contains 30–40 genes, many of which have not been well characterized. A small percentage of affected individuals have shorter deletions in the same region. This condition is described as a contiguous gene deletion syndrome because it results from the loss of many genes that are close together.

INHERITANCE PATTERN OF DIGEORGE SYNDROME

The inheritance of DiGeorge syndrome is considered autosomal dominant because a deletion in one copy of chromosome 22 in each cell is sufficient to cause the condition. Most cases of DiGeorge syndrome are not inherited. However, the deletion occurs most often as a random event during the formation of reproductive cells (eggs or sperm) or in early fetal development. Affected people typically have no history of the disorder in their family though they can pass the condition to their children. In about 10 percent of cases, a person with this condition inherits the deletion in chromosome 22 from a parent. In inherited cases, other family members may be affected as well.[1]

---

[1] MedlinePlus, "22q11.2 Deletion Syndrome," National Institutes of Health (NIH), December 1, 2019. Available online. URL: https://medlineplus.gov/genetics/condition/22q112-deletion-syndrome. Accessed April 19, 2023.

Chapter 17 | Hyperimmunoglobulin E Syndrome

WHAT IS HYPERIMMUNOGLOBULIN E SYNDROME?

Autosomal dominant hyperimmunoglobulin E syndrome (AD-HIES), formerly known as "Job syndrome," is a condition that affects several body systems, particularly the immune system. Recurrent infections are common in people with this condition. Affected individuals tend to have frequent bouts of pneumonia, which are caused by certain kinds of bacteria that infect the lungs and cause inflammation. Inflammation is a normal immune system response to injury and foreign invaders (such as bacteria). However, excessive inflammation can damage body tissues. Recurring pneumonia often results in the formation of air-filled cysts (pneumatoceles) in the lungs. Frequent skin infections and an inflammatory skin disorder called "eczema" are also very common in AD-HIES. These skin problems cause rashes, blisters, accumulations of pus (abscesses), open sores, and scaling.

For unknown reasons, people with AD-HIES have abnormally high levels of an immune system protein called "immunoglobulin E" (IgE) in the blood. IgE normally triggers an immune response against foreign invaders in the body, particularly parasitic worms, and is involved in allergies. However, IgE is not needed for these roles in people with AD-HIES, and it is unclear why affected individuals have such high levels of the protein without having allergies.

AD-HIES also affects other parts of the body, including the bones and teeth. Many people with AD-HIES have skeletal abnormalities such as an unusually large range of joint movement (hyperextensibility), an abnormal curvature of the spine (scoliosis), reduced bone density (osteopenia), and a tendency for bones to fracture easily. A common dental abnormality in this condition is that the primary (baby) teeth do not fall out at the usual time during childhood but are retained as the adult teeth grow in. Other signs and symptoms of AD-HIES can include abnormalities of the arteries that supply blood to the heart muscle (coronary arteries), distinctive facial features, and structural abnormalities of the brain, which do not affect a person's intelligence.

Other Names of This Condition
- AD-HIES
- autosomal dominant HIES
- autosomal dominant hyper-IgE recurrent infection syndrome
- autosomal dominant hyperimmunoglobulin E recurrent infection syndrome
- autosomal dominant Job syndrome
- Buckley syndrome
- Job syndrome
- Job's syndrome
- Job-Buckley syndrome
- STAT3 deficiency
- STAT3-deficient hyper IgE syndrome

FREQUENCY OF HYPERIMMUNOGLOBULIN E SYNDROME
Autosomal dominant hyperimmunoglobulin E syndrome is rare, affecting fewer than 1 per million people worldwide.

CAUSES OF HYPERIMMUNOGLOBULIN E SYNDROME
Mutations in the *STAT3* gene cause most cases of AD-HIES. This gene provides instructions for making a protein that plays important roles in several body systems. To carry out its roles, the STAT3 protein attaches to deoxyribonucleic acid (DNA) and helps

control the activity of particular genes. In the immune system, the STAT3 protein regulates genes that are involved in the maturation of immune system cells, especially certain types of T cells. T cells and other immune system cells help control the body's response to foreign invaders such as bacteria and fungi.

Changes in the *STAT3* gene alter the structure and function of the STAT3 protein, impairing its ability to control the activity of other genes. A shortage of functional STAT3 blocks the maturation of T cells (specifically a subset known as "T_h17 cells") and other immune cells. The resulting immune system abnormalities make people with AD-HIES highly susceptible to infections, particularly bacterial and fungal infections of the lungs and skin. The STAT3 protein is also involved in the formation of cells that build and break down bone tissue, which could help explain why *STAT3* gene mutations lead to the skeletal and dental abnormalities character-istic of this condition. It is unclear how *STAT3* gene mutations lead to increased IgE levels.

Mutations in the *ZNF341* gene cause a disorder similar to AD-HIES but with a different pattern of inheritance. When the *STAT3* gene is involved, one altered copy of the gene is sufficient to cause the disorder (which is known as "autosomal dominant inheritance"). In contrast, when the *ZNF341* gene is involved, both copies of the gene are altered (which is known as "autosomal reces-sive inheritance").

The *ZNF341* gene provides instructions for making a protein that appears to control the activity of the *STAT3* gene. *ZNF341* gene mutations, which prevent production of functional ZNF341 protein, result in a shortage of STAT3 protein, leading to immune system problems similar to those caused by *STAT3* gene mutations. AD-HIES is thought to be caused by mutations in other genes that have not been definitively linked to the condition.

INHERITANCE OF HYPERIMMUNOGLOBULIN E SYNDROME

Autosomal dominant hyperimmunoglobulin E syndrome has an autosomal dominant pattern of inheritance, which means one copy of the altered gene in each cell is sufficient to cause the disorder. In about half of cases caused by *STAT3* gene mutations, an affected person inherits the mutation from one affected parent. The other half result from new mutations in the gene and occur in people with no history of the disorder in their family.

A similar condition caused by mutations in the *ZNF341* gene has an autosomal recessive pattern of inheritance, which means both copies of the gene in each cell have mutations. The parents of an individual with an autosomal recessive condition each carry one copy of the mutated gene, but they typically do not show signs and symptoms of the condition.[1]

---

[1] MedlinePlus, "Autosomal Dominant Hyper-IgE Syndrome," National Institutes of Health (NIH), August 1, 2019. Available online. URL: https://medlineplus.gov/genetics/condition/autosomal-dominant-hyper-ige-syndrome. Accessed April 21, 2023.

Chapter 18 | X-Linked Hyperimmunoglobulin M Syndrome

WHAT IS X-LINKED HYPERIMMUNOGLOBULIN M SYNDROME?

X-linked hyperimmunoglobulin M (hyper-IgM) syndrome is a condition that affects the immune system and occurs almost exclusively in males. People with this disorder have abnormal levels of proteins called "antibodies" or "immunoglobulins." Antibodies help protect the body against infection by attaching to specific foreign particles and germs, marking them for destruction. There are several classes of antibodies, and each one has a different function in the immune system. Although the name of this condition implies that affected individuals always have high levels of immunoglobulin M (IgM), some people have normal levels of this antibody. People with X-linked hyper-IgM syndrome have low levels of the following three other classes of antibodies:

- immunoglobulin G (IgG)
- immunoglobulin A (IgA)
- immunoglobulin E (IgE)

The lack of certain antibody classes makes it difficult for people with this disorder to fight off infections.

Individuals with X-linked hyper-IgM syndrome begin to develop frequent infections in infancy and early childhood. Common infections include pneumonia, sinus infections (sinusitis), and ear infections (otitis). Infections often cause these children to have chronic diarrhea, and they fail to gain weight and grow at the expected rate (failure to thrive). Some people with X-linked hyper-IgM syndrome have low levels of white blood cells (WBCs) called "neutrophils" (neutropenia). Affected individuals may develop autoimmune disorders, neurologic complications from brain and spinal cord (central nervous system (CNS)) infections, liver disease, and gastrointestinal tumors. They also have an increased risk of lymphoma, which is a cancer of immune system cells.

CAUSES OF X-LINKED HYPERIMMUNOGLOBULIN M SYNDROME

Variants (also known as "mutations") in the *CD40LG* gene cause X-linked hyper-IgM syndrome. This gene provides instructions for making a protein called "CD40 ligand," which is found on the surface of immune system cells known as "T cells." The CD40 ligand attaches like a key in a lock to its receptor protein, which is located on the surface of immune system cells called "B cells." B cells are involved in the production of antibodies, and initially, they are able to make only IgM antibodies. When the CD40 ligand and its receptor protein are connected, they trigger a series of chemical signals that instruct the B cell to start making IgG, IgA, or IgE antibodies.

INHERITANCE OF X-LINKED HYPERIMMUNOGLOBULIN M SYNDROME

This condition is inherited in an X-linked recessive pattern. The gene associated with this condition is located on the X chromosome, which is one of the two sex chromosomes. In males (who have only one X chromosome), one altered copy of the gene in each cell is sufficient to cause the condition. In females (who have two X chromosomes), a variant would have to occur in both copies of the gene to cause the disorder. Because it is unlikely that females will have two altered copies of this gene, males are affected by X-linked recessive disorders much more frequently than females. A characteristic of X-linked inheritance is that fathers cannot pass X-linked traits to their sons.[1]

---

[1] MedlinePlus, "X-Linked Hyper IgM Syndrome," National Institutes of Health (NIH), February 6, 2023. Available online. URL: https://medlineplus.gov/genetics/condition/x-linked-hyper-igm-syndrome. Accessed April 21, 2023.

Chapter 19 | Immune Dysregulation, Polyendocrinopathy, Enteropathy, X-Linked Syndrome

WHAT IS IMMUNE DYSREGULATION, POLYENDOCRINOPATHY, ENTEROPATHY, X-LINKED SYNDROME?

Immune dysregulation, polyendocrinopathy, enteropathy, X-linked (IPEX) syndrome primarily affects males and is caused by problems with the immune system. The immune system normally protects the body from foreign invaders, such as bacteria and viruses, by recognizing and attacking these invaders and clearing them from the body. However, the immune system can malfunction and attack the body's own tissues and organs instead, which is known as "autoimmunity." IPEX syndrome is characterized by the development of multiple autoimmune disorders in affected individuals. Although IPEX syndrome can affect many different areas of the body, autoimmune disorders involving the intestines, skin, and hormone-producing (endocrine) glands occur most often. IPEX syndrome can be life-threatening in early childhood.

Almost all individuals with IPEX syndrome develop a disorder of the intestines called "autoimmune enteropathy." Autoimmune enteropathy occurs when certain cells in the intestines are destroyed by a person's immune system. It causes severe diarrhea, which is usually the first symptom of IPEX syndrome. Autoimmune enteropathy typically begins in the first few months of life. It can cause failure to gain weight and grow at the expected rate (failure to thrive) and general wasting and weight loss (cachexia).

People with IPEX syndrome frequently develop inflammation of the skin, called "dermatitis." Eczema is the most common type of dermatitis that occurs in this syndrome, and it causes abnormal patches of red, irritated skin. Other skin disorders that cause similar symptoms are sometimes present in IPEX syndrome.

The term "polyendocrinopathy" is used in IPEX syndrome because individuals can develop multiple disorders of the endocrine glands. Type 1 diabetes mellitus (DM) is an autoimmune condition involving the pancreas and is the most common endocrine disorder present in people with IPEX syndrome. It usually develops within the first few months of life and prevents the body from properly controlling the amount of sugar in the blood. Autoimmune thyroid disease may also develop in people with IPEX syndrome. The thyroid gland is a butterfly-shaped organ in the lower neck that produces hormones. This gland is commonly underactive (hypothyroidism) in individuals with this disorder but may become overactive (hyperthyroidism).

Individuals with IPEX syndrome typically develop other types of autoimmune disorders in addition to those that involve the intestines, skin, and endocrine glands. Autoimmune blood disorders are common; about half of affected individuals have low levels of red blood cells (RBCs; anemia), platelets (thrombocytopenia), or certain white blood cells (WBCs; neutropenia) because these cells are attacked by the immune system. In some individuals, IPEX syndrome involves the liver and kidneys.

Other Names of This Condition
- autoimmunity-immunodeficiency syndrome, X-linked
- diabetes mellitus, congenital insulin-dependent, with fatal secretory diarrhea
- diarrhea, polyendocrinopathy, fatal infection syndrome, X-linked

- enteropathy, autoimmune, with hemolytic anemia and polyendocrinopathy
- IDDM-secretory diarrhea syndrome
- immunodeficiency, polyendocrinopathy, and enteropathy, X-linked
- insulin-dependent diabetes mellitus secretory diarrhea syndrome
- IPEX syndrome
- polyendocrinopathy, immune dysfunction, and diarrhea, X-linked
- X-linked autoimmunity-allergic dysregulation syndrome
- XLAAD

FREQUENCY OF IMMUNE DYSREGULATION, POLYENDOCRINOPATHY, ENTEROPATHY, X-LINKED SYNDROME

Immune dysregulation, polyendocrinopathy, enteropathy, X-linked syndrome is a rare disorder that affects an estimated 1 in 1.6 million people.

CAUSES OF IMMUNE DYSREGULATION, POLYENDOCRINOPATHY, ENTEROPATHY, X-LINKED SYNDROME

Mutations in the *FOXP3* gene cause IPEX syndrome. The protein produced from this gene is a transcription factor, which means that it attaches (binds) to specific regions of deoxyribonucleic acid (DNA) and helps control the activity of particular genes. This protein is essential for the production and normal function of certain immune cells called "regulatory T cells." Regulatory T cells play an important role in controlling immune responses and preventing autoimmune disorders. Mutations in the *FOXP3* gene impair the normal function of regulatory T cells, making it difficult for the body to turn off immune responses when they are not needed. Normal body tissues and organs are attacked, causing the multiple autoimmune disorders that develop in people with IPEX syndrome.

INHERITANCE OF IMMUNE DYSREGULATION, POLYENDOCRINOPATHY, ENTEROPATHY, X-LINKED SYNDROME

Immune dysregulation, polyendocrinopathy, enteropathy, X-linked syndrome is inherited in an X-linked recessive pattern. The *FOXP3* gene is located on the X chromosome, which is one of the two sex chromosomes. In males (who have only one X chromosome), one altered copy of the gene in each cell is sufficient to cause the condition. In females (who have two X chromosomes), a mutation must be present in both copies of the gene to cause the disorder. Males are affected by X-linked recessive disorders much more frequently than females. A characteristic of X-linked inheritance is that fathers cannot pass X-linked traits to their sons.

Some people have conditions that appear identical to IPEX syndrome, but they do not have mutations in the *FOXP3* gene. These conditions do not follow an X-linked inheritance pattern, and females can be affected. Such conditions are classified as IPEX-like syndromes.[1]

---

[1] MedlinePlus, "Immune Dysregulation, Polyendocrinopathy, Enteropathy, X-Linked Syndrome," National Institutes of Health (NIH), May 1, 2017. Available online. URL: https://medlineplus.gov/genetics/condition/immune-dysregulation-polyendocrinopathy-enteropathy-x-linked-syndrome. Accessed April 21, 2023.

Chapter 20 | Leukocyte Adhesion Deficiency Type 1

Leukocyte adhesion deficiency (LAD) type 1 is a disorder that causes the immune system to malfunction, resulting in a form of immunodeficiency. Immunodeficiencies are conditions in which the immune system is not able to protect the body effectively from foreign invaders such as viruses, bacteria, and fungi. Starting from birth, people with LAD type 1 develop serious bacterial and fungal infections.

One of the first signs of LAD type 1 is a delay in the detachment of the umbilical cord stump after birth. In newborns, the stump normally falls off within the first two weeks of life, but in infants with LAD type 1, this separation usually occurs at three weeks or later. In addition, affected infants often have inflammation of the umbilical cord stump (omphalitis) due to a bacterial infection.

In LAD type 1, bacterial and fungal infections most commonly occur on the skin and mucous membranes such as the moist lining of the nose and mouth. In childhood, people with this condition develop severe inflammation of the gums (gingivitis) and other tissue around the teeth (periodontitis), which often results in the loss of both primary and permanent teeth. These infections often spread to cover a large area. A hallmark of LAD type 1 is the lack of pus formation at the sites of infection. In people with this condition, wounds are slow to heal, which can lead to additional infection.

Life expectancy in individuals with LAD type 1 is often severely shortened. Due to repeat infections, affected individuals may not survive past infancy.

CAUSES OF LEUKOCYTE ADHESION DEFICIENCY

Mutations in the *ITGB2* gene cause LAD type 1. This gene provides instructions for making one part (the β2 subunit) of at least four different proteins known as "β2 integrins." Integrins that contain the β2 subunit are found embedded in the membrane that surrounds white blood cells (leukocytes). These integrins help leukocytes gather at sites of infection or injury, where they contribute to the immune response. β2 integrins recognize signs of inflammation and attach (bind) to proteins called "ligands" on the lining of blood vessels. This binding leads to the linkage (adhesion) of the leukocyte to the blood vessel wall. Signaling through the β2 integrins triggers the transport of the attached leukocyte across the blood vessel wall to the site of infection or injury.

ITGB2 gene mutations that cause LAD type 1 lead to the production of a β2 subunit that cannot bind with other subunits to form β2 integrins. Leukocytes that lack these integrins cannot attach to the blood vessel wall or cross the vessel wall to contribute to the immune response. As a result, there is a decreased response to injury and foreign invaders, such as bacteria and fungi, resulting in frequent infections, delayed wound healing, and other signs and symptoms of this condition.

INHERITANCE PATTERN OF LEUKOCYTE ADHESION DEFICIENCY

This condition is inherited in an autosomal recessive pattern, which means both copies of the gene in each cell have mutations. The parents of an individual with an autosomal recessive condition each carry one copy of the mutated gene, but they typically do not show signs and symptoms of the condition.[1]

---

[1] MedlinePlus, "Leukocyte Adhesion Deficiency Type 1," National Institutes of Health (NIH), April 1, 2014. Available online. URL: https://medlineplus.gov/genetics/condition/leukocyte-adhesion-deficiency-type-1. Accessed April 21, 2023.

Chapter 21 | **PLCG2- Associated Antibody Deficiency and Immune Dysregulation**

PLCG2-associated antibody deficiency and immune dysregulation (PLAID) and PLAID-like diseases are rare, inherited immune disorders with overlapping features. PLAID is caused by mutations in the *PLCG2* gene, which is involved in the activity of specific immune cells, including B cells, natural killer cells, and myeloid cells. PLAID-like diseases refer to disorders that resemble PLAID, but mutations in *PLCG2* have not been identified. Mutations in other genes that regulate immune activity along with *PLCG2* are likely responsible, and research on PLAID-like diseases is ongoing.

People with PLAID experience cold urticaria, an allergic response of the skin to cold temperatures, from infancy.

Additionally, some individuals with PLAID can develop a burn-like rash at birth in areas most likely to be exposed to cold temperatures, such as the nose. People with PLAID may also have recurrent bacterial infections, autoimmune symptoms and an increased likelihood of developing an autoimmune disorder, and a burning sensation in the throat when eating cold foods.

No treatments that target the underlying cause of PLAID and PLAID-like diseases exist, so people with PLAID are advised to avoid allergic triggers by warming rapidly after showers, avoiding drafts, and toweling off sweat. Antihistamines are used to treat allergic reactions. The allergic response to cold likely results from abnormal activation of immune cells at low temperatures. The National Institute of Allergy and Infectious Diseases (NIAID) researchers have shown that immune cells from PLAID patients are abnormally activated by cold temperatures. In the future, it may be possible to develop therapies that target the *PLCG2* defect to restore normal immune function.[1]

[1] "PLCG2-Associated Antibody Deficiency and Immune Dysregulation (PLAID)," National Institute of Allergy and Infectious Diseases (NIAID), April 22, 2019. Available online. URL: www.niaid.nih.gov/diseases-conditions/plcg2-associated-antibody-deficiency-and-immune-dysregulation-plaid. Accessed April 21, 2021.

Chapter 22 |
Severe Combined Immunodeficiency

WHAT IS SEVERE COMBINED IMMUNODEFICIENCY?

Severe combined immunodeficiency (SCID) is a group of rare disorders caused by mutations in different genes involved in the development and function of infection-fighting immune cells. Infants with SCID appear healthy at birth but are highly susceptible to severe infections. The condition is fatal, usually within the first or second year of life, unless infants receive immune-restoring treatments, such as transplants of blood-forming stem cells, gene therapy, or enzyme therapy. More than 80 percent of SCID infants do not have a family history of the condition. However, the development of a newborn screening test has made it possible to detect SCID before symptoms appear, helping ensure that affected infants receive lifesaving treatments.[1]

WHAT DO YOU KNOW ABOUT THE IMMUNE SYSTEM AND SEVERE COMBINED IMMUNODEFICIENCY?

Lymphocytes, a type of white blood cell (WBC), are made from blood-forming precursor, or "stem," cells in the bone marrow. Some lymphocyte precursors move to the thymus gland, where they become T cells. Others remain in the bone marrow where they mature into B cells and natural killer cells. Each specialized type

---

[1] "Severe Combined Immunodeficiency (SCID)," National Institute of Allergy and Infectious Diseases (NIAID), April 4, 2019. Available online. URL: www.niaid.nih.gov/diseases-conditions/severe-combined-immunodeficiency-scid. Accessed April 21, 2023.

of cell is responsible for a particular immune response. Normally, T cells encourage other immune cells to respond to foreign substances as well as directly combat certain viral and fungal infections. B cells become antibody-producing cells. The antibodies attack foreign substances, or antigens, that mark invading viruses, bacteria, and fungi.

"Severe combined immunodeficiency," or "SCID," is a term applied to a group of inherited disorders characterized by defects in both T and B cell responses, hence the term combined. The most common type of SCID is called "XSCID" because the mutated gene, which normally produces a receptor for activation signals on immune cells, is located on the X chromosome. Another form of SCID is caused by a deficiency of adenosine deaminase (ADA) normally produced by a gene on chromosome 20.

The classic symptoms of SCID include an increased susceptibility to a variety of infections, including ear infections (acute otitis media (AOM)), pneumonia or bronchitis, oral thrush (a type of yeast that multiplies rapidly, creating white, sore areas in the mouth), and diarrhea. Because children with SCID experience multiple infections, they fail to grow and gain weight as expected (i.e., failure to thrive). Children with untreated SCID rarely live past the age of two.

HOW COMMON IS SEVERE COMBINED IMMUNODEFICIENCY?
There is no central record of how many babies are diagnosed with SCID in the United States each year, but the best estimate is somewhere around 40–100. So SCID is a rare condition. On the other hand, researchers have no clear idea of how many babies are not diagnosed and die of SCID-related infections each year. The actual number of cases could be higher.

If a baby exhibits any of the following persistent symptoms within the first year of life, he or she should be evaluated for SCID or other types of immune deficiency syndromes:
- eight or more ear infections
- two or more cases of pneumonia
- infections that do not resolve with antibiotic treatment for two or more months
- failure to gain weight or grow normally
- infections that require intravenous antibiotic treatment

- deep-seated infections, such as pneumonia that affects an entire lung or an abscess in the liver
- persistent thrush in the mouth or throat
- a family history of immune deficiency or infant deaths due to infections

WHAT IS X-LINKED SEVERE COMBINED IMMUNODEFICIENCY?

X-linked severe combined immunodeficiency (XSCID) is caused by mutations in a gene on the X chromosome called "*IL2RG*." This gene creates a key part of a receptor on the surface of a lymphocyte, which, when activated by chemical messengers called "cytokines," transmits information that directs lymphocytes to mature, proliferate, and mobilize to fight infection. The defective part of the lymphocyte receptor is called the "common" gamma chain because it is a common component of lymphocyte receptors for several types of cytokines, including the interleukin-2 (IL-2) receptor. Thus, it is a critical component for mobilizing the body's defenses against infection.

Because females have two X chromosomes, if they have a mutation that disrupts the *IL2RG* gene on one X chromosome, they still have a spare normal gene on the other X chromosome that can compensate for the mutation. Thus, they have normal immune systems. However, since males have only one X chromosome and one Y chromosome, they do not have a spare *IL2RG* gene. A male with a defect in his only *IL2RG* gene produces immune cells that are missing the γc part of their receptors. Because the receptors cannot respond to stimulation, immune dysfunction and SCID set in. XSCID affects only males and is the most common type of SCID. Therefore, the overall incidence of SCID is higher in males than in females.

WHAT IS ADENOSINE DEAMINASE DEFICIENCY SEVERE COMBINED IMMUNODEFICIENCY?

Adenosine deaminase deficiency SCID, commonly called "ADA SCID," is a very rare genetic disorder. It is caused by a mutation in the gene that encodes a protein called "ADA." This ADA protein is an essential enzyme needed by all body cells to produce new deoxyribonucleic acid (DNA). This enzyme also breaks down toxic metabolites that otherwise accumulate to harmful levels that kill lymphocytes. People afflicted with this disease often have to take antibiotics and supplemental infusions of antibodies to protect themselves from serious infections. They can also receive ADA injections given once or twice a week. ADA SCID is lethal without treatment.

HOW IS SEVERE COMBINED IMMUNODEFICIENCY DIAGNOSED?
Early diagnosis of SCID is rare because doctors do not routinely count each type of WBC in newborns. As a result, the average age at which babies are diagnosed with SCID is just over six months, usually because of recurrent infections and failure to thrive. Blood tests for SCID typically reveal significantly lower-than-normal levels of T cells and a lack of germ-fighting antibodies. Even if B cells are present in the blood of SCID patients, they do a poor job of producing antibodies. Low antibody levels and lack of specific antibodies after vaccination or a natural infection are characteristic features of SCID.

IS THERE ANY EFFECTIVE TREATMENT FOR SEVERE COMBINED IMMUNODEFICIENCY?
The most effective treatment for SCID is the transplantation of blood-forming stem cells from the bone marrow of a healthy person. Bone marrow stem cells can live for a long time by renewing themselves as needed and can also produce a continuous supply of healthy immune cells. A bone marrow transplant from a tissue-matched sister or brother offers the greatest chance of curing SCID. However, most patients do not have a matched sibling donor, so transplants from a parent or unrelated matched donor are often performed. These latter types of transplants succeed less often than transplants from matched, related donors. All transplants done in the first three months of life have the highest success rate.[2]

---

[2] "About Severe Combined Immunodeficiency," National Human Genome Research Institute (NHGRI), June 2, 2014. Available online. URL: www.genome.gov/Genetic-Disorders/Severe-Combined-Immunodeficiency. Accessed April 21, 2023.

Chapter 23 | Wiskott-Aldrich Syndrome

WHAT IS WISKOTT-ALDRICH SYNDROME?

Wiskott-Aldrich syndrome is characterized by abnormal immune system function (immune deficiency), eczema (an inflammatory skin disorder characterized by abnormal patches of red, irritated skin), and a reduced ability to form blood clots. This condition primarily affects males.

Individuals with Wiskott-Aldrich syndrome have microthrombocytopenia, which is a decrease in the number and size of blood cells involved in clotting (platelets). This platelet abnormality, which is typically present from birth, can lead to easy bruising, bloody diarrhea, or episodes of prolonged bleeding following nosebleeds or minor trauma. Microthrombocytopenia can also lead to small areas of bleeding just under the surface of the skin, resulting in purplish spots called "purpura," or variably sized rashes made up of tiny red spots called "petechiae." In some cases, particularly if a bleeding episode occurs within the brain, prolonged bleeding can be life-threatening.

Wiskott-Aldrich syndrome is also characterized by abnormal or nonfunctional immune system cells known as "white blood cells" (WBCs). Changes in WBCs lead to an increased risk of several immune and inflammatory disorders in people with Wiskott-Aldrich syndrome. These immune problems vary in severity and include increased susceptibility to infection from bacteria, viruses, and fungi. People with Wiskott-Aldrich syndrome are at greater risk of developing autoimmune disorders, such as rheumatoid arthritis (RA), vasculitis, or hemolytic anemia. These disorders

159

occur when the immune system malfunctions and attacks the body's own tissues and organs.

CAUSES OF WISKOTT-ALDRICH SYNDROME

Mutations in the *WAS* gene cause Wiskott-Aldrich syndrome. The *WAS* gene provides instructions for making a protein called "WASP." This protein is found in all blood cells. WASP is involved in relaying signals from the surface of blood cells to the actin cytoskeleton, which is a network of fibers that make up the cell's structural framework. WASP signaling triggers the cell to move and attach to other cells and tissues (adhesion). In WBCs, this signaling allows the actin cytoskeleton to establish interactions between cells and the foreign invaders that they target (immune synapses).

WAS gene mutations that cause Wiskott-Aldrich syndrome lead to a lack of any functional WASP. Loss of WASP signaling disrupts the function of the actin cytoskeleton in developing blood cells. WBCs that lack WASP have a decreased ability to respond to their environment and form immune synapses. As a result, WBCs are less able to respond to foreign invaders, causing many of the immune problems related to Wiskott-Aldrich syndrome. Similarly, a lack of functional WASP in platelets impairs their development, leading to reduced size and early cell death.

INHERITANCE OF WISKOTT-ALDRICH SYNDROME

This condition is inherited in an X-linked pattern. A condition is considered X-linked if the mutated gene that causes the disorder is located on the X chromosome, one of the two sex chromosomes in each cell. In males, who have only one X chromosome, a mutation in the only copy of the gene in each cell is sufficient to cause the condition. In females, who have two copies of the X chromosome, one altered copy of the gene in each cell can lead to less severe features of the condition or may cause no signs or symptoms at all. A characteristic of X-linked inheritance is that fathers cannot pass X-linked traits to their sons.[1]

---

[1] MedlinePlus, "Wiskott-Aldrich Syndrome," National Institutes of Health (NIH), December 1, 2019. Available online. URL: https://medlineplus.gov/genetics/condition/wiskott-aldrich-syndrome. Accessed April 21, 2023.

Chapter 24 | X-Linked Agammaglobulinemia

WHAT IS X-LINKED AGAMMAGLOBULINEMIA?

X-linked agammaglobulinemia (XLA) is a condition that affects the immune system and occurs almost exclusively in males. It is part of a group of disorders called "primary immunodeficiencies" (or inborn errors of immunity), in which part of the immune system does not function as it should. People with XLA have very few B cells, which are specialized white blood cells (WBCs) that help protect the body against infection. B cells can mature into cells that produce special proteins called "antibodies" or "immunoglobulins." Antibodies attach to specific foreign particles and germs, marking them for destruction. Individuals with XLA are more susceptible to infections because their body makes very few antibodies.

Children with XLA are usually healthy for the first one or two months of life because they are protected by antibodies acquired before birth from their mother. After this time, the maternal antibodies are cleared from the body, and the affected child begins to develop recurrent infections. Children with XLA generally take longer to recover from infections, and infections often occur again, even in children who are taking antibiotic medications.

The most common bacterial infections that occur in people with XLA are lung infections (pneumonia and bronchitis), ear infections (otitis), pink eye (conjunctivitis), and sinus infections (sinusitis). Infections that cause chronic diarrhea are also common. Recurrent infections can lead to organ damage. Treatments that replace antibodies can help prevent infections, improving the quality of life (QOL) for people with XLA.

CAUSES OF X-LINKED AGAMMAGLOBULINEMIA

Variants (also called "mutations") in the *BTK* gene cause XLA. This gene provides instructions for making the BTK protein, which is important for the development of B cells and the normal functioning of the immune system. Most variants in the *BTK* gene prevent the production of any BTK protein. The absence of functional BTK protein blocks B cell development and leads to a lack of antibodies. Without antibodies, the immune system cannot properly respond to foreign invaders and prevent infection.

INHERITANCE OF X-LINKED AGAMMAGLOBULINEMIA

This condition is inherited in an X-linked recessive pattern. The gene associated with this condition is located on the X chromosome, which is one of the two sex chromosomes. In males (who have only one X chromosome), one altered copy of the gene in each cell is sufficient to cause the condition. In females (who have two X chromosomes), a variant would have to occur in both copies of the gene to cause the disorder. Because it is unlikely that females will have two altered copies of this gene, males are affected by X-linked recessive disorders much more frequently than females.

An affected person's mother may carry one altered copy of the *BTK* gene. Individuals with only one altered copy of this gene do not have the immune system abnormalities associated with XLA, but they can pass the altered gene to their children. Fathers cannot pass X-linked traits to their sons, but they can pass them to their daughters.

About half of the affected individuals do not have a family history of XLA. In most of these cases, the affected individual has a new variant in the *BTK* gene that was not inherited from a parent.[1]

---

[1] MedlinePlus, "X-Linked Agammaglobulinemia," National Institutes of Health (NIH), March 17, 2023. Available online: https://medlineplus.gov/genetics/condition/x-linked-agammaglobulinemia. Accessed April 21, 2023.

Chapter 25 | X-Linked Immunodeficiency with Magnesium Defect, Epstein-Barr Virus Infection, and Neoplasia

WHAT IS X-LINKED IMMUNODEFICIENCY WITH MAGNESIUM DEFECT, EPSTEIN-BARR VIRUS INFECTION, AND NEOPLASIA?

X-linked immunodeficiency with magnesium defect, Epstein-Barr virus (EBV) infection, and neoplasia (typically known by the acronym XMEN) is a disorder that affects the immune system in males. In XMEN, certain types of immune system cells called "T cells" are reduced in number or do not function properly. Normally, these cells recognize foreign invaders, such as viruses, bacteria, and fungi, and are then turned on (activated) to attack these invaders in order to prevent infection and illness. Because males with XMEN do not have enough functional T cells, they have frequent infections, such as ear infections, sinus infections, and pneumonia.

In particular, affected individuals are vulnerable to EBV. EBV is a very common virus that infects more than 90 percent of the general population and, in most cases, goes unnoticed. Normally, after initial infection, EBV remains in the body for the rest of a person's life. However, the virus is generally inactive (latent) because it is controlled by T cells. In males with XMEN, however, the T cells cannot control the virus, and EBV infection can lead to cancers of immune system cells (lymphomas). The EBV infection itself usually does not cause any other symptoms in males with XMEN, and affected individuals may not come to medical attention until they develop lymphoma.

CAUSES OF X-LINKED IMMUNODEFICIENCY WITH MAGNESIUM DEFECT, EPSTEIN-BARR VIRUS INFECTION, AND NEOPLASIA

X-linked immunodeficiency with magnesium defect, Epstein-Barr virus infection, and neoplasia is caused by mutations in the *MAGT1* gene. This gene provides instructions for making a protein called a "magnesium transporter," which moves charged atoms (ions) of magnesium (Mg^{2+}) into certain T cells. Specifically, the magnesium transporter produced from the *MAGT1* gene is active in CD8+ T cells, which are especially important in controlling viral infections such as EBV. These cells normally take in magnesium when they detect a foreign invader, and the magnesium is involved in activating the T cell's response.

Mutations in the *MAGT1* gene impair the magnesium transporter's function, reducing the amount of magnesium that gets into T cells. This magnesium deficiency prevents the efficient activation of the T cells from targeting EBV and other infections. Uncontrolled EBV infection increases the likelihood of developing lymphoma.

INHERITANCE OF X-LINKED IMMUNODEFICIENCY WITH MAGNESIUM DEFECT, EPSTEIN-BARR VIRUS INFECTION, AND NEOPLASIA

This condition is inherited in an X-linked recessive pattern. The gene associated with this condition is located on the X chromosome, which is one of the two sex chromosomes. In males (who have only one X chromosome), one altered copy of the gene in each cell is sufficient to cause the condition. In females (who have two X chromosomes), a mutation would have to occur in both copies of the gene to cause the disorder. Because it is unlikely that females will have two altered copies of this gene, males are affected by X-linked recessive disorders much more frequently than females. A characteristic of X-linked inheritance is that fathers cannot pass X-linked traits to their sons.[1]

---

[1] MedlinePlus, "X-Linked Immunodeficiency with Magnesium Defect, Epstein-Barr Virus Infection, and Neoplasia," National Institutes of Health (NIH), June 1, 2014. Available online. URL: https://medlineplus.gov/genetics/condition/x-linked-immunodeficiency-with-magnesium-defect-epstein-barr-virus-infection-and-neoplasia. Accessed April 21, 2023.

Chapter 26 | X-Linked Lymphoproliferative Disease

WHAT IS X-LINKED LYMPHOPROLIFERATIVE DISEASE?

X-linked lymphoproliferative (XLP) disease is a disorder of the immune system and blood-forming cells that is found almost exclusively in males. More than half of individuals with this disorder experience an exaggerated immune response to the Epstein-Barr virus (EBV). EBV is a very common virus that eventually infects most humans. In some people, it causes infectious mononucleosis (commonly known as "mono"). Normally, after initial infection, EBV remains in certain immune system cells (lymphocytes) called "B cells." However, the virus is generally inactive (latent) because it is controlled by other lymphocytes called "T cells" that specifically target EBV-infected B cells.

People with XLP disease may respond to EBV infection by producing abnormally large numbers of T cells, B cells, and other lymphocytes called "macrophages." This proliferation of immune cells often causes a life-threatening reaction called "hemophagocytic lymphohistiocytosis." Hemophagocytic lymphohistiocytosis causes fever, destroys blood-producing cells in the bone marrow, and damages the liver. The spleen, heart, kidneys, and other organs and tissues may also be affected. In some individuals with XLP disease, hemophagocytic lymphohistiocytosis or related symptoms may occur without EBV infection.

165

About one-third of people with XLP disease experience dys-gammaglobulinemia, which means they have abnormal levels of some types of antibodies. Antibodies (also known as "immuno-globulins") are proteins that attach to specific foreign particles and germs, marking them for destruction. Individuals with dys-gammaglobulinemia are prone to recurrent infections. Cancers of immune system cells (lymphomas) occur in about one-third of people with XLP disease. Without treatment, most people with XLP survive only into childhood. Death usually results from hemophagocytic lymphohistiocytosis.

XLP disease can be divided into two types based on its genetic cause and pattern of signs and symptoms: XLP1 (also known as "classic XLP") and XLP2. People with XLP2 have not been known to develop lymphoma, are more likely to develop hemophago-cytic lymphohistiocytosis without EBV infection, usually have an enlarged spleen (splenomegaly), and may also have inflammation of the large intestine (colitis). Some researchers believe that these individuals should actually be considered to have a similar but separate disorder rather than a type of XLP disease.

Other Names of This Condition
- Duncan disease
- Epstein-Barr virus–induced lymphoproliferative disease in males
- familial fatal Epstein-Barr infection
- Purtilo syndrome
- severe susceptibility to EBV infection
- severe susceptibility to infectious mononucleosis
- X-linked lymphoproliferative syndrome
- XLP

FREQUENCY OF X-LINKED LYMPHOPROLIFERATIVE DISEASE
Classic XLP, or XLP1, is estimated to occur in about 1 per million males worldwide. XLP2 is less common, occurring in about 1 per 5 million males.

CAUSES OF X-LINKED LYMPHOPROLIFERATIVE DISEASE

Mutations in the *SH2D1A* and *XIAP* genes cause XLP disease. *SH2D1A* gene mutations cause XLP1, and *XIAP* gene mutations cause XLP2. The *SH2D1A* gene provides instructions for making a protein called "signaling lymphocyte activation molecule" (SLAM) associated protein (SAP). This protein is involved in the functioning of lymphocytes that destroy other cells (cytotoxic lymphocytes) and is necessary for the development of specialized T cells called "natural killer T cells." The SAP protein also helps control immune reactions by triggering self-destruction (apoptosis) of cytotoxic lymphocytes when they are no longer needed.

Some *SH2D1A* gene mutations impair SAP function. Others result in an abnormally short protein that is unstable or nonfunctional or prevent any SAP from being produced. The loss of functional SAP disrupts proper signaling in the immune system and may prevent the body from controlling the immune reaction to EBV infection. In addition, lymphomas may develop when defective lymphocytes are not properly destroyed by apoptosis.

The *XIAP* gene provides instructions for making a protein that helps protect cells from undergoing apoptosis in response to certain signals. *XIAP* gene mutations can lead to an absence of XIAP protein or decrease the amount of XIAP protein that is produced. It is unknown how a lack of XIAP protein results in the signs and symptoms of XLP disease or why features of this disorder differ somewhat between people with *XIAP* and *SH2D1A* gene mutations.

INHERITANCE PATTERN OF X-LINKED LYMPHOPROLIFERATIVE DISEASE

This condition is generally inherited in an X-linked recessive pattern. The genes associated with this condition are located on the X chromosome, which is one of the two sex chromosomes. In males (who have only one X chromosome), one altered copy of an associated gene in each cell is sufficient to cause the condition. A characteristic of X-linked inheritance is that fathers cannot pass X-linked traits to their sons.

In females (who have two X chromosomes), a mutation usually has to occur in both copies of the gene to cause the disorder. Because it is unlikely that females will have two altered copies of an associated gene, males are affected by X-linked recessive disorders much more frequently than females. However, in rare cases, a female carrying one altered copy of the *SH2D1A* or *XIAP* gene in each cell may develop signs and symptoms of this condition.[1]

[1] MedlinePlus, "X-Linked Lymphoproliferative Disease," National Institutes of Health (NIH), May 17, 2021. Available online. URL: https://medlineplus.gov/genetics/condition/x-linked-lymphoproliferative-disease. Accessed April 21, 2023.

Part 3 | Secondary Immunodeficiency Diseases

Chapter 27 | Understanding Secondary Immunodeficiencies

Secondary immunodeficiencies are conditions where the immune system becomes weaker due to external factors that are not directly related to the immune system itself. These factors include environmental agents, malnutrition, the effects caused by medications, and various other conditions.

These immunodeficiencies are acquired and more prevalent when compared to primary immunodeficiencies, which are genetic and present from birth. Secondary immunodeficiencies can affect the immune system differently, making the body more susceptible to diseases and infections.

Secondary immunodeficiencies are one of the major causes of adult infections, and they can be transient or persistent. In some cases, the immune system may recover once the cause of the immunodeficiency is treated. However, in other cases, the immunodeficiency may be chronic and require ongoing management.

CAUSES OF SECONDARY IMMUNODEFICIENCIES

Secondary immunodeficiencies have many causes, including infectious agents, drugs, metabolic diseases, and environmental conditions. Worldwide, malnutrition ranks as one of the primary causes of secondary immunodeficiencies. In underdeveloped countries, up to 50 percent of the population suffers from malnutrition, leaving them vulnerable to infections and compromised health.

Other common causes of secondary immunodeficiency include radiation therapy or chemotherapy, chronic diseases, aging, severe burns, and infections caused by human immunodeficiency virus (HIV). Leukemia, a cancer that begins in the bone marrow, can also lead to a type of secondary immunodeficiency called "hypogammaglobulinemia."

Some drugs prescribed to manage autoimmune conditions have the potential to weaken the immune system, thereby raising the likelihood of contracting infections. Chronic infections, such as HIV/acquired immunodeficiency syndrome (AIDS), can also lead to secondary immunodeficiency disorders. The virus attacks a specific type of blood cells called "white blood cells" (WBCs) that help the body fight off infections and bacteria by multiplying. However, over time, HIV reduces the number of these WBCs, making the body more susceptible to different diseases.

SYMPTOMS OF SECONDARY IMMUNODEFICIENCIES

The symptoms of secondary immunodeficiencies vary widely depending on the severity of the external factors and the individual's susceptibility to infections.

Some common symptoms observed in individuals with secondary immunodeficiencies include recurrent infections, delayed wound healing, opportunistic infections (OIs), recurrent inflammation, and allergic reactions. People with secondary immunodeficiencies may experience a higher frequency of infections, such as respiratory tract infections (RTIs), urinary tract infections (UTIs), skin infections, sinus infections, ear infections, and gastrointestinal infections (GIs).

The symptoms of each immunodeficiency disorder vary and can be acute or chronic. Acute symptoms occur suddenly and are short-lived, while chronic symptoms persist over a long period. It is essential to understand how to recognize the symptoms of secondary immunodeficiencies, seek prompt medical attention, and receive proper treatment.

DIAGNOSIS OF SECONDARY IMMUNODEFICIENCIES

Individuals on chronic medication regimes for inflammatory illnesses with abnormal immune system test results provide firsthand clues in diagnosing secondary immunodeficiency. Before and after immune system suppression, health-care providers evaluate factors such as lymphocyte subsets, immunoglobulin levels, and inflammatory markers to diagnose secondary immunodeficiencies. To formulate the best treatment based on the diagnosis, they consider criteria such as age, gender, medical history, and drugs used.

TREATMENT FOR SECONDARY IMMUNODEFICIENCIES

The best way to treat secondary immunodeficiencies is to identify the underlying cause and treat the primary condition that causes the immune system to weaken. For example, the WBC count can be normalized from a deficient level in an HIV patient by undergoing therapies such as highly active antiretroviral therapy (HAART) and antiviral treatments, thus increasing their life span. Secondary immunodeficiency may require a bone marrow transplant in certain instances. This is a common treatment option for those with certain types of cancer or genetic disorders that affect the bone marrow's ability to produce healthy blood cells. The transplant can replace the damaged bone marrow with healthy stem cells, which can help restore the immune system.

PREVENTION OF SECONDARY IMMUNODEFICIENCIES

Some preventive measures can help strengthen the immune system and reduce the risk of secondary immunodeficiencies. The immune system can be boosted or strengthened by adopting healthy practices such as getting enough sleep, exercising regularly, and consuming a balanced and nutritious diet. If you are susceptible to having a weakened immune system, it is crucial to talk to your health-care provider about your lifestyle habits and make any necessary adjustments. Additionally, avoiding sharing needles and practicing safe sex can help protect against HIV, a major cause of secondary immunodeficiency.

For individuals with diabetes, managing blood sugar levels is essential because poorly controlled blood sugar can weaken the immune system. When the WBCs, which play a crucial role in fighting infections, do not function properly, it can increase the risk of infections.

Nutrition also plays a vital role in preventing secondary immunodeficiency disorders. When a person does not get enough essential nutrients, it can weaken their immune system, making them more prone to infections, especially if they are on medications that lower their immune response. It is recommended to seek advice from a health-care provider or a nutrition expert to get the right nutrients for a strong immune system. Overall, taking care of your health and following preventive measures can help maintain a healthy immune system and prevent secondary immunodeficiency disorders.

References

Chinen, Javier and Shearer, William T. "Secondary Immunodeficiencies, including HIV Infection," National Center for Biotechnology Information (NCBI), February 2010. Available online. URL: www.ncbi.nlm.nih.gov/pmc/articles/PMC6151868. Accessed April 28, 2023.

Manhães, Isabella, et al. "Secondary Immunodeficiency: A Difficult Diagnosis in Clinical Practice," *The Journal of Allergy and Clinical Immunology*, 145, no. 2 (2020). https://doi.org/10.1016/j.jaci.2019.12.251.

Nguyen-Luu, Nha Uyen. "Secondary Immunodeficiency," The Association of Allergists and Immunologists of Québec, January 16, 2011. Available online. URL: https://allerg.qc.ca/Information_allergique/6_2_secondaire_en.html. Accessed April 28, 2023.

Tuano, Karen S.; Seth, Neha and Chinen, Javier. "Secondary Immunodeficiencies: An Overview," *Annals of Allergy, Asthma & Immunology*, 127, no. 6 (2021): 617–626. https://doi.org/10.1016/j.anai.2021.08.413.

Weishaupt, Jeffrey. "What to Know about Secondary Immunodeficiency Disorders?" WebMD, November 9, 2021. Available online. URL: www.webmd.com/hiv-aids/what-to-know-secondary-immunodeficiency-disorders. Accessed April 28, 2023.

Chapter 28 | **Acquired Immunodeficiency Syndrome**

WHAT IS ACQUIRED IMMUNODEFICIENCY SYNDROME?

Acquired immunodeficiency syndrome (AIDS) is the final stage of infection with human immunodeficiency virus (HIV). It happens when the body's immune system is badly damaged because of the virus. Not everyone with HIV develops AIDS.

HIV harms your immune system by destroying a type of white blood cell (WBC) that helps your body fight infection. This puts you at risk of other infections and diseases.

HOW DOES HUMAN IMMUNODEFICIENCY VIRUS SPREAD?

Human immunodeficiency virus is spread through certain body fluids from a person who has HIV. This can happen:

- by having unprotected vaginal or anal sex with a person who has HIV ("Unprotected" means not using condoms or medicine to treat or prevent HIV. This is the most common way that it spreads.)
- by sharing drug needles
- through contact with the blood of a person with HIV
- from mother to baby during pregnancy, childbirth, or breastfeeding

WHO IS AT RISK OF HUMAN IMMUNODEFICIENCY VIRUS INFECTION?

Anyone can get HIV, but certain groups have a higher risk of getting it:

- people who have another sexually transmitted disease (STD)
- people who inject drugs with shared needles
- gay and bisexual men
- Black/African Americans and Hispanic/Latino Americans who make up a higher proportion of new HIV diagnoses and people with HIV, compared to other races and ethnicities
- people who engage in risky sexual behaviors, such as not using condoms or medicine to prevent or treat HIV

Factors such as stigma, discrimination, income, education, and geographic region can also affect people's risk of HIV.

WHAT ARE THE SYMPTOMS OF HUMAN IMMUNODEFICIENCY VIRUS INFECTION?

The first signs of HIV infection may be flu-like symptoms:

- chills
- fatigue
- fever
- mouth ulcers
- muscle aches
- night sweats (heavy sweating during sleep)
- rash
- sore throat
- swollen lymph nodes

These symptoms may come and go within two to four weeks. This stage is called "acute HIV infection."

If the infection is not treated, it becomes a chronic HIV infection. Often, there are no symptoms during this stage. If it is not treated, eventually, the virus will weaken your body's immune system. Then the infection will progress to AIDS. This is the late stage of HIV infection. Because your immune system is badly damaged, your body cannot fight off other infections, called "opportunistic infections" (OIs). OIs are infections that happen more frequently or are more severe in people who have weakened immune systems.

Some people may not feel sick during the earlier stages of HIV infection. So the only way to know for sure whether you have HIV is to get tested.

HOW DO YOU KNOW IF YOU HAVE HUMAN IMMUNODEFICIENCY VIRUS INFECTION?

A blood test can tell if you have an HIV infection. Your healthcare provider can do the test, or you can use a home testing kit. You can also use the Centers for Disease Control and Prevention (CDC) Testing Locator (https://gettested.cdc.gov) to find free testing websites.

WHAT ARE THE TREATMENTS FOR HUMAN IMMUNODEFICIENCY VIRUS INFECTION?

There is no cure for HIV infection, but it can be treated with medicines. This is called "antiretroviral therapy" (ART). ART can make HIV infection a manageable chronic condition. It also reduces the risk of spreading the virus to others.

Most people with HIV live long and healthy lives if they get ART as soon as possible and stay on it. It is also important to take care of yourself. Making sure that you have the support you need, living a healthy lifestyle, and getting regular medical care can help you enjoy a better quality of life (QOL).

CAN HUMAN IMMUNODEFICIENCY VIRUS INFECTION BE PREVENTED?

You can reduce the risk of getting or spreading HIV by:
- getting tested for HIV
- choosing less risky sexual behaviors, which includes limiting the number of sexual partners you have and using latex condoms every time you have sex (If

you or your partner is allergic to latex, you can use polyurethane condoms.)
- getting tested and treated for STDs
- not injecting drugs
- talking to your health-care provider about medicines to prevent HIV with the following:
  - **Pre-exposure prophylaxis (PrEP).** This medicine is for people who do not already have HIV but are at very high risk of getting it. PrEP is daily medicine that can reduce this risk.
  - **Post-exposure prophylaxis (PEP).** This medicine is for people who have possibly been exposed to HIV. It is only for emergency situations. PEP must be started within 72 hours after a possible exposure to HIV.[1]

---

[1] MedlinePlus, "HIV," National Institutes of Health (NIH), February 14, 2023. Available online. URL: https://medlineplus.gov/hiv.html. Accessed April 21, 2023.

Chapter 29 | **Opportunistic Infections**

WHAT ARE OPPORTUNISTIC INFECTIONS?

- Opportunistic infections (OIs) are illnesses that occur more frequently and are more severe in people with weakened immune system.
- OIs are less common in people with human immunodeficiency virus (HIV) because of effective HIV treatment.
- But some people with HIV still develop OIs because:
  - they may not know they have HIV
  - they may not be on HIV treatment
  - their HIV treatment may not be working properly

WHAT ARE COMMON OPPORTUNISTIC INFECTIONS?
Candidiasis

- Candidiasis is caused by infection with a fungus called "*Candida*."
- Candidiasis can affect the skin, nails, and mucous membranes throughout the body.
- People with HIV often have trouble with *Candida*, especially in the mouth and vagina.
- Candidiasis is only considered an OI when it causes severe or persistent infections in the mouth or vagina or when it develops in the esophagus (swallowing tube) or lower respiratory tract, such as the trachea and bronchi (breathing tube), or deeper lung tissue.

Invasive Cervical Cancer

- Cervical cancer starts within the cervix (the lower part of the uterus at the top of the vagina) and spreads (becomes invasive) to other parts of the body.
- Cervical cancer can be prevented by having your healthcare provider perform regular examinations of the cervix.

Coccidioidomycosis

- This illness is caused by the fungus *Coccidioides*.
- It is sometimes called "valley fever," "desert fever," or "San Joaquin Valley fever."
- People can get it by breathing in fungal spores.
- The disease is especially common in hot, dry regions of the southwestern United States, Central America, and South America.

Cryptococcosis

- This illness is caused by infection with the fungus *Cryptococcus neoformans*.
- The fungus typically enters the body through the lungs and can cause pneumonia.
- Cryptococcosis usually affects the lungs or the central nervous system (the brain and spinal cord), but it can also affect other parts of the body.

Cryptosporidiosis

- Cryptosporidiosis (Crypto) is a diarrheal disease caused by a tiny parasite called "*Cryptosporidium*."
- Symptoms include abdominal cramps and severe, chronic, watery diarrhea.

Cystoisosporiasis

- Cystoisosporiasis is formerly known as "isosporiasis."
- This infection is caused by the parasite *Cystoisospora belli* (formerly known as "*Isospora belli*").
- Cystoisosporiasis can enter the body through contaminated food or water.

- Symptoms include diarrhea, fever, headache, abdominal pain, vomiting, and weight loss.

Cytomegalovirus

- Cytomegalovirus (CMV) can infect multiple parts of the body and cause pneumonia, gastroenteritis (especially abdominal pain caused by infection of the colon), encephalitis (infection) of the brain, and sight-threatening retinitis (infection of the retina at the back of the eye).
- People with CMV retinitis have difficulty with vision that worsens over time. CMV retinitis is a medical emergency because it can cause blindness if not treated promptly.

Encephalopathy (Human Immunodeficiency Virus Related)

- This brain disorder can occur as part of acute HIV infection or can result from chronic HIV infection.
- Its exact cause is unknown, but it is thought to be related to infection of the brain with HIV and the resulting inflammation.

Herpes Simplex Virus

- Herpes simplex virus (HSV) is a common virus that causes no major problems for most people.
- HSV is usually acquired sexually or passed from mother to child during birth.
- In most people with healthy immune systems, HSV is usually latent (inactive).
- Stress, trauma, other infections, or suppression of the immune system (such as by HIV) can reactivate the latent virus, and symptoms can return.
- HSV can cause painful cold sores (sometimes called "fever blisters") in or around the mouth or painful ulcers on or around the genitals or anus.
- In people with severely damaged immune systems, HSV can also cause infection of the bronchus (breathing tube), pneumonia (infection of the lungs), and esophagitis (infection of the esophagus or swallowing tube).

Histoplasmosis

- Histoplasmosis is caused by the fungus "*Histoplasma*."
- *Histoplasma* most often develops in the lungs and produces symptoms similar to the flu or pneumonia.
- People with severely damaged immune systems can get a very serious form of the disease called "progressive disseminated histoplasmosis." This form of histoplasmosis can last a long time and spread to other parts of the body.

Kaposi Sarcoma

- Kaposi sarcoma (KS) is caused by a virus called "Kaposi sarcoma herpesvirus (KSHV)" or "human herpesvirus 8" (HHV-8).
- KS causes small blood vessels to grow abnormally and can occur anywhere in the body.
- KS appears as firm pink or purple spots on the skin that can be raised or flat.
- KS can be life-threatening when it affects organs inside the body, such as the lung, lymph nodes, or intestines.

Lymphoma

- Lymphoma refers to cancer of the lymph nodes and other lymphoid tissues in the body.
- There are many kinds of lymphomas. Some types, such as non-Hodgkin lymphoma and Hodgkin lymphoma, are associated with HIV.

Tuberculosis

- Tuberculosis (TB) is caused by a bacterium called "*Mycobacterium tuberculosis*."
- TB can spread through the air when a person with TB coughs, sneezes, or speaks. Breathing in the bacteria can lead to infection in the lungs.
- Symptoms of TB in the lungs include cough, tiredness, weight loss, fever, and night sweats.

Mycobacterium avium Complex

- *Mycobacterium avium* complex (MAC) is caused by infection with different types of mycobacterium: MAC, *Mycobacterium intracellulare*, or *Mycobacterium kansasii*.
- These bacteria live in our environment, including in soil and dust particles.
- Infections with these bacteria spread throughout the body and can be life-threatening in people with weakened immune systems.

Pneumocystis pneumonia

- *Pneumocystis pneumonia* (PCP) is a lung infection caused by the fungus *Pneumocystis jirovecii*.
- PCP occurs in people with weakened immune systems.
- The first signs of infection are difficulty breathing, high fever, and dry cough.

Pneumonia

- Pneumonia is an infection in one or both lungs.
- Many germs, including bacteria, viruses, and fungi, can cause pneumonia.
- Symptoms include a cough (with mucous), fever, chills, and trouble breathing.
- In people with immune systems severely damaged by HIV, one of the most common and life-threatening causes of pneumonia is an infection with the bacteria *Streptococcus pneumoniae*, also called "*Pneumococcus.*" People with HIV should get a vaccine to prevent infection with *Streptococcus pneumoniae*.

Progressive Multifocal Leukoencephalopathy

- This rare brain and spinal cord disease is caused by the John Cunningham (JC) virus.
- It is seen almost exclusively in people whose immune systems have been severely damaged by HIV.
- Symptoms may include loss of muscle control, paralysis, blindness, speech problems, and an altered mental state.
- This disease often progresses rapidly and may be fatal.

Salmonella Septicemia

- *Salmonella* are bacteria that typically enter the body through eating or drinking contaminated food or water.
- Infection with *Salmonella* (called "salmonellosis") can affect anyone and usually causes nausea, vomiting, and diarrhea.
- *Salmonella* septicemia is a severe form of infection in which the bacteria circulate through the whole body and exceeds the immune system's ability to control it.

Toxoplasmosis

- This infection is caused by the parasite *Toxoplasma gondii*.
- The parasite is carried by warm-blooded animals, such as cats, rodents, and birds, and is released in their feces (stool).
- People can develop it by inhaling dust or eating food contaminated with the parasite.
- Toxoplasma can also occur in commercial meats, especially red meats and pork, but rarely poultry.
- Infection can occur in the lungs, retina of the eye, heart, pancreas, liver, colon, testes, and brain.
- Although cats can transmit toxoplasmosis, litter boxes can be changed safely by wearing gloves and washing hands thoroughly with soap and water afterward.
- All raw red meats that have not been frozen for at least 24 hours should be cooked through to an internal temperature of at least 150 °F (65.56 °C).

HOW CAN YOU PREVENT OPPORTUNISTIC INFECTIONS?

Taking HIV medicine is the best way to prevent getting OIs. HIV medicine can keep your immune system strong and healthy. If you develop an OI, talk to your health-care provider about how to treat it.[1]

---

[1] "AIDS and Opportunistic Infections," Centers for Disease Control and Prevention (CDC), May 20, 2021. Available online. URL: www.cdc.gov/hiv/basics/livingwithhiv/opportunisticinfections.html. Accessed April 21, 2023.

Chapter 30 | Malnutrition and Infection

Malnutrition is caused by the body consuming too few or too many nutrients, which can damage cell function and structure. It can lead to health problems such as losing weight, stunted growth, muscle wasting, obesity, and poor health. Malnutrition is widely classified into the following two types:
- **Micronutrient-dependent malnutrition**. This occurs when an individual's diet lacks essential micronutrients, such as minerals and vitamins.
- **Macronutrient-dependent malnutrition**. This is caused by a deficiency or excess of one or more macronutrients, such as carbohydrates, proteins, fats, and water.

Moreover, taking excessive micronutrients and macronutrients can weaken the immune system, affecting people of all ages.

MALNUTRITION AND INFECTION

Malnutrition and infection are inextricably related, with malnutrition increasing the likelihood and severity of infections. Malnutrition can weaken the immune system by suppressing immunological responses and making people more susceptible to infections. Malnutrition can also exacerbate metabolic and non-communicable diseases and damage immune systems.

Diet directly impacts the immune system's ability to combat infections and inflammation. When individuals eat a lot of processed foods, they do not get sufficient essential vitamins and minerals, present in whole foods, their bodies need to stay healthy. As a result, their body's natural defense system becomes weaker, making it harder for them to fight off infections because their immune system is not strong enough. This makes them more likely to fall sick.

TYPES OF INFECTIONS RELATED TO MALNUTRITION

The immune system requires adequate nutrition to function well. Infections can interfere with how the body absorbs, processes, and moves nutrients. However, a lack of necessary nutrients (malnutrition) can harm the immune system, leading to more frequent or severe infections and illnesses. Malnourished people are more susceptible to major system infection categories, including the following:

- **Respiratory**. Malnourished individuals are likely to become ill due to the colonization of pathogenic germs in the respiratory system.
- **Gastrointestinal**. Viral and bacterial gastroenteritis or intestinal helminth (parasitic worm) infections can cause diarrhea. If diarrhea lasts for an extended period, it will cause severe malnutrition and may hinder growth.
- **Systemic**. Bloodstream infections, such as tuberculosis, malaria, and visceral leishmaniasis, are among the most lethal complications of severe acute malnutrition, with high mortality rates, especially in children suffering from septic shock.

Malnutrition raises the likelihood and severity of these infections. Tuberculosis can cause pneumonia in those who are severely malnourished. This implies that their bodies do not have enough resources to fight infections, making them more susceptible to pneumonia. Pneumonia leads to other respiratory infections that damage the lungs and make breathing difficult. Also, malnutrition, sickness, and decreased immunity promote the spread of opportunistic infections such as noma, a bacterial infection that causes mutilating orofacial gangrene.

Malaria, a parasitic infection, can cause growth retardation. Furthermore, if people do not consume enough protein and energy, they can become sicker from malaria and even die more easily. Taking zinc or vitamin A supplements has been shown in studies to help reduce the severity of malaria infections.

Intestinal parasitism and malnutrition frequently coexist and impede an individual's ability to obtain sufficient nutrients from meals. Soil-transmitted parasites substantially influence individuals' nutritional status.

MANAGEMENT AND PREVENTION OF INFECTION DUE TO MALNUTRITION

Malnutrition is a worldwide problem that cannot be ignored. Malnutrition raises the risk of infections produced by viruses, bacteria, and protozoa, which can result in diseases and, ultimately, death. Recovering from infections necessitates many nutrients, which can be difficult for malnourished people to obtain.

Cost-effective solutions are required to address this issue. Having a healthy diet that is filled with nutrients can make the gut stronger and help the body fight off infections and diseases. When someone gets sick, their body's ability to use energy and protein is affected, so it is important to adjust their diet to provide the necessary nutrients during the illness.

To effectively tackle the harmful cycle of long-term malnutrition and infection, it is crucial for researchers from diverse disciplines, including biomedicine, to focus their efforts together. Collaboration between public health officials and researchers is essential in developing practical solutions to address the issue of malnutrition.

References

Foolchand, Ashmika; Ghazi, Terisha and Chuturgoon, Anil A. "Malnutrition and Dietary Habits Alter the Immune System Which May Consequently Influence SARS-CoV-2 Virulence: A Review," Multidisciplinary Digital Publishing Institute (MDPI), February 28,

2022. Available online. URL: www.mdpi.com/1422-0067/23/5/2654. Accessed May 2, 2023.

Goodluck, Ohanube A. K.; Ojong, Agimogim Kelvin and Chinaza, Ikeagwulonu Richard. "Malnutrition: The Tripple Burden and the Immune System," IntechOpen, October 1, 2022. Available online. URL: www.intechopen. com/online-first/83915. Accessed May 3, 2023.

Ibrahim, Marwa K., et al. "Impact of Childhood Malnutrition on Host Defense and Infection," *American Society for Microbiology Journals*, 30, no. 4 (2017): 919–971. https://doi.org/10.1128/CMR.00119-16.

Macallan, Derek. "Infection and Malnutrition," *Medicine*, 37, no. 10 (2009): 525–528. https://doi. org/10.1016/j.mpmed.2009.07.005.

Schaible, Ulrich E. and Kaufmann, Stefan H. E. "Malnutrition and Infection: Complex Mechanisms and Global Impacts," National Center for Biotechnology Information (NCBI), May 1, 2007. Available online. URL: www.ncbi.nlm.nih. gov/pmc/articles/PMC1858706. Accessed May 3, 2023.

Stephensen, Charles. "Primer on Immune Response and Interface with Malnutrition," *Nutrition and Infectious Diseases* (2020): 83–110. https://doi. org/10.1007/978-3-030-56913-6_3.

Walson, Judd L. and Berkley, James A. "The Impact of Malnutrition on Childhood Infections," National Center for Biotechnology Information (NCBI), April 26, 2018. Available online. URL: www.ncbi.nlm.nih.gov/pmc/ articles/PMC6037284. Accessed May 3, 2023.

Chapter 31 | Chemotherapy-Induced Neutropenia

WHAT IS NEUTROPENIA?

Neutropenia is a decrease in the number of white blood cells (WBCs). These cells are the body's main defense against infection. Neutropenia is common after receiving chemotherapy and increases your risk of infections.

WHY DOES CHEMOTHERAPY CAUSE NEUTROPENIA?

These cancer-fighting drugs work by killing fast-growing cells in the body—both good and bad. These drugs kill cancer cells as well as healthy WBC.

HOW DO YOU KNOW IF YOU HAVE NEUTROPENIA?

Your doctor or nurse will tell you. Because neutropenia is common after receiving chemotherapy, your doctor may draw some blood to look for neutropenia.

WHEN WILL YOU BE MOST LIKELY TO HAVE NEUTROPENIA?

Neutropenia often occurs between 7 and 12 days after you receive chemotherapy. This period can be different depending on the chemotherapy you get. Your doctor or nurse will let you know exactly when your WBC count is likely to be at its lowest. You should carefully watch for signs and symptoms of infection during this time.

HOW CAN YOU PREVENT NEUTROPENIA?

There is not much you can do to prevent neutropenia from occurring, but you can decrease your risk of getting an infection while your WBC count is low.[1]

_____

[1] "Neutropenia and Risk for Infection," Centers for Disease Control and Prevention (CDC), November 2, 2022. Available online. URL: www.cdc.gov/cancer/preventinfections/neutropenia.htm. Accessed April 26, 2023.

Chapter 32 | **Infections and Cancer in Transplant Recipients**

IMMUNOSUPPRESSION

Many people who receive organ transplants take medications to suppress the immune system so the body will not reject the organ. These "immunosuppressive" drugs make the immune system less able to detect and destroy cancer cells or fight off infections that cause cancer. Infection with human immunodeficiency virus (HIV) also weakens the immune system and increases the risk of certain cancers.

Research has shown that transplant recipients are at increased risk of a large number of different cancers. Some of these cancers can be caused by infectious agents, whereas others are not. The four most common cancers among transplant recipients and that occur more commonly in these individuals than in the general population are non-Hodgkin lymphoma (NHL) and cancers of the lung, kidney, and liver. NHL can be caused by Epstein-Barr virus (EBV) infection, and liver cancer can be caused by chronic infection with the hepatitis B virus (HBV) and hepatitis C virus (HCV). Lung and kidney cancers are not generally thought to be associated with infection.

People with HIV/acquired immunodeficiency syndrome (AIDS) also have increased risks of cancers that are caused by infectious agents, including EBV; human herpesvirus 8 (HHV-8), or Kaposi sarcoma–associated virus (KSHV); HBV and HCV, which cause liver cancer; and human papillomavirus, which causes cervical, anal, oropharyngeal, and other cancers.

INFECTIOUS AGENTS

Certain infectious agents, including viruses, bacteria, and parasites, can cause cancer or increase the risk that cancer will form. Some viruses can disrupt signaling that normally keeps cell growth and proliferation in check. Also, some infections weaken the immune system, making the body less able to fight off other cancer-causing infections. And some viruses, bacteria, and parasites also cause chronic inflammation, which may lead to cancer.

Most of the viruses that are linked to an increased risk of cancer can be passed from one person to another through blood and/or other body fluids. You can lower your risk of infection by getting vaccinated, not having unprotected sex, and not sharing needles.

Epstein-Barr Virus

EBV, a type of herpes virus, causes mononucleosis as well as certain types of lymphoma and cancers of the nose and throat. EBV is most commonly transmitted by contact with saliva, such as through kissing or by sharing toothbrushes or drinking glasses. It can also be spread by sexual contact, blood transfusions, and organ transplantation. EBV infection is lifelong. More than 90 percent of people worldwide will be infected with EBV during their lifetime, and most do not develop any symptoms. There is no vaccine to prevent EBV infection and no specific treatment for EBV infection. New research shows that EBV may lead to cancer by causing breaks in human deoxyribonucleic acid (DNA).

Helicobacter pylori

Helicobacter pylori (H. pylori) is a type of bacterium that can cause noncardia gastric cancer (a type of stomach cancer) and a type of lymphoma in the stomach lining, gastric mucosa–associated lymphoid tissue (MALT) lymphoma. It can also cause stomach ulcers. The bacterium is thought to spread through consumption of contaminated food or water and direct mouth-to-mouth contact.

The CDC estimates that approximately two-thirds of the world's population harbor *H. pylori*, with infection rates much higher in developing countries than in developed nations. In most populations, the bacterium is first acquired during childhood. If you have stomach problems, see a doctor. Infection with *H. pylori* can be detected and treated with antibiotics.

Hepatitis B Virus and Hepatitis C Virus

Chronic infections with HBV or HCV can cause liver cancer. Both viruses can be transmitted via blood (e.g., by sharing needles or through blood transfusions) and from mother to baby at birth. In addition, HBV can be transmitted via sexual contact.

Since the 1980s, infants in the United States and most other countries have been routinely vaccinated against HBV infection. Experts recommend that adults who have not been vaccinated against HBV and are at increased risk of HBV infection get vaccinated as soon as possible. Vaccination is especially important for health-care workers and other professionals who come into contact with human blood.

The U.S. Centers for Disease Control and Prevention (CDC) also recommends that everyone in the United States born from 1945 to 1965, and other populations at increased risk of HCV infection, be tested for HCV. Although there is not currently a vaccine against HCV, new therapies can cure people of HCV infection. If you think you may be at risk of HBV or HCV infection, ask your doctor about being tested. These infections do not always cause symptoms, but tests can show whether you have the virus. If so, your doctor may suggest treatment. Also, your doctor can tell you how to keep from infecting other people.

Human Immunodeficiency Virus

HIV is the virus that causes AIDS. HIV does not cause cancer itself, but infection with HIV weakens the immune system and makes the body less able to fight off other infections that cause cancer. People infected with HIV have increased risks of a number of cancers, especially Kaposi sarcoma, lymphomas (including both

NHL and Hodgkin disease), and cancers of the cervix, anus, lung, liver, and throat.

HIV can be transmitted via blood and through sexual contact. Men who have unprotected sex with other men and people who share needles for injection drug use are at the highest risk of acquiring HIV infection; heterosexual individuals who have unprotected sex with multiple partners are at the next highest risk.

People can be infected with HIV for years before they begin to develop symptoms. If you think you may be at risk of HIV infection, ask your doctor about being tested. If you test positive, your doctor can prescribe highly effective antiviral treatment and can tell you how to keep from infecting other people.

Human Papillomaviruses

Infections with high-risk types of human papillomavirus (HPV) cause nearly all cervical cancers. They also cause most anal cancers and many oropharyngeal, vaginal, vulvar, and penile cancers. High-risk HPVs spread easily through direct sexual contact, including vaginal, oral, and anal sex. Several vaccines have been developed that prevent infection with the types of HPV that cause most HPV-associated cancers. In the United States, experts recommend that children be vaccinated at age 11 or 12, but children as young as 9 and adults as old as 26 can also be vaccinated.

Cervical cancer screening can be used to detect signs of HPV infections in the cervix. Although HPV infections themselves cannot be treated, the cervical abnormalities that these infections can cause over time can be treated.

Human T-Cell Leukemia/Lymphoma Virus Type 1

Human T-cell leukemia/lymphoma virus type 1 (HTLV-1) can cause an aggressive type of NHL called "adult T-cell leukemia/lymphoma" (ATLL). This virus spreads via blood (by sharing needles or through transfusions), through sexual contact, and from mother to child in the womb or via breastfeeding. Infection with this virus is more common in Japan, Africa, the Caribbean, and South America than in the United States. Most people with HTLV-1 infection do not have any symptoms or develop the disease.

Blood is routinely screened for HTLV-1 in the United States. There is no vaccine to prevent infection with this virus and no treatment if you are infected. If you think you may be at risk of HTLV-1 infection, ask your doctor about being tested. If you test positive, your doctor can tell you how to keep from infecting other people and monitor you for HTLV 1–induced disease.

Kaposi Sarcoma–Associated Herpesvirus

KSHV (or HHV-8) can cause Kaposi sarcoma. KSHV can also cause primary effusion lymphoma and multicentric Castleman disease.

This herpesvirus is most commonly spread through saliva. It can also be spread through organ or bone marrow transplantation, and there is some evidence that it can be spread by blood transfusion although this risk is minimized by practices followed in the United States such as blood storage and removal of white cells.

KSHV infection is generally limited to certain populations, and the way KSHV is spread varies among these populations. In sub-Saharan Africa and certain regions of Central and South America, where KSHV infection is relatively common, it is believed to spread by contact with saliva among family members. In Mediterranean countries (such as Italy, Greece, Israel, and Saudi Arabia), where KSHV infection is present at intermediate levels, it is thought to spread by contact among children and by ill-defined routes among adults. Finally, in regions where KSHV infection is uncommon, such as the United States and Northern Europe, it appears to be mostly transmitted sexually, especially among men who have sex with men.

Most people infected with KSHV do not develop cancer or show any symptoms although those who also have HIV infection or are immunosuppressed for other reasons are more likely to develop KSHV-caused diseases. There is no vaccine to prevent KSHV infection and no therapy to treat the infection. Men who have sex with men may be advised to avoid oral–anal contact (including the use of saliva as a personal lubricant). And people who are infected with

HIV can lower their risk of KSHV-related complications by using antiretroviral therapy.

Merkel Cell Polyomavirus

Merkel cell polyomavirus (MCPyV) can cause Merkel cell carcinoma, a rare type of skin cancer. Most adults are infected with MCPyV, with transmission most likely occurring through casual direct (i.e., skin-to-skin) or indirect (i.e., touching a surface that an infected person has touched) contact in early childhood. The risk of Merkel cell carcinoma is greatly increased in elderly people and in younger adults who are infected with HIV or are immunosuppressed for other reasons. Infection does not generally cause symptoms, and there are no treatments for MCPyV.

Opisthorchis viverrini

This parasitic flatworm (fluke), which is found in Southeast Asia, can cause cholangiocarcinoma (cancer of the bile ducts in the liver). People become infected when they eat raw or undercooked freshwater fish that contain the larvae. Antiparasitic drugs are used to treat the infection.

Schistosoma hematobium

This parasitic flatworm (fluke), which lives in certain types of freshwater snails found in Africa and the Middle East, can cause bladder cancer. People become infected when infectious free-swimming flatworm larvae burrow into the skin that has come into contact with contaminated freshwater. Antiparasitic drugs are used to treat the infection.[1]

[1] "Immunosuppression," National Cancer Institute (NCI), April 29, 2015. Available online. URL: www.cancer.gov/about-cancer/causes-prevention/risk/immunosuppression. Accessed May 8, 2023.

Part 4 | **Autoimmune Diseases**

Chapter 33 | **Autoimmune Disorders of Blood**

Chapter Contents

Section 33.1 | Autoimmune Hemolytic Anemia

Autoimmune hemolytic anemia (AIHA) occurs when your immune system makes antibodies that attack your red blood cells (RBCs). This causes a drop in the number of RBCs, leading to hemolytic anemia. Symptoms may include unusual weakness and fatigue with tachycardia and breathing difficulties, jaundice, dark urine, and/or splenomegaly. AIHA can be primary (idiopathic) or result from an underlying disease or medication. The condition may develop gradually or occur suddenly. There are two main types of AIHA: warm antibody hemolytic anemia and cold antibody hemolytic anemia. Treatment may include corticosteroids such as prednisone, splenectomy, immunosuppressive drugs, and/or blood transfusions.

SYMPTOMS OF AUTOIMMUNE HEMOLYTIC ANEMIA

The human phenotype ontology (HPO) provides the following list of features that have been reported in people with this condition. If available, the list includes a rough estimate of how common a feature is (its frequency). Frequencies are based on a specific study and may not be representative of all studies (refer to Table 33.1).

Table 33.1. Autoimmune Hemolytic Anemia

Signs and Symptoms	Approximate Number of Patients (%; When Available)
Autoimmunity	90
Hemolytic anemia	90
Migraine	90
Muscle weakness	90
Pallor	90
Respiratory insufficiency	90

Table 33.1. Continued

Signs and Symptoms	Approximate Number of Patients (%; When Available)
Abnormality of the liver	50
Lymphoma	50
Abdominal pain	7.5
Abnormality of temperature regulation	7.5
Abnormality of urine homeostasis	7.5
Arrhythmia	7.5
Congestive heart failure	7.5
Splenomegaly	7.5
Abnormality of metabolism/homeostasis	—
Autoimmune hemolytic anemia	—
Autosomal recessive inheritance	—

CAUSES OF AUTOIMMUNE HEMOLYTIC ANEMIA

In about half of cases, the cause of AIHA cannot be determined (idiopathic or primary). This condition can also be caused by or occur with another disorder (secondary) or rarely occur following the use of certain drugs (such as penicillin) or after a person has a blood and marrow stem cell transplant. Secondary causes of AIHA include:

- autoimmune diseases, such as lupus
- chronic lymphocytic leukemia (CLL)
- non-Hodgkin lymphoma (NHL) and other blood cancers
- Epstein-Barr virus (EBV)
- cytomegalovirus
- mycoplasma pneumonia
- hepatitis
- human immunodeficiency virus (HIV)

INHERITANCE OF AUTOIMMUNE HEMOLYTIC ANEMIA

In many cases, the cause of AIHA remains unknown. Some researchers believe that there are multiple factors involved, including genetic and environmental influences (multifactorial). In a very small number of cases, AIHA appears to run in families. In these cases, it appears to follow an autosomal recessive pattern of inheritance.

PROGNOSIS OF AUTOIMMUNE HEMOLYTIC ANEMIA

The outlook depends on the underlying cause of the disease and whether symptoms are managed appropriately and in a timely manner. Death as a result of AIHA is rare.[1]

Section 33.2 | Immune Thrombocytopenia

WHAT IS IMMUNE THROMBOCYTOPENIA?

Immune thrombocytopenia (ITP) is a type of platelet disorder. In ITP, your blood does not clot as it should because you have a low platelet count. Platelets are tiny blood cells that are made in the bone marrow. When you are injured, platelets stick together to form a plug that seals your wound. This plug is called a "blood clot." When you have a low platelet count, you may have trouble stopping bleeding.

ITP can be acute (short-term) or chronic (long-term). Acute ITP often lasts less than six months. It mainly occurs in children—both boys and girls—and is the most common type of ITP. Chronic ITP lasts six months or longer and mostly affects adults. However, some teens and children do get this type of ITP. Chronic ITP affects women two to three times more often than it affects men.

---

[1] Genetic and Rare Diseases Information Center (GARD), "Autoimmune Hemolytic Anemia," National Center for Advancing Translational Sciences (NCATS), March 9, 2016. Available online. URL: https://rarediseases.info.nih.gov/diseases/5870/autoimmune-hemolytic-anemia. Accessed May 9, 2023.

WHAT ARE THE SYMPTOMS OF IMMUNE THROMBOCYTOPENIA?

Immune thrombocytopenia may not cause any symptoms. However, ITP can cause bleeding that is hard to stop. This bleeding can be inside your body, underneath your skin, or from your skin. Signs of bleeding may include the following:

- petechiae, which are small, flat red spots under the skin caused by blood leaking from blood vessels
- purpura, which is bleeding in your skin that can cause red, purple, or brownish-yellow spots
- clotted or partially clotted blood under your skin (called a "hematoma") that looks or feels like a lump
- nosebleeds or bleeding from your gums
- blood in your urine or stool
- heavy menstrual bleeding
- extreme tiredness

WHAT CAUSES IMMUNE THROMBOCYTOPENIA?

Immune thrombocytopenia is caused by problems with your immune system. Normally, your immune system helps your body fight off infections and diseases. In ITP, however, your immune system attacks and destroys your body's platelets by mistake. You may also make fewer platelets. Why this happens is not known. Some things that can raise your risk of ITP include the following:

- antibiotics, antiviral medicines, or medicines to treat inflammation
- viral or bacterial infections, which can trigger your immune system to start destroying your platelets
- vaccines, such as the measles, mumps, and rubella (MMR) vaccine, which, rarely, can raise the risk of ITP, especially in children

HOW IS IT DIAGNOSED?

To diagnose ITP, your provider will ask about your medical and family history. They will also ask about your symptoms and do a physical exam to look for signs of bleeding. Your provider may order one or more of the following blood tests:

- **Complete blood count (CBC)**. This test measures your platelet count and the number of other blood cells in your blood.
- **Blood smear**. For this test, some of your blood is put on a slide. A microscope is used to look at your platelets.
- **Bone marrow tests**. These tests check whether your bone marrow is healthy. You may need this test to confirm that you have ITP and not another platelet disorder, especially if your treatment is not working.

You may also have a blood test to check for the antibodies that attack platelets.

If you are at risk for human immunodeficiency virus (HIV), hepatitis C, or *Helicobacter pylori*, your provider may screen you for these infections, which might be linked to ITP.

HOW IS IMMUNE THROMBOCYTOPENIA TREATED?

For most children and adults, ITP is not a serious condition. Acute ITP in children often goes away on its own within a few weeks or months and does not return. For a small number of children, ITP does not go away on its own, and the child may need treatment.

Chronic ITP varies from person to person and can last for many years. Even people who have serious types of chronic ITP can live for decades. Most people who have chronic ITP can stop treatment at some point and maintain a safe platelet count.

Treatment depends on your platelet count and whether you have any symptoms. In mild cases, you may not need any treatment, and your provider will monitor your condition to make sure that your platelet count does not become too low. If you need treatment, your treatment plan may include medicines and procedures. If your ITP was caused by an infection, treating the infection may help increase your platelet count and lower your risk of bleeding problems.

Medicines

Medicines are often used as the first treatment for both children and adults.

Corticosteroids, such as prednisone and dexamethasone, are commonly used to treat ITP. These medicines help increase your platelet count. However, steroids have many side effects. Some people relapse (get worse) when treatment ends. Other medicines used to raise the platelet count include the following:

- eltrombopag
- immune globulin
- rituximab
- romiplostim

Removal of Your Spleen (Splenectomy)

Doctors can surgically remove your spleen if necessary. The spleen is an organ in your upper left abdomen. It makes antibodies that help fight infections. In ITP, these antibodies destroy platelets by mistake.

Removing your spleen may raise your risk of infections. Before you have the surgery, your doctor may give you vaccines to help prevent infections. They will explain what steps you can take to help avoid infections and what symptoms to watch for.

Platelet Transfusions

Some people who have ITP with serious bleeding may need to have a platelet transfusion. This is done in a hospital. Some people will need platelet transfusions before having surgery.

For a platelet transfusion, donor platelets from a blood bank are injected into your bloodstream. This increases your platelet count for a short time.[2]

[2] "Immune Thrombocytopenia (ITP)," National Heart, Lung, and Blood Institute (NHLBI), March 24, 2022. Available online. URL: www.nhlbi.nih.gov/health/immune-thrombocytopenia. Accessed May 9, 2023.

Section 33.3 | Pernicious Anemia

WHAT IS PERNICIOUS ANEMIA?

Pernicious anemia is a condition in which the body cannot make enough healthy red blood cells (RBCs) because it does not have enough vitamin B_{12}. Vitamin B_{12} is a nutrient found in some foods. The body needs this nutrient to make healthy RBCs and to keep its nervous system working properly.

People who have pernicious anemia cannot absorb enough vitamin B_{12} from food. This is because they lack intrinsic factor, a protein made in the stomach. A lack of this protein leads to vitamin B_{12} deficiency.

Other conditions and factors can also cause vitamin B_{12} deficiency. Examples include infections, surgery, medicines, and diet. Technically, the term "pernicious anemia" refers to vitamin B_{12} deficiency due to a lack of intrinsic factor. Often though, vitamin B_{12} deficiency due to other causes is also called "pernicious anemia."

SIGNS, SYMPTOMS, AND COMPLICATIONS OF PERNICIOUS ANEMIA

A lack of vitamin B_{12} (vitamin B_{12} deficiency) causes the signs and symptoms of pernicious anemia. Without enough vitamin B_{12}, your body cannot make enough healthy RBCs, which causes anemia.

Some of the signs and symptoms of pernicious anemia apply to all types of anemia. Other signs and symptoms are specific to a lack of vitamin B_{12}.

Signs and Symptoms of Anemia

The most common symptom of all types of anemia is fatigue (tiredness). Fatigue occurs because your body does not have enough RBCs to carry oxygen to its various parts.

A low RBC count can also cause shortness of breath, dizziness, headache, coldness in your hands and feet, pale or yellowish skin, and chest pain.

A lack of RBCs also means that your heart has to work harder to move oxygen-rich blood through your body. This can lead to irregular heartbeats called "arrhythmias," heart murmur, an enlarged heart, or even heart failure.

Signs and Symptoms of Vitamin B$_{12}$ Deficiency

A vitamin B$_{12}$ deficiency may lead to nerve damage. This can cause tingling and numbness in your hands and feet, muscle weakness, and loss of reflexes. You may also feel unsteady, lose your balance, and have trouble walking. Vitamin B$_{12}$ deficiency can cause weakened bones and may lead to hip fractures.

Severe vitamin B$_{12}$ deficiency can cause neurological problems, such as confusion, dementia, depression, and memory loss.

Other symptoms of vitamin B$_{12}$ deficiency involve the digestive tract. These symptoms include nausea (feeling sick to your stomach) and vomiting, heartburn, abdominal bloating and gas, constipation or diarrhea, loss of appetite, and weight loss. An enlarged liver is another symptom.

A smooth, thick, red tongue is also a sign of vitamin B$_{12}$ deficiency and pernicious anemia.

Infants who have vitamin B$_{12}$ deficiency may have poor reflexes or unusual movements, such as face tremors. They may have trouble feeding due to tongue and throat problems. They may also be irritable. If vitamin B$_{12}$ deficiency is not treated, these infants may have permanent growth problems.

CAUSES OF PERNICIOUS ANEMIA

Pernicious anemia is caused by a lack of intrinsic factor or other causes, such as infections, surgery, medicines, or diet.

Lack of Intrinsic Factor

Intrinsic factor is a protein made in the stomach. It helps your body absorb vitamin B$_{12}$. In some people, an autoimmune response causes a lack of intrinsic factor. An autoimmune response occurs if the body's immune system makes antibodies (proteins) that mistakenly attack and damage the body's tissues or cells.

In pernicious anemia, the body makes antibodies that attack and destroy the parietal cells. These cells line the stomach and make intrinsic factor. Why this autoimmune response occurs is not known.

As a result of this attack, the stomach stops making intrinsic factor. Without intrinsic factor, your body cannot move vitamin B_{12} through the small intestine, where it is absorbed. This leads to vitamin B_{12} deficiency.

A lack of intrinsic factor can also occur if you have had part or all of your stomach surgically removed. This type of surgery reduces the number of parietal cells available to make intrinsic factor.

Rarely, children are born with an inherited disorder that prevents their bodies from making intrinsic factor. This disorder is called "congenital pernicious anemia."

Other Causes

Pernicious anemia also has other causes besides a lack of intrinsic factor. Malabsorption in the small intestine and a diet lacking vitamin B_{12} both can lead to pernicious anemia.

Malabsorption in the Small Intestine

Sometimes, pernicious anemia occurs because the body's small intestine cannot properly absorb vitamin B_{12}. This may be the result of the following:

- **Too many of the wrong kinds of bacteria in the small intestine**. This is a common cause of pernicious anemia in older adults. The bacteria use up the available vitamin B_{12} before the small intestine can absorb it.
- **Diseases that interfere with vitamin B_{12} absorption**. One example is celiac disease. This is a genetic disorder in which your body cannot tolerate a protein called "gluten." Another example is Crohn's disease, an inflammatory bowel disease (IBD). Human

immunodeficiency virus (HIV) may also interfere with vitamin B_{12} absorption.

- **Certain medicines that alter bacterial growth or prevent the small intestine from properly absorbing vitamin B_{12}.** Examples include antibiotics and certain diabetes and seizure medicines.
- **Surgery.** It involves the surgical removal of part or all of the small intestine.
- **A tapeworm infection.** The tapeworm feeds off of vitamin B_{12}. Eating undercooked, infected fish may cause this type of infection.

Diet Lacking Vitamin B_{12}

Some people get pernicious anemia because they do not have enough vitamin B_{12} in their diets. This cause of pernicious anemia is less common than other causes.

Good food sources of vitamin B_{12} include:

- breakfast cereals with added vitamin B_{12}
- meats such as beef, liver, poultry, and fish
- eggs and dairy products (such as milk, yogurt, and cheese)
- foods fortified with vitamin B_{12}, such as soy-based beverages and vegetarian burgers

Strict vegetarians who do not eat any animal or dairy products and do not take a vitamin B_{12} supplement are at risk for pernicious anemia.

Breastfed infants of strict vegetarian mothers are also at risk for pernicious anemia. These infants can develop anemia within months of being born. This is because they have not had enough time to store vitamin B_{12} in their bodies. Doctors treat these infants with vitamin B_{12} supplements.

Other groups, such as the elderly and people who suffer from alcoholism, may also be at risk for pernicious anemia. These people may not get the proper nutrients in their diets.

RISK FACTORS OF PERNICIOUS ANEMIA

Pernicious anemia is more common in people of Northern European and African descent than in other ethnic groups.

Older people are also at higher risk for the condition. This is mainly due to a lack of stomach acid and intrinsic factor, which prevents the small intestine from absorbing vitamin B_{12}. As people grow older, they tend to make less stomach acid.

Pernicious anemia can also occur in younger people and other populations. You are at higher risk for pernicious anemia if you:

- have a family history of the condition
- have had part or all of your stomach surgically removed (The stomach makes intrinsic factor that helps your body absorb vitamin B_{12}.)
- have an autoimmune disorder that involves the endocrine glands, such as Addison disease, type 1 diabetes, Graves disease, or vitiligo
- have had part or all of your small intestine (where vitamin B_{12} is absorbed) surgically removed
- have certain intestinal diseases or other disorders that may prevent your body from properly absorbing vitamin B_{12}, for example, Crohn's disease, intestinal infections, and HIV
- take medicines that prevent your body from properly absorbing vitamin B_{12}, for example, medicines such as antibiotics and certain seizure medicines
- are a strict vegetarian who does not eat any animal or dairy products and does not take a vitamin B_{12} supplement or if you eat poorly overall

PREVENTION OF PERNICIOUS ANEMIA

You cannot prevent pernicious anemia caused by a lack of intrinsic factor. Without intrinsic factor, you would not be able to absorb vitamin B_{12} and will develop pernicious anemia.

Although uncommon, some people develop pernicious anemia because they do not get enough vitamin B_{12} in their diets. Eating foods high in vitamin B$_{12}$ can help prevent low vitamin B$_{12}$ levels. Good food sources of vitamin B$_{12}$ include:

- breakfast cereals with added vitamin B$_{12}$
- meats such as beef, liver, poultry, and fish
- eggs and dairy products (such as milk, yogurt, and cheese)
- foods fortified with vitamin B$_{12}$, such as soy-based beverages and vegetarian burgers

If you are a strict vegetarian, talk with your doctor about having your vitamin B$_{12}$ level checked regularly.

Vitamin B$_{12}$ is also found in multivitamins and B complex vitamin supplements. Doctors may recommend supplements for people at risk for vitamin B$_{12}$ deficiency, such as strict vegetarians or people who have had stomach surgery.

Older adults may have trouble absorbing vitamin B$_{12}$. Thus, doctors may recommend that older adults eat foods fortified with vitamin B$_{12}$ or take vitamin B$_{12}$ supplements.

DIAGNOSIS OF PERNICIOUS ANEMIA

Your doctor will diagnose pernicious anemia based on your medical and family histories, a physical exam, and test results.

Your doctor will want to find out whether the condition is due to a lack of intrinsic factor or another cause. He or she will also want to find out the severity of the condition, so it can be properly treated.

TREATMENT FOR PERNICIOUS ANEMIA

Doctors treat pernicious anemia by replacing the missing vitamin B$_{12}$ in the body. People who have pernicious anemia may need lifelong treatment.

The goals of treating pernicious anemia include:

- preventing or treating the anemia and its signs and symptoms
- preventing or managing complications, such as heart and nerve damage

- treating the cause of the pernicious anemia (if a cause can be found)

Specific Types of Treatment

Pernicious anemia is usually easy to treat with vitamin B_{12} shots or pills.

If you have severe pernicious anemia, your doctor may recommend shots first. Shots are usually given in a muscle every day or every week until the level of vitamin B_{12} in your blood increases. After your vitamin B_{12} blood level returns to normal, you may get a shot only once a month.

For less severe pernicious anemia, your doctor may recommend large doses of vitamin B_{12} pills. A vitamin B_{12} nose gel and spray are also available. These products may be useful for people who have trouble swallowing pills, such as older people who have had strokes.

Your signs and symptoms may begin to improve within a few days after you start treatment. Your doctor may advise you to limit your physical activity until your condition improves.

If your pernicious anemia is caused by something other than a lack of intrinsic factor, you may get treatment for the cause (if a cause can be found). For example, your doctor may prescribe medicines to treat a condition that prevents your body from absorbing vitamin B_{12}.

LIVING WITH PERNICIOUS ANEMIA

With proper treatment, people who have pernicious anemia can recover, feel well, and live normal lives. If you have complications of pernicious anemia, such as nerve damage, early treatment may help reverse the damage.

Ongoing Care

If you have pernicious anemia, you may need lifelong treatment. See your doctor regularly for checkups and ongoing care. Take vitamin B_{12} supplements as your doctor advises. This may help prevent symptoms and complications.

During your follow-up visits, your doctor may check for signs of vitamin B_{12} deficiency. He or she may also adjust your treatment as needed. If you have pernicious anemia, you are at higher risk for stomach cancer. See your doctor regularly, so he or she can check for this complication.

Also, tell your family members, especially your children and brothers and sisters, that you have pernicious anemia. Pernicious anemia can run in families, so they may have a higher risk for the condition.[3]

[3] "Pernicious Anemia," National Heart, Lung, and Blood Institute (NHLBI), December 22, 2017. Available online. URL: www.nhlbi.nih.gov/health-topics/pernicious-anemia. Accessed May 9, 2023.

Chapter 34 | **Autoimmune Disorders of Blood Vessels**

Chapter Contents

Section 34.1 | Antiphospholipid Syndrome

WHAT IS ANTIPHOSPHOLIPID SYNDROME?

Antiphospholipid syndrome is a disorder characterized by an increased tendency to form abnormal blood clots (thromboses) that can block blood vessels. This clotting tendency is known as "thrombophilia." In antiphospholipid syndrome, thromboses can develop in nearly any blood vessel in the body. If a blood clot forms in the vessels in the brain, blood flow is impaired and can lead to stroke. Antiphospholipid syndrome is an autoimmune disorder. Autoimmune disorders occur when the immune system attacks the body's own tissues and organs.

Women with antiphospholipid syndrome are at increased risk of complications during pregnancy. These complications include pregnancy-induced high blood pressure (preeclampsia), an under-developed placenta (placental insufficiency), early delivery, or pregnancy loss (miscarriage). In addition, women with antiphospholipid syndrome are at greater risk of having a thrombosis during pregnancy than at other times during their lives. At birth, infants of mothers with antiphospholipid syndrome may be small and underweight.

A thrombosis or pregnancy complication is typically the first sign of antiphospholipid syndrome. This condition usually appears in early adulthood to mid-adulthood but can begin at any age.

Other signs and symptoms of antiphospholipid syndrome that affect blood cells and vessels include a reduced amount of cells involved in blood clotting called "platelets" (thrombocytopenia), a shortage of red blood cells (RBCs; anemia) due to their premature breakdown (hemolysis), and a purplish skin discoloration (livedo reticularis) caused by abnormalities in the tiny blood vessels of the skin. In addition, affected individuals may have open sores (ulcers) on the skin, migraine headaches, or heart disease. Many people with antiphospholipid syndrome also have other autoimmune disorders such as systemic lupus erythematosus (SLE).

Rarely do people with antiphospholipid syndrome develop thromboses in multiple blood vessels throughout their body. These thromboses block blood flow in affected organs, which impairs

217

their function and ultimately causes organ failure. These individuals are said to have catastrophic antiphospholipid syndrome (CAPS). CAPS typically affects the kidneys, lungs, brain, heart, and liver and is fatal in over half of affected individuals. Less than 1 percent of individuals with antiphospholipid syndrome develop CAPS.

Other Names of This Condition
- antiphospholipid syndrome
- antiphospholipid antibody syndrome
- Hughes syndrome

FREQUENCY OF ANTIPHOSPHOLIPID SYNDROME
Antiphospholipid syndrome is estimated to affect 1 in 2,000 people. This condition may be responsible for up to 1 percent of all thromboses. It is estimated that 20 percent of individuals younger than age 50 who have a stroke have antiphospholipid syndrome. About 10–15 percent of people with systemic lupus erythematosus have antiphospholipid syndrome. Similarly, 10–15 percent of women with recurrent miscarriages likely have this condition. Approximately 70 percent of individuals diagnosed with antiphospholipid syndrome are female.

CAUSES OF ANTIPHOSPHOLIPID SYNDROME
The genetic cause of antiphospholipid syndrome is unknown. This condition results from the presence of three abnormal immune proteins (antibodies) in the blood. The antibodies that cause antiphospholipid syndrome are called "lupus anticoagulant," "anticardiolipin," and "anti-B2 glycoprotein I." These antibodies are referred to as antiphospholipid antibodies. People with this condition can test positive for one, two, or all three antiphospholipid antibodies in their blood. Antibodies normally attach (bind) to specific foreign particles and germs, marking them for destruction, but the antibodies in antiphospholipid syndrome attack normal human proteins. When these antibodies attach to proteins, the proteins change shape and attach to other molecules and receptors on the surface of

cells. Attaching to cells, particularly immune cells, turns on (activates) the blood clotting pathway and other immune responses.

The production of the antiphospholipid antibodies may coincide with exposure to foreign invaders, such as viruses and bacteria, that are similar to normal human proteins. Exposure to these foreign invaders may cause the body to produce antibodies to fight the infection, but because the invaders are so similar to the body's own proteins, the antibodies also attack the human proteins. Similar triggers may occur during pregnancy when a woman's physiology, particularly her immune system, adapts to accommodate the developing fetus. These changes during pregnancy may explain the high rate of affected females.

Certain genetic variations (polymorphisms) in a few genes have been found in people with antiphospholipid syndrome and may predispose individuals to produce the specific antibodies known to contribute to the formation of thromboses. However, the contribution of these genetic changes to the development of the condition is unclear.

People who repeatedly test positive for any of the antiphospholipid antibodies but have not had a thrombosis or recurrent miscarriages are said to be antiphospholipid carriers. These individuals are at greater risk of developing a thrombosis than the general population. The risk is especially high in people who test positive for all three antiphospholipid antibodies (triple-positive).

INHERITANCE OF ANTIPHOSPHOLIPID SYNDROME

Most cases of antiphospholipid syndrome are sporadic, which means they occur in people with no history of the disorder in their family. Rarely does the condition has been reported to run in families; however, it does not have a clear pattern of inheritance. Multiple genetic and environmental factors likely play a part in determining the risk of developing antiphospholipid syndrome.[1]

---

[1] MedlinePlus, "Antiphospholipid Syndrome," National Institutes of Health (NIH), July 11, 2022. Available online. URL: https://medlineplus.gov/genetics/condition/antiphospholipid-syndrome. Accessed May 10, 2023.

Section 34.2 | **Behçet Disease**

WHAT IS BEHÇET DISEASE?

Behçet disease is an inflammatory condition that affects many parts of the body. The health problems associated with Behçet disease result from widespread inflammation of blood vessels (vasculitis). This inflammation most commonly affects small blood vessels in the mouth, genitals, skin, and eyes.

Painful mouth sores called "aphthous ulcers" are usually the first sign of Behçet disease. These sores can occur on the lips, tongue, inside the cheeks, the roof of the mouth, the throat, and the tonsils. The ulcers look like common canker sores, and they typically heal within one to two weeks. About 75 percent of all people with Behçet disease develop similar ulcers on the genitals. These ulcers occur most frequently on the scrotum in men and on the labia in women.

Behçet disease can also cause painful bumps and sores on the skin. Most affected individuals develop pus-filled bumps that resemble acne. These bumps can occur anywhere on the body. Some affected people also have red, tender nodules called "erythema nodosum." These nodules usually develop on the legs but can also occur on the arms, face, and neck.

Inflammation of the eye, called "uveitis," is found in more than half of people with Behçet disease. Eye problems are more common in younger people with the disease and affect men more often than women. Uveitis can result in blurry vision and extreme sensitivity to light (photophobia). Rarely, inflammation can also cause eye pain and redness. If untreated, the eye problems associated with Behçet disease can lead to blindness.

Joint involvement is also common in Behçet disease. Often this affects one joint at a time, with each affected joint becoming swollen and painful and then getting better.

Less commonly, Behçet disease can affect the brain and spinal cord (central nervous system (CNS)), gastrointestinal tract, large blood vessels, heart, lungs, and kidneys. CNS abnormalities can lead to headaches, confusion, personality changes, memory loss, impaired speech, and problems with balance and movement. The involvement of the gastrointestinal tract can lead to a hole in the wall of the intestine (intestinal perforation), which can cause serious infection and may be life-threatening.

The signs and symptoms of Behçet disease usually begin in a person's twenties or thirties although they can appear at any age. Some affected people have relatively mild symptoms that are limited to sores in the mouth and on the genitals. Others have more severe symptoms affecting various parts of the body, including the eyes and the vital organs. The features of Behçet disease typically come and go over a period of months or years. In most affected individuals, the health problems associated with this disorder improve with age.

Other Names of This Condition
- Adamantiades-Behcet disease (ABD)
- Behcet disease
- Behcet syndrome
- Behcet triple symptom complex
- Behcet's syndrome
- malignant aphthosis
- old silk route disease
- triple symptom complex

FREQUENCY OF BEHÇET DISEASE
Behçet disease is most common in Mediterranean countries, the Middle East, Japan, and other parts of Asia. However, it has been found in populations worldwide.

The highest prevalence of Behçet disease has been reported in northern Turkey, where the disorder affects up to 420 in 100,000 people. The disorder is rare in northern European countries and the United States, where it generally affects fewer than 1 in 100,000 people.

CAUSES OF BEHÇET DISEASE
The cause of Behçet disease is unknown. The condition probably results from a combination of genetic and environmental factors, most of which have not been identified. However, a particular

variation in the *HLA-B* gene has been associated with the risk of developing Behçet disease.

The *HLA-B* gene provides instructions for making a protein that plays an important role in the immune system. The *HLA-B* gene is part of a family of genes called the "human leukocyte antigen (HLA) complex." The HLA complex helps the immune system distinguish the body's own proteins from proteins made by foreign invaders (such as viruses and bacteria). The *HLA-B* gene has many different normal variations, allowing each person's immune system to react to a wide range of foreign proteins. A variation of the *HLA-B* gene called "*HLA-B51*" increases the risk of developing Behçet disease by about a factor of six although the mechanism is not well understood. One-third to two-thirds of people with Behçet disease have the *HLA-B51* variation, but most people with this version of the *HLA-B* gene never develop the disorder.

Other genetic and environmental factors likely contribute to the risk of Behçet disease. Researchers are studying several genes related to immune system function. It also appears likely that environmental factors, such as certain bacterial or viral infections, play a role in triggering the disease in people who are at risk. However, the influence of genetic and environmental factors on the development of this complex disorder remains unclear.

INHERITANCE PATTERN OF BEHÇET DISEASE

Most cases of Behçet disease are sporadic, which means they occur in people with no history of the disorder in their family. A small percentage of all cases have been reported to run in families; however, the condition does not have a clear pattern of inheritance.[2]

---

[2] MedlinePlus, "Behçet Disease," National Institutes of Health (NIH), June 1, 2017. Available online. URL: https://medlineplus.gov/genetics/condition/behcet-disease. Accessed May 10, 2023.

Section 34.3 | Polyarteritis Nodosa

WHAT IS POLYARTERITIS NODOSA?

Polyarteritis nodosa (PAN) is a blood vessel disease characterized by inflammation of small and medium-sized arteries (vasculitis), preventing them from bringing oxygen and food to organs. Most cases occur in the fourth or fifth decade of life although it can occur at any age. PAN most commonly affects vessels related to the skin, joints, peripheral nerves, gastrointestinal tract, heart, eyes, and kidneys. Symptoms are caused by damage to affected organs and may include fever, fatigue, weakness, loss of appetite, weight loss, muscle and joint aches, rashes, numbness, and abdominal pain. The underlying cause of PAN is unknown. Treatment involves medicines to suppress inflammation and the immune system, including steroids.

SYMPTOMS OF POLYARTERITIS NODOSA

The human phenotype ontology (HPO) provides the list of features (refer to Table 34.1) that have been reported in people with this condition. If available, the list includes a rough estimate of how common a feature is and its frequency. Frequencies are based on a specific study and may not be representative of all studies.

Table 34.1. Polyarteritis Nodosa

Signs and Symptoms	Approximate Number of Patients (%; When Available)
Abdominal pain	90
Abnormal pyramidal signs	90
Abnormality of temperature regulation	90
Aneurysm	90
Arthralgia	90
Asthma	90
Cutis marmorata	90

Table 34.1. Continued

Signs and Symptoms	Approximate Number of Patients (%; When Available)
Edema of the lower limbs	90
Hemiplegia/hemiparesis	90
Hypertensive crisis	90
Hypertrophic cardiomyopathy	90
Migraine	90
Myalgia	90
Nephropathy	90
Orchitis	90
Paresthesia	90
Polyneuropathy	90
Renal insufficiency	90
Skin rash	90
Subcutaneous hemorrhage	90
Vasculitis	90
Weight loss	90
Arrhythmia	50
Behavioral abnormality	50
Coronary artery disease	50
Gangrene	50
Gastrointestinal hemorrhage	50
Gastrointestinal infarctions	50
Leukocytosis	50
Seizures	50
Skin ulcer	50

Table 34.1. Continued

Signs and Symptoms	Approximate Number of Patients (%; When Available)
Urticaria	50
Abnormality of extrapyramidal motor function	7.5
Abnormality of the pericardium	7.5
Abnormality of the retinal vasculature	7.5
Acrocyanosis	7.5
Arterial thrombosis	7.5
Arthritis	7.5
Ascites	7.5
Autoimmunity	7.5
Congestive heart failure	7.5
Encephalitis	7.5
Hemobilia	7.5
Inflammatory abnormality of the eye	7.5
Malabsorption	7.5
Myositis	7.5
Osteolysis	7.5
Osteomyelitis	7.5
Pancreatitis	7.5
Retinal detachment	7.5
Ureteral stenosis	7.5

CAUSES OF POLYARTERITIS NODOSA

The exact cause of PAN is not known, and in most cases, no predisposing cause has been found (it is idiopathic). Many scientists believe that it is an autoimmune disease. Research has suggested that an abnormal immune response to an initial infection may

225

trigger the development of PAN. However, the reasons that many smaller arteries and capillaries are spared are not understood.

Hepatitis B virus (HBV), hepatitis C, and hairy cell leukemia have been associated with some cases of PAN. In one report from France, HBV accounted for a third of the cases of PAN. HBV-related PAN typically occurs within four months after the onset of HBV infection. PAN has also been seen in drug abusers (particularly those using amphetamines). It has also appeared to occur as an allergic reaction to some drugs and vaccines.

The specific symptoms of PAN are due to ischemia or infarction of tissues and organs. Thickening of the walls of affected vessels causes narrowing of the inside of the vessels, reducing blood flow and predisposing to blood clots in affected vessels.

TREATMENT FOR POLYARTERITIS NODOSA

There is no cure for PAN, but the disease and its symptoms can be managed. The goal of treatment is to prevent disease progression and further organ damage. The exact treatment depends on the severity of each person. While many people do well with treatment, relapses can occur.

When the cause of PAN is unknown (idiopathic), treatment involves corticosteroids and immunosuppressive medications. If there are no serious neurologic, renal, gastrointestinal, or heart symptoms, corticosteroids may initially be sufficient. For severe diseases with these symptoms, cyclophosphamide may also be used. Hypertension should be treated aggressively.

When PAN is related to hepatitis B, treatment often involves steroids, antiviral medications, and sometimes plasma exchange (also called "plasmapheresis").

PROGNOSIS OF POLYARTERITIS NODOSA

There is no known description of the average life expectancy for individuals with PAN. However, one study examined the overall mortality of a group of individuals with this condition. Mortality is a measure of the proportion of individuals in a group who die in a given time period. Of 348 individuals with PAN, approximately

20 percent had died within five years of initial diagnosis and treatment; approximately 32 percent had died within 10 years. Only a third of these deaths were directly caused by severe symptoms of PAN. Factors that increased the risk of death included being older than 65 years, being recently diagnosed with high blood pressure (hypertension), or having gastrointestinal symptoms that required surgery at the time of diagnosis (e.g., abdominal pain, internal bleeding, pancreatitis, cholecystitis, and appendicitis).[3]

Section 34.4 | Vasculitis

WHAT IS VASCULITIS?

Vasculitis, also known as "angiitis" or "arteritis," includes a group of rare conditions that can take place when swelling affects the walls of your blood vessels. Swelling is your body's response to tissue injury. Autoimmune disorders or diseases that make your body attack itself, infections, and trauma are some examples of potential causes of swelling in the blood vessels. Swelling in the blood vessels can lead to serious problems, including organ damage and aneurysms, a bulge in the wall of a blood vessel.

There are many different types of vasculitis, and it can affect any of the blood vessels in the body. With vasculitis, you may experience general symptoms, such as fever, weight loss, tiredness, pain, and rash. You may have other symptoms depending on the part of the body that is affected and if the vasculitis is serious. If you are diagnosed with vasculitis, medicine can help improve your symptoms and help you avoid flares and complications. If vasculitis responds to treatment, it can go into remission, a period of time when the disease is not active.

---

[3] Genetic and Rare Diseases Information Center (GARD), "Polyarteritis Nodosa," National Center for Advancing Translational Sciences (NCATS), January 23, 2017. Available online. URL: https://rarediseases.info.nih.gov/diseases/7360/polyarteritis-nodosa. Accessed May 10, 2023.

TYPES OF VASCULITIS

The following are a few types of vasculitis:

- **Antiglomerular basement membrane disease**. This disease affects blood vessels in the lungs and kidneys.
- **Behçet disease**. It can cause damage to many areas of your body.
- **Buerger disease**. It is also known as "thromboangiitis obliterans" and usually affects blood flow to the arms and legs.
- **Central nervous system (CNS) vasculitis**. Also called "primary angiitis," this type of vasculitis affects the blood vessels in the CNS, or the brain and spinal cord. This type of vasculitis may also occur as the result of another type of vasculitis.
- **Cogan syndrome**. This syndrome is an autoimmune disorder associated with a particular type of vasculitis that affects the whole body.
- **Cryoglobulinemic vasculitis**. This vasculitis affects the small blood vessels. It prevents proper blood flow and causes pain and damage to the skin, joints, peripheral nerves, kidneys, and liver.
- **Eosinophilic granulomatosis with polyangiitis**. Also known as "Churg-Strauss syndrome," this disease often affects the respiratory tract.
- **Giant cell arteritis**. This type mostly affects the aorta or its major branches. The condition often affects the temporal artery in the head.
- **Granulomatosis with polyangiitis**. It usually affects the nose and throat area, lungs, and kidneys.
- **Hypersensitivity vasculitis**. It affects the skin. This condition is also known as "allergic vasculitis," "cutaneous vasculitis," or "leukocytoclastic vasculitis."
- **Hypocomplementemic urticarial vasculitis**. This vasculitis is associated with swelling in the small blood vessels and low levels of complement proteins, which affect the body's ability to develop defenses against infection.

- **Immunoglobulin A (IgA) vasculitis**. Also known as "Henoch-Schönlein purpura," this type is one of the most common types of vasculitis in children but can also affect adults. It develops when IgA, which is a type of antibody that usually helps defend the body against infections, builds up in blood vessels in the skin, joints, intestines, and kidneys.
- **Kawasaki disease**. It is a rare childhood disease that develops when the walls of the blood vessels throughout the body swell. Kawasaki disease is also known as "mucocutaneous lymph node syndrome."
- **Microscopic polyangiitis**. This vasculitis type affects small blood vessels, often including those in the kidneys and lungs.
- **Polyarteritis nodosa (PAN)**. It is a type of vasculitis that causes swelling and damage, most often to medium-sized arteries. PAN may cause muscle pain or symptoms related to the stomach or intestines, such as heartburn.
- **Takayasu arteritis**. It most often affects the aorta and its branches. The condition can also affect medium-sized arteries.

SYMPTOMS OF VASCULITIS

The symptoms of vasculitis vary depending on which type of vasculitis you have, the organs involved, and whether your condition is serious. Some people may have few symptoms. Other people may become very sick.

Sometimes, the symptoms develop slowly over months. The symptoms may also develop very quickly over days or weeks. Some people have general symptoms, such as:

- tiredness
- fever
- general aches and pains
- loss of appetite
- weight loss

Inflammation from vasculitis can block normal blood flow, which may damage parts of the body. Serious problems depend on which parts of the body are damaged, and they can be life-threatening. They include the following:

- aneurysm or aortic dissection
- arrhythmia
- coronary heart disease
- deep vein thrombosis, a type of venous thromboembolism
- heart attack
- high blood pressure
- low blood pressure
- kidney disease
- myocarditis, a type of heart inflammation
- stroke and transient ischemic attack (TIA, which, also known as a "mini-stroke," occurs if blood flow to a part of the brain is blocked only for a short time)

CAUSES OF VASCULITIS

Vasculitis occurs when your immune system hurts your blood vessels by mistake. What causes this to happen is not fully known, but when it occurs, your blood vessels swell and can narrow or close off. Rarely, the blood vessel wall may weaken, causing it to expand or bulge. This bulge is known as an "aneurysm."

WHAT ARE THE RISK FACTORS OF VASCULITIS?
Age

Vasculitis can happen at any age. However, some types of vasculitis are more common among people of certain ages.

- **Buerger disease**. This disease usually affects men younger than 45 who smoke or have smoked.
- **IgA vasculitis**. This vasculitis is diagnosed more often in children than in adults.
- **Giant cell arteritis**. This type affects adults 50 years and older and is most common in people who are in their 70s and 80s.

- **Kawasaki disease**. This disease affects only children and is most common under the age of five.

Family History
The following types of vasculitis may run in families:
- Behçet disease
- granulomatosis with polyangiitis
- Kawasaki disease

Lifestyle Habits
- Smoking raises your risk of vasculitis.
- Using illegal drugs, such as cocaine, also raises your risk.

Medicines
The risk of vasculitis is higher if you take certain medicines, including the following:
- **Hydralazine**. It is used to treat high blood pressure.
- **Levamisole**. This medicine is used for infections but is also added to most cocaine.
- **Propylthiouracil**. This medicine is used to treat some thyroid disorders.
- **Tumor necrosis factor (TNF) inhibitors**. These are drugs used as a treatment for some immune diseases.

Other Medical Conditions
- autoimmune disorders, such as lupus, rheumatoid arthritis (RA), and scleroderma
- hepatitis B or C, infections that sometimes trigger vasculitis inflammation
- lymphoma, a cancer of the blood

Race or Ethnicity
- Behçet disease is most common in Turkey and is relatively common in other countries in the Mediterranean, the

Middle East, Central Asia, China, and Japan. It is relatively uncommon in Northern and Western Europe and the United States.

- Giant cell arteritis is most common in Scandinavia and Minnesota.
- Kawasaki disease is more common among children of Japanese descent.

Sex
- Behçet disease is more common in men in some countries and more common in women in other countries.
- Buerger disease is more common in men.
- Giant cell arteritis affects women two to four times more often than men.
- Microscopic polyangiitis affects men slightly more often than women.

DIAGNOSIS OF VASCULITIS
Your health-care provider may be able to diagnose the type of vasculitis that you have and how serious it is. Depending on your symptoms, your provider may recommend you see a specialist for more tests or procedures.

Which Specialists Can Diagnose Vasculitis?
- cardiologists (the doctors who specialize in the heart)
- dermatologists (the doctors who specialize in skin)
- infectious disease specialists (the doctors who are experts in the diagnosis and treatment of infections)
- nephrologists (the doctors who specialize in the kidneys)
- neurologists (the doctors who specialize in the brain and nervous system)
- ophthalmologists (the doctors who specialize in eyes)
- pulmonologists (the doctors who specialize in the lungs)

- rheumatologists (the doctors who specialize in joints, muscles, and autoimmune diseases)
- urologists (the doctors who specialize in the urinary tract and urogenital system)

Diagnostic Tests and Procedures

Diagnosis of vasculitis can be difficult. Some types of vasculitis cannot be diagnosed with a test. Instead, your provider will diagnose you based on your symptoms or order tests or procedures.

- **Biopsy.** A biopsy collects a small sample of your tissue from a specific blood vessel or an organ. A pathologist, someone with special training in laboratory results, will study the sample for specific signs of swelling and tissue damage.
- **Blood tests**. These tests detect levels of certain blood cells and antibodies in your blood.
- **Chest x-ray**. A chest x-ray finds out whether vasculitis is affecting your lungs or your large arteries, such as the aorta or the arteries in the lungs.
- **Computed tomography (CT) scan**. This test looks for signs of granulomatosis with polyangiitis.
- **Echocardiography**. This is an ultrasound test to learn how well the heart is working.
- **Pathergy test**. A pathergy test diagnoses Behçet disease. In this test, a needle pricks the skin, and sometimes, a small amount of saline solution may be injected. The test is positive if a red bump or ulcer develops after two days.
- **Coronary angiography**. This is a procedure that looks at your blood vessels for damage, inflammation, blockages, or aneurysms.
- **Positron emission tomography (PET) scan**. This is a type of nuclear scan that detects inflammation in the blood vessels.
- **Ultrasound**. This looks for signs of inflammation in your blood vessels or organs.
- **Urinalysis**. This test checks for kidney damage.

233

TREATMENT FOR VASCULITIS

The goal of treatment is usually to reduce inflammation. People who have mild vasculitis may find relief with over-the-counter (OTC) pain medicines. For severe vasculitis, you may receive prescription medicines. With treatment, vasculitis can go into remission, which is a period of time when you do not have symptoms.

Medicine

OTC pain medicines can relieve symptoms of mild vasculitis. For more serious cases, your provider may prescribe the following medicines:

- **Corticosteroids**. These medicines reduce swelling in your blood vessels. For some types of vasculitis, you will need steroids for months or years. Corticosteroids can affect your bone density and raise your blood sugar and blood pressure levels.
- **Dual endothelin receptor antagonists**. These block the action of a chemical called "endothelin" that can reduce blood flow.
- **Immunomodulators**. Immunomodulators, such as colchicine, reduce the swelling that causes symptoms. Possible side effects can include gastrointestinal problems.
- **Immunosuppressive medicines**. Medicines, such as cyclosporine and mycophenolate mofetil (MMF), suppress or weaken the immune system. Possible side effects include an increased risk of infection and birth defects.
- **Interferon therapy**. This therapy blocks and reduces swelling. Interferons are molecules that the immune system normally makes, but they have also been developed as medicines.
- **Interleukin antagonists**. These reduce swelling by blocking a protein in the body that causes the swelling.
- **Intravenous immunoglobulin (IVIG)**. This is a treatment that helps control the body's immune response. This medicine also fights infection by introducing purified antibodies from healthy donors

into the bloodstream. Some people may have a strong negative immune response to IVIG.

- **Monoclonal antibodies**. These antibodies suppress the immune system. Possible side effects include fever-like symptoms, stomach pain, and allergic reactions.
- **Nonsteroidal anti-inflammatory drugs (NSAIDs)**. NSAIDs reduce swelling in the body. One possible side effect is increased bleeding.
- **Phosphodiesterase inhibitors**. These medications increase blood flow by blocking the action of a particular enzyme in the body. Possible side effects include headaches, heart palpitations, upset stomach, nausea, and vomiting.
- **TNF inhibitors**. These drugs suppress the immune system by blocking a protein called "tumor necrosis factor alpha."

Procedures or Surgery

- **Plasmapheresis**. During this procedure, blood plasma is removed and then replaced to lower plasma antibody levels.
- **Surgical bypass of the blood vessels**. This surgical procedure may help restore blood flow to some areas in case of Buerger disease. Surgery to treat vasculitis is rare.

CAN VASCULITIS BE PREVENTED?

Some types of vasculitis cannot be prevented, as they are caused by autoimmune disorders. However, depending on what caused the vasculitis, some types can be prevented from flaring up. Medicines may be used to reduce the symptoms of vasculitis.

- Anticlotting medicines treat blood clots or prevent blood clots from forming. You may need them if you have an aneurysm.
- Beta-blockers lower blood pressure. You may need them if you have an aneurysm.
- Statins control or lower high blood cholesterol levels.

Healthy lifestyle changes may also be recommended.
- Adopt a heart-healthy lifestyle.
- Avoid illegal drugs, including cocaine. If you use illegal or street drugs, ask your provider how to get help to stop. You can also call the National Helpline of the Substance Abuse and Mental Health Services Administration (SAMHSA) at 800-662-HELP.
- Quit smoking and tobacco. Visit the Smoking and Your Heart (www.nhlbi.nih.gov/health/heart/smoking) and Your Guide to a Healthy Heart of the National Heart, Lung, and Blood Institute web page (NHLBI; www.nhlbi.nih.gov/resources/your-guide-healthy-heart). Although these resources focus on heart health, they include basic information about how to quit smoking. For free help and support to quit smoking, you may call the Smoking Quitline of the National Cancer Institute (NCI) at 877-44U-QUIT (877-448-7848).

LIVING WITH VASCULITIS

After you are diagnosed with vasculitis, it is important to follow your treatment plan. Your provider may recommend additional follow-up care and medicines to avoid problems.

Receive Routine Follow-Up Care

- Talk to your provider about any new symptoms and other changes in your health, including side effects of your medicines.
- Your provider will monitor you regularly to check for side effects from medicines used to treat vasculitis, such as corticosteroids.
- If you had Kawasaki disease as a child, you will need follow-up heart testing throughout your life.

Monitor Your Condition

To monitor your condition, your provider may recommend the following regular monitoring tests or procedures:

- blood tests to look for abnormal levels of certain blood cells and antibodies
- cardiac magnetic resonance imaging (MRI) to look for heart and vascular problems caused by vasculitis
- a chest x-ray to look for any problems in the lungs, heart, and large blood vessels, such as an aortic aneurysm
- echocardiography (echo) or electrocardiography (EKG) to look for heart problems caused by vasculitis
- myocardial perfusion imaging to measure the blood supply to your heart, which can also be used to look for heart problems caused by vasculitis
- a PET scan to check for aneurysms or heart problems caused by vasculitis

Plan for a Healthy Pregnancy

Most women who have vasculitis have no problems during pregnancy. However, vasculitis can raise the risk for the mother and baby.

- If you had Kawasaki disease or another type of vasculitis as a child, tell your provider that you are planning to become pregnant. They will want to monitor you for heart problems during pregnancy.
- Some medicines given to people who have vasculitis can be dangerous to a developing baby; be sure your provider knows what you are taking. Medicines may need to be adjusted during pregnancy. Do not stop taking medicine without first talking with your provider.
- Vasculitis raises your risk for high blood pressure during pregnancy. Your blood pressure should be monitored closely.

How Can You Prevent Vasculitis Flares?

After vasculitis is treated and goes into remission, you may have flares, which are repeat occurrences or worsening of symptoms. You may have different symptoms from when you first had vasculitis. Taking medicines and adopting healthy lifestyle changes to treat other health conditions you have, such as high blood pressure or cholesterol, can help prevent flare-ups. Part of the goal of vasculitis treatment is avoiding flares.

- Flares may be treated with some of the same medicines used for your initial treatment, including corticosteroids.
- If your vasculitis goes into remission, your provider may carefully stop your medicines. However, you will still need to be monitored for flares.

Learn the Warning Signs of Serious Complications and Have a Plan

An aneurysm can lead to a more serious problem, such as a dissection or rupture, which is a tear in the blood vessel wall. Vasculitis can also lead to other serious heart and blood vessel problems, such as heart attack or stroke.

If you think that you or someone else is having symptoms of one of these conditions, call 911 right away. Every minute matters.[4]

---

[4] "Vasculitis," National Heart, Lung, and Blood Institute (NHLBI), March 24, 2022. Available online. URL: www.nhlbi.nih.gov/health/vasculitis. Accessed May 10, 2023.

Chapter 35 | Autoimmune Disorders of Connective Tissues, Bone, and Joints

Chapter Contents

WHAT IS ANKYLOSING SPONDYLITIS?

Ankylosing spondylitis is a type of arthritis that causes inflammation in the joints and ligaments of the spine. Normally, the joints and ligaments in the spine help us move and bend. If you have ankylosing spondylitis, over time, the inflammation in the joints and tissues of the spine can cause stiffness. In severe cases, this may cause the vertebrae (bones in the spine) to fuse (grow together). When the vertebrae fuse, it can lead to a rigid and inflexible spine.

Many people with ankylosing spondylitis have mild episodes of back pain and stiffness that come and go. But others have severe, ongoing pain with loss of flexibility in the spine. In addition, other symptoms may develop if other areas of the body—such as the hips, ribs, shoulders, knees, ankles, and feet—are affected by the disease.

There is no cure for ankylosing spondylitis. Doctors recommend treatments that may include exercise and medications to help manage pain, control inflammation, improve posture and body position, and slow the progression of the disease. With treatment, most people with ankylosing spondylitis can have productive lives.

WHO GETS ANKYLOSING SPONDYLITIS?

Anyone can get ankylosing spondylitis; however, certain factors may increase your risk of developing the disease. These factors include the following:

- **Family history and genetics**. If you have a family history of ankylosing spondylitis, you are more likely to develop the disease.
- **Age**. Most people develop symptoms of ankylosing spondylitis before age 45. However, some people develop the disease when they are children or teens.
- **Other conditions**. People who have Crohn's disease, ulcerative colitis, or psoriasis may be more likely to develop the disease.

SYMPTOMS OF ANKYLOSING SPONDYLITIS

The most common symptom of ankylosing spondylitis is lower back and/or hip pain and stiffness. Over time, the symptoms may progress to other areas of the spine. The pain typically worsens during periods of rest or inactivity, which may cause some people to experience more pain during the middle of the night or after prolonged sitting. Usually, moving and exercise can help improve pain.

Symptoms of ankylosing spondylitis vary from person to person. Some people have mild episodes of pain that come and go, while others will have chronic, severe pain. The symptoms of ankylosing spondylitis, whether mild or severe, may worsen in "flares" and improve during periods of remission.

Because the disease can affect other areas of the body, other symptoms may develop and may include the following:

- pain, stiffness, and inflammation in other joints, such as the ribs, shoulders, knees, or feet
- difficulty taking deep breaths if the joints connecting the ribs are affected
- vision changes and eye pain due to uveitis, which is inflammation of the eye
- fatigue, or feeling very tired
- loss of appetite and weight loss
- skin rashes
- abdominal pain and loose bowel movements

CAUSES OF ANKYLOSING SPONDYLITIS

Researchers do not know the cause of ankylosing spondylitis. However, studies show that both genes and environment may lead to the development of the disease. Researchers know that the *HLA-B27* gene increases the risk of developing ankylosing spondylitis, but this does not mean you will get the disease if you have the gene. Many people have the gene and never develop ankylosing spondylitis, which tells researchers that environmental factors also play a role.

Researchers continue to discover many other gene variations that may cause the disease; however, *HLA-B27* is the primary gene that increases your risk of developing ankylosing spondylitis.

DIAGNOSIS OF ANKYLOSING SPONDYLITIS

To diagnose ankylosing spondylitis, your doctor will ask you about your medical history and perform a physical exam. Your doctor may order imaging studies and lab tests to help confirm a diagnosis.

Medical and Family History

Your doctor may ask about your medical and family history, including questions such as:
- How long have you had pain?
- Where is your pain?
- What makes the pain better or worse?
- Does anyone in your family have a history of back pain, joint pain, or arthritis?

Physical Exam

A physical exam may include the following:
- examining your joints, including your spine, pelvis, heels, and chest
- watching how you move and bend in different directions, checking for flexibility
- asking you to breathe deeply to check for rib stiffness and inflammation

Imaging Studies

Your doctor may order the following imaging studies to help diagnose ankylosing spondylitis:
- **X-rays.** They help doctors see joint changes. However, you may have the disease for years before the changes show on x-rays. Doctors may use x-rays to monitor the progression of the disease or to rule out other causes of joint pain.
- **Magnetic resonance imaging (MRI).** MRI uses energy from a powerful magnet to produce signals that create a series of cross-sectional images. These images or "slices" are analyzed by a computer to produce an

image of the joint. MRI can help diagnose ankylosing spondylitis in the early stages of the disease.

Your doctor may use both x-rays and MRIs to follow the progression of your disease.

Lab Tests

At this time, no single test diagnoses ankylosing spondylitis. Your doctor may order a blood test to check for the *HLA-B27* gene, which is present in most people with the disease. You may have the *HLA-B27* gene and never develop ankylosing spondylitis, but it can give doctors more information when making a diagnosis.

TREATMENT FOR ANKYLOSING SPONDYLITIS

There is no cure for ankylosing spondylitis; however, your doctor will work with you to help manage the disease. The goals of treatment include the following:
- Relieve symptoms.
- Help maintain proper posture.
- Slow the progression of the disease.

In most cases, treatment includes medication and physical therapy. Sometimes, people in critical condition of the disease need surgery to repair joint damage.

Medications

Most people with ankylosing spondylitis take medications, which may include one or more of the following:
- Over-the-counter (OTC) anti-inflammatory medications to relieve pain and inflammation are commonly used to treat ankylosing spondylitis.
- Biologic medications target specific immune messages and interrupt the signal, helping to decrease or stop inflammation. These medications may be prescribed if your disease is unresponsive to other treatments.

- Janus kinase (JAK) inhibitors may also be prescribed if your disease is unresponsive to other treatments. These medications send messages to specific cells to stop inflammation from inside the cell.
- Corticosteroids can help decrease inflammation and provide some pain relief. They are usually injected into the joint. Because they are potent drugs, your doctor will determine how much and how many injections you should receive to achieve the desired benefit.

Physical Therapy

Your doctor may recommend physical therapy to help:
- relieve pain
- strengthen back and neck muscles
- improve core and abdominal muscle strength because these muscles provide support for your back
- improve posture
- maintain and improve flexibility in joints

A physical therapist can recommend the best sleeping positions and an exercise program. Because your symptoms may worsen when inactive or at rest, it is important to stay active and exercise regularly.

Surgery

If you have severe joint damage and you are unable to participate in your daily activities, your doctor may recommend surgery. Surgery is not for everyone. You and your doctor can discuss the options and choose what is right for you.

Your doctor will consider the following before recommending surgery:
- your overall health
- the condition of the affected bone or joint
- the risks and benefits of the surgery

Types of surgery may include joint repairs and joint replacements. Rarely, some people may have surgery to correct or straighten the spine or repair fractures (breaks) in the vertebrae.

Who Treats Ankylosing Spondylitis?

Diagnosing and treating ankylosing spondylitis may require a team of health-care professionals that may include the following:

- rheumatologists, who specialize in arthritis and other diseases of the bones, joints, and muscles
- dermatologists, who specialize in conditions of the skin, hair, and nails
- gastroenterologists, who specialize in conditions of the digestive system
- mental health professionals, who help people cope with difficulties in the home and workplace that may result from their medical conditions
- nurse educators, who specialize in helping people understand their overall condition and set up their treatment plans
- occupational therapists, who teach ways to protect joints, minimize pain, perform activities of daily living, and conserve energy
- ophthalmologists, who specialize in conditions of the eye
- orthopedic surgeons, who specialize in the treatment and surgery of bone and joint diseases
- physiatrists (physical, medicine, and rehabilitation specialists), who supervise exercise programs
- physical therapists, who help improve joint function
- primary care doctors, such as family physicians or internal medicine specialists, who coordinate care between the different health providers and treat other problems as they arise
- psychologists or social workers, who help with psychosocial challenges caused by medical conditions

LIVING WITH ANKYLOSING SPONDYLITIS

Research shows that people who take part in their own care report less pain and make fewer doctor visits. They also enjoy a better quality of life (QOL).

Self-care can help you play a role in managing your ankylosing spondylitis and improving your health. You can:

- learn about the disease and its treatments
- communicate well with your health-care team, so you can have more control over your disease
- reach out for support to help cope with the physical, emotional, and mental effects of ankylosing spondylitis

Participating in your care can help build confidence in your ability to perform day-to-day activities, allowing you to lead a full, active, and independent life.

The following lifestyle changes and activities can help improve your ability to function on your own and maintain a positive outlook:

- **Exercise**. Exercise is important for maintaining healthy and strong muscles, preserving joint mobility, and maintaining flexibility. In addition to an exercise program, your doctor may recommend low-impact exercises, such as water exercise programs. Talk to your health-care providers before beginning any exercise program. Exercise can help:
  - improve your sleep
  - decrease pain
  - keep a positive attitude
  - maintain a healthy weight
- **Posture**. Another important thing you can do for yourself is to practice good posture. Your physical therapist and doctors can give you tips and exercises to help maintain and improve your posture. Practicing good posture can help you avoid some of the complications that can occur with ankylosing spondylitis.
- **Support or assistive devices**. Using a cane or walker can help you move around safely, provide stability, and lower pain. If you have trouble bending due to spine stiffness, try using a device to grab or pick up items.
- **Monitoring of symptoms**. It is important to monitor your symptoms for any changes or the development of

new symptoms. Understanding your symptoms and how they may change can help you and your doctor manage your pain when you have a flare.

- **Stress management**. The emotions you may feel because of your disease, along with any pain, physical limitations, and the unpredictable nature of flares, can increase your stress level. Although there is no evidence that stress plays a role in your disease, it can make living with ankylosing spondylitis more difficult. Ways to cope with stress can include the following:
  - using relaxation techniques such as deep breathing, meditating, or listening to quiet sounds or music
  - trying movement exercise programs, such as yoga and tai chi
- **Mental health management**. If you feel alone, anxious, or depressed about having ankylosing spondylitis, talk to your doctor or mental health professional. Keep the lines of communication open. Talk to family and friends about your disease. You may find it helpful to join an online or community support group.
- **Healthy diet**. A healthy diet is good for everyone, and it may be very helpful if you have ankylosing spondylitis. There is no specific diet for people with ankylosing spondylitis, but keeping a healthy weight is important. It reduces stress on painful joints.
- **Quit smoking**. If you smoke, quit. Ankylosing spondylitis is more severe in people who smoke, and smoking blunts the effect of treatment. In addition, if you have ankylosing spondylitis in the chest or ribs, smoking can compromise your lung function even more. Smoking is also a risk factor for the progression of the disease.[1]

---

[1] "Ankylosing Spondylitis," National Institute of Arthritis and Musculoskeletal and Skin Diseases (NIAMS), February 2020. Available online. URL: www.niams.nih.gov/health-topics/ankylosing-spondylitis. Accessed May 10, 2023.

Section 35.2 | **Juvenile Rheumatoid Arthritis**

WHAT IS JUVENILE IDIOPATHIC ARTHRITIS?

Like adults, children can develop arthritis. The most common type of chronic, or long-lasting, arthritis that affects children is called "juvenile idiopathic arthritis" (JIA). JIA broadly refers to several different chronic disorders involving inflammation of joints (arthritis), which can cause joint pain, swelling, warmth, stiffness, and loss of motion. The various forms of JIA have different features, such as the pattern of joints involved and inflammation of other parts of the body besides the joints. JIA may last a limited time, such as a few months or years, but in some cases, it is a lifelong disease that requires treatment into adulthood.

JIA is "idiopathic," meaning that its origins are not understood. While the exact causes of JIA are unknown, it begins when the immune system becomes overactive and creates inflammation. With treatment, most children achieve periods of wellness (remission), and sometimes, the disease goes away permanently with no further need for medications. It is important to see a doctor early if your child has swollen or stiff joints because delaying therapy can lead to joint damage, a lesser response to treatment, and other problems.

WHO GETS JUVENILE IDIOPATHIC ARTHRITIS?

By definition, JIA begins in children and adolescents before the 16th birthday. Most types of the disease are more frequent in girls, but enthesitis-related JIA, a form of the disease that involves inflammation of the places where ligaments and tendons (flexible bands of tissue) attach to bones, is more common in boys. Systemic JIA, a rare type of JIA that features fever and rash, affects boys and girls equally. Children of all races and ethnic backgrounds can get the disease.

It is very rare for more than one member of a family to have JIA, but children with a family member with chronic arthritis, including JIA, are at a slightly increased risk of developing it. Having a family member with psoriasis is a risk factor for a form of JIA called "psoriatic JIA."

TYPES OF JUVENILE IDIOPATHIC ARTHRITIS

There are multiple types of JIA, each with distinct features. Generally, they all share arthritic symptoms of joint pain, swelling, warmth, and stiffness that last at least six weeks. The types are as follows:

- **Oligoarticular JIA.** This is the most common and mildest form, affecting four or fewer joints. It is considered persistent if symptoms continue for six months or longer and extended if five or more joints become involved after six months of illness. Commonly affected joints are knees or ankles. A form of eye inflammation called "chronic (long-lasting) uveitis" can develop in children with this form of JIA. About half of the children with JIA have this type.
- **Polyarticular JIA (rheumatoid factor (RF) negative).** This is the second most common type, affecting five or more joints in the first six months. Tests for RF are negative. The RF blood test checks for autoimmune disease, especially rheumatoid arthritis, which is an adult form of arthritis. Some of these children develop chronic uveitis.
- **Polyarticular JIA (RF positive).** A child with this type has arthritis in five or more joints during the first six months of the disease. Tests for RF, a marker for autoimmune disease, are positive. It tends to occur in preteen and teenage girls, and it appears to be essentially the same as adult rheumatoid arthritis.
- **Enthesitis-related JIA.** This form of JIA involves both arthritis and enthesitis. Enthesitis happens when inflammation occurs where a ligament or tendon attaches to a bone. The most common locations for enthesitis are the knees, heels, and bottoms of the feet. Arthritis is usually in the hips, knees, ankles, and feet, but the sacroiliac joints (at the base of the back) and spinal joints can also become inflamed. Some children get episodes of acute anterior uveitis, a sudden onset of inflammation of the front of the eye. Unlike most other

forms of JIA, enthesitis-related JIA is more common in boys.

- **Psoriatic JIA.** Children with this type have psoriasis, a skin condition, as well as inflammation of the joints. The skin condition usually appears first, but sometimes, painful, stiff joints are the first sign, with the skin disease occurring years later. Pitted fingernails and dactylitis (swollen fingers or toes) are also signs of the disease.
- **Systemic JIA.** Systemic means the disease can affect the whole body, not just a specific organ or joint. Systemic JIA usually starts with fever and rash that come and go over the span of at least two weeks. In many cases, the joints become inflamed, but sometimes not until long after the fever goes away and sometimes not at all if treatment is started quickly. In severe forms, inflammation can develop in and around organs, such as the spleen, lymph nodes, liver, and linings of the heart and lungs. Systemic JIA affects boys and girls with equal frequency.
- **Undifferentiated arthritis.** This category includes children who have symptoms that do not fit into any of the other types or that fit into more than one type.

SYMPTOMS OF JUVENILE IDIOPATHIC ARTHRITIS

Symptoms of JIA vary depending on the type, but all forms share persistent joint pain, swelling, warmth, and stiffness that are typically worse in the morning and after a nap or prolonged sitting. The pain may limit movement of the affected joint although many children, especially younger ones, will not complain of pain. One of the earliest signs may be limping in the morning due to disease in one or both legs. The symptoms of JIA may go through cycles, flaring for a few weeks or months followed by periods when they go into remission. Some children have just one or two flares and never have symptoms again, while others have many flares or symptoms that never fully go away.

Besides joint problems, the inflammation associated with JIA can cause other symptoms, including the following:

- **Eye inflammation**. Uveitis (inflammation of the front and middle parts of the eye) often occurs in children with JIA. It usually starts within a few years after the JIA diagnosis, but in a small fraction of children, it appears before the joint symptoms or many years afterward. The type of JIA that a child has may cause the development of different types of uveitis.
  - Children with oligoarticular JIA, especially when it begins at an early age, can have chronic (long-lasting) uveitis that has mild or no symptoms. Children with polyarticular JIA without RF or with psoriatic JIA are also at risk.
  - Children with enthesitis-related JIA and some children with psoriatic JIA can have episodes of acute anterior uveitis, which has a sudden onset and causes eye pain, eye redness, and sensitivity to light.

If left untreated, uveitis can lead to eye problems such as cataracts, glaucoma, and vision loss, so it is important for children with JIA to have frequent eye exams.

- **Skin changes**. Depending on the type of JIA a child has, he or she may develop skin changes.
  - Children with systemic JIA who have fevers can get a light red or pink rash that comes and goes.
  - Children with psoriatic JIA can develop scaly red patches of skin. Psoriatic JIA can also cause pitted nails and dactylitis (swollen fingers or toes).
  - Children with polyarticular JIA with RF can get small bumps or nodules on parts of the body that receive pressure, such as from sitting.
- **Fever**. Patients with systemic JIA typically have daily fevers when the disease begins or flares. The fever usually appears in the evening, and the rash may move from one part of the body to another, usually happening with the fever. Patients with other types of JIA do not generally develop fevers.

- **Growth problems**. Inflammation in children with any type of JIA can lead to growth problems. Depending on the severity of the disease and the joints involved, bones near inflamed joints may grow too quickly or too slowly. This can cause one leg or arm to be longer than the other or can result in a small or misshapen chin. Overall growth may also be slowed if the disease is severe. Growth normally improves when inflammation is well-controlled through treatment.

CAUSES OF JUVENILE IDIOPATHIC ARTHRITIS

In JIA, the body's immune system—which normally helps fight off infections and heal cuts and wounds—mistakenly attacks some of its own healthy cells and tissues. The result is inflammation, marked by pain, swelling, warmth, and stiffness. Inflammation from JIA can damage the joints, eyes, or other affected organs. Scientists do not know why the immune system attacks healthy tissues in children with JIA, but they believe that a complex mix of genes and environmental factors is involved.

While the origin of the immune system's overreaction in JIA is unknown, scientists have identified some of the molecules that contribute to inflammation in some forms of the disease. It is now known that three molecules—tumor necrosis factor alpha (TNF-α), interleukin-6 (IL-6), and interleukin-1 (IL-1)—are involved in creating inflammation in the joints of many children with JIA. This has led to new therapies that specifically target these molecules.

DIAGNOSIS OF JUVENILE IDIOPATHIC ARTHRITIS

There is no single test that doctors can use to diagnose JIA. However, they may suspect that a child has the disease if he or she is younger than age 16 and has unexplained joint pain, stiffness, or swelling that has lasted for at least six weeks. Doctors usually diagnose JIA by ruling out other conditions that have similar features.

The process doctors use involves the following.

Medical History and Physical Exam

During the examination, the doctors usually do the following:

- Ask about your child's symptoms and when they began. They may also want to know about your child's family medical history because autoimmune diseases such as JIA can run in families.
- Check your child's joints and skin.
- Watch your child's movements for signs of trouble walking, climbing onto the examination table, moving the neck, or raising or closing the hands.
- Shine a small light into your child's eyes to look for eye problems that stem from uveitis (inflammation of the middle part of the eye), such as glaucoma or cataracts.
- Check the lymph nodes and abdomen for signs of swelling or sensitivity.

Lab Tests

The doctors may order blood tests for the following:

- **Erythrocyte sedimentation rate (ESR or "sed rate") and C-reactive protein (CRP).** These blood tests are measures of inflammation, or so-called inflammatory markers. They are often high in children with systemic JIA and may be elevated in children with other forms of JIA as well. But they are not specific for JIA and may also be elevated for an unrelated reason such as an infection. In cases where inflammatory markers are elevated because of JIA, doctors can use these tests to monitor if treatments are working.
- **Autoantibodies**. Antibodies are molecules made by the immune system—for example, in response to infections. Autoantibodies are antibodies that target one's own cells and tissues. Autoantibodies that may be found in children with JIA include the following:
  - **Antinuclear antibody (ANA)**. An autoantibody directed against substances in the cell nucleus, ANA is found in many children with JIA, but children without JIA may also test positive. Those who test

positive for ANA are at higher risk of developing eye inflammation and need to follow up more frequently with an eye doctor.

- **RF and anti-cyclic citrullinated peptide (CCP) antibodies**. These autoantibodies are rarely detected in children with JIA. When present, they usually correspond to a diagnosis of RF-positive polyarticular JIA.
- *HLA-B27*. This gene is a risk factor for enthesitis-related JIA. However, some children who have enthesitis-related JIA test negative for *HLA-B27*, and not all those who test positive have, or will ever develop, the disease.
- **Other lab tests**. Doctors may also order a basic panel of tests, including liver and kidney function tests, as well as a complete blood count (CBC). The CBC can tell if your child has anemia (low levels of red blood cells (RBC)), which can occur in people with systemic JIA or other chronic inflammatory disorders.

Imaging Studies

The doctors may order the following:

- **X-rays**. They use a small amount of radiation to assess the structure of bones. They are often the first type of imaging study the doctor orders because they help rule out other causes of joint pain, such as a fracture, infection, or tumor. As JIA progresses, x-rays can show if there is damage to the joint.
- **Ultrasounds**. They rely on high-frequency sound waves and are a noninvasive way to visualize joints without using radiation. Unlike x-rays, they can detect fluid and inflammation, which typically occur before any damage can be seen on x-rays.
- **Magnetic resonance imaging (MRI)**. MRI is a highly sensitive tool for visualizing the joints. MRIs use large magnets to create detailed, three-dimensional images of the joints, including inflammation, cartilage, and bone.

The diagnostic process will determine if your child has JIA and, if so, identify the type he or she has. It will also provide information to help doctors best treat the disease.

TREATMENT FOR JUVENILE IDIOPATHIC ARTHRITIS

The goals of treatment are to:
- control inflammation
- reduce pain and stiffness
- prevent joint and organ damage
- preserve and improve joint function
- promote physical and psychosocial growth and development
- achieve remission (little or no disease activity or symptoms)
- allow for full engagement with normal activities (e.g., school, work, sports, social life, family life)

Most children with JIA need a combination of medicines and a healthy lifestyle, including a balanced diet and exercise, to reach these goals. The specific treatment plan will depend on the child's age, the type of JIA, and other factors, such as disease severity. In general, doctors will treat the disease aggressively early on, tapering off medications once remission is reached.

Medications

The types of medications your child may be prescribed include the following:
- **Anti-inflammatory and pain medications**. These can help alleviate pain and swelling from inflammation. They are often prescribed by the doctor, but some are also available over the counter.
- **Disease-modifying antirheumatic drugs (DMARDs)**. These oral medications suppress the immune system on a broad level, helping to prevent the progression of the disease and saving the joints

from permanent damage. Depending on the drug, they may be taken by mouth or given as injections under the skin. DMARDs are sometimes combined with biologic response modifiers.

- **Biologic response modifiers.** By blocking specific immune signals that cause inflammation, biologic response modifiers help prevent the progression of JIA, achieve remission, and protect against permanent damage. Depending on the drug, they may be given as injections under the skin or intravenously. These drugs are sometimes combined with oral DMARDs. If doctors prescribe drugs in this class, they are usually inhibitors of TNF-α, IL-1, or IL-6, molecules that are known to promote inflammation in JIA.
- **Corticosteroids**. When injected into an affected joint, these strong inflammation-fighting drugs usually bring fast relief though it is not always long-lasting. In certain situations, they are given by mouth or intravenously, especially for systemic JIA and occasionally to alleviate severe symptoms from other types of JIA. Because they are powerful drugs with many possible side effects, doctors typically prescribe the lowest dose of steroids necessary and taper off as quickly as possible.

Physical Therapy
Physical therapy can be an important part of JIA treatment. The doctor may recommend physical therapy to help:
- relieve pain
- improve and maintain range of motion in affected joints
- strengthen muscles
- prevent injury from sports or other physical activities

A physical therapist can also teach pain-reducing techniques and develop a home exercise program for your child.

Routine Monitoring and Ongoing Care

Regular medical care is important because your doctor can do the following:

- Monitor how well the treatment is working.
- Adjust the treatment as needed. If a medication is not working well or if there are side effects, the doctor may try a different dosage, a different medicine, or a combination of medicines. If the treatment is working very well and the disease is well controlled, the doctor may discuss options for tapering or stopping medicines.

Who Treats Juvenile Idiopathic Arthritis?

Treating JIA typically requires a team approach that involves several different health-care providers. JIA is primarily treated by:

- pediatric rheumatologists, who specialize in treating arthritis and other diseases in children that involve the joints, bones, muscles, and immune system.

Other members of your child's health-care team may include the following:

- mental health professionals, who can help children cope with difficulties at home and school that may result from their medical condition
- occupational therapists, who teach ways to protect joints, minimize pain, perform activities of daily living, and conserve energy
- ophthalmologists, who diagnose and treat diseases of the eyes
- orthopedists, who specialize in the treatment of and surgery for bone and joint diseases or injuries
- pediatricians, who provide routine medical care for children
- physical therapists, who help improve joint function
- rheumatology nurses, who may serve as the main point of contact with your doctor's office about appointments, tests, medications, and instructions

- social workers, who can help your child and your family deal with lifestyle changes caused by arthritis and find resources and can serve as a liaison with your child's school, working with school-based staff to address any issues

LIVING WITH JUVENILE IDIOPATHIC ARTHRITIS

Juvenile idiopathic arthritis affects the entire family; all family members must cope with the special challenges of the disease. Having JIA can strain your child's participation in social and after-school activities and make schoolwork more difficult. Nevertheless, it is important to treat your child as normally as possible.

Certain activities can help improve children's ability to function on their own and maintain a positive outlook. These include the following:

- **Managing medical care**. Ensure that your child receives appropriate medical care and that you and your child follow the doctor's instructions. Learn as much as you can about the disease and its treatment. Many treatment options are available, and because JIA is different in each child, what works for one may not work for another. If the medications that the doctor prescribes do not relieve symptoms or if they cause unpleasant side effects, you and your child should discuss other choices with the doctor. It can be helpful to keep a day-to-day record of your child's symptoms and side effects of medications. Being prepared for doctors' appointments can help reduce the anxiety associated with them.
- **Balance rest and exercise**. Your child should have more rest when JIA is active and more exercise when it is not. Rest helps decrease active joint inflammation, pain, and fatigue. In general, shorter rest breaks every now and then are more helpful than long times spent in bed. During symptom-free periods, many doctors encourage playing team sports and other physical activities, which help maintain strong muscles, joint mobility, and

flexibility while providing social interactions with other children. Swimming is especially helpful because it uses many muscles and joints without stressing the joints. Exercise can also help:

- improve sleep
- decrease pain
- keep a positive attitude
- maintain a healthy weight[2]

Section 35.3 | Lambert-Eaton Myasthenic Syndrome

WHAT IS LAMBERT-EATON MYASTHENIC SYNDROME?

Lambert-Eaton myasthenic syndrome (LEMS) is a disorder of the neuromuscular junction—the place where nerve and muscle cells meet to help activate a person's muscles. LEMS is caused by a disruption of electrical impulses between the two kinds of cells.

LEMS is an autoimmune condition. Normally, the body's immune system protects the body from infection and disease. In autoimmune conditions, the immune system attacks the body's own tissues by mistake.

The disruption of electrical impulses is associated with antibodies produced as a consequence of this autoimmunity. Symptoms include muscle weakness, a tingling sensation in the affected areas, fatigue, and dry mouth. LEMS is closely associated with cancer, in particular small-cell lung cancer. More than half of the individuals diagnosed with LEMS also develop small-cell lung cancer. LEMS may appear up to three years before the cancer is diagnosed.

TREATMENT FOR LAMBERT-EATON MYASTHENIC SYNDROME

There is no cure for LEMS. The U.S. Food and Drug Administration (FDA) has approved amifampridine tablets (Firdapse) to treat

[2] "Juvenile Idiopathic Arthritis (JIA)," National Institute of Arthritis and Musculoskeletal and Skin Diseases (NIAMS), May 2021. Available online. URL: www.niams.nih.gov/health-topics/juvenile-arthritis. Accessed May 10, 2023.

LEMS in adults and amifampridine (Ruzurgi) tablets in children aged 6 to less than 17 years of age. Another treatment is directed at decreasing the autoimmune response (through the use of steroids, plasmapheresis, or high-dose intravenous immunoglobulin) or improving the transmission of the disrupted electrical impulses by giving drugs such as diaminopyridine (DAP) or pyridostigmine bromide (Mestinon). For patients with small-cell lung cancer, treatment of the cancer is the first priority.

PROGNOSIS OF LAMBERT-EATON MYASTHENIC SYNDROME

The prognosis for individuals with LEMS varies. Those with LEMS not associated with malignancy have a benign overall prognosis. Generally, the presence of cancer determines prognosis.

HOW CAN YOU OR YOUR LOVED ONE HELP IMPROVE CARE FOR PEOPLE WITH A LAMBERT-EATON MYASTHENIC SYNDROME?

Consider participating in a clinical trial, so clinicians and scientists can learn more about the LEMS and related disorders. Clinical research uses human volunteers to help researchers learn more about a disorder and perhaps find better ways to safely detect, treat, or prevent disease.

All types of volunteers are needed—those who are healthy or may have an illness or disease—of all different ages, sexes, races, and ethnicities to ensure that study results apply to as many people as possible and that treatments will be safe and effective for everyone who will use them.

For information about participating in clinical research, visit the web page of the National Institutes of Health (NIH) Clinical Research Trials and You (www.nih.gov/health-information/nih-clinical-research-trials-you). Learn about clinical trials currently looking for people with LEMS at Clinicaltrials.gov (https://clinicaltrials.gov).[3]

---

[3] "Lambert-Eaton Myasthenic Syndrome," National Institute of Neurological Disorders and Stroke (NINDS), January 20, 2023. Available online. URL: www.ninds.nih.gov/health-information/disorders/lambert-eaton-myasthenic-syndrome. Accessed May 10, 2023.

Section 35.4 | **Multiple Sclerosis**

WHAT IS MULTIPLE SCLEROSIS?

Multiple sclerosis (MS) is the most common disabling neurological disease of young adults with symptom onset generally occurring between the ages of 20 and 40. In MS, the immune system cells that normally protect us from viruses, bacteria, and unhealthy cells mistakenly attack myelin in the central nervous system (CNS; brain, optic nerves, and spinal cord). Myelin is a substance that makes up the protective sheath (myelin sheath) that coats nerve fibers (axons).

MS is a chronic disease that affects people differently. A small number of people with MS will have a mild course with little to no disability, whereas others will have a steadily worsening disease that leads to increased disability over time. Most people with MS, however, will have short periods of symptoms followed by long stretches of relative quiescence (inactivity or dormancy), with partial or full recovery. The disease is rarely fatal, and most people with MS have a normal life expectancy.

Myelin and the Immune System

MS attacks axons in the CNS protected by myelin, which are commonly called "white matter." MS also damages the nerve cell bodies, which are found in the brain's gray matter, as well as the axons themselves in the brain, spinal cord, and optic nerves that transmit visual information from the eye to the brain. As the disease progresses, the outermost layer of the brain, called the "cerebral cortex," shrinks in a process known as "cortical atrophy."

The term "multiple sclerosis" refers to the distinctive areas of scar tissue (sclerosis—also called "plaques" or "lesions") that result from the attack on myelin by the immune system. These plaques are visible using magnetic resonance imaging (MRI). Plaques can be as small as a pinhead or as large as a golf ball. The symptoms of MS depend on the severity of the inflammatory reaction as well as the location and extent of the plaques, which primarily appear in the brain stem, cerebellum (involved with balance and coordination of movement, among other functions), spinal cord, optic nerves, and the white matter around the brain ventricles (fluid-filled cavities).

SIGNS AND SYMPTOMS OF MULTIPLE SCLEROSIS

The natural course of MS is different for each person, which makes it difficult to predict. The onset and duration of MS symptoms usually depend on the specific type but may begin over a few days and go away quickly or develop more slowly and gradually over many years. The following are the four main types of MS, named according to the progression of symptoms over time:

- **Relapsing-remitting MS**. Symptoms in this type come in the form of attacks. In between attacks, people recover or return to their usual level of disability. When symptoms occur in this form of MS, it is called an "attack," a "relapse," or an "exacerbation." The periods of disease inactivity between MS attacks are referred to as remission. Weeks, months, or even years may pass before another attack occurs, followed again by a period of inactivity. Most people with MS are initially diagnosed with this form of the disease.
- **Secondary-progressive MS**. People with this form of MS usually have had a previous history of MS attacks but then start to develop gradual and steady symptoms and deterioration in their function over time. Most individuals with severe relapsing-remitting MS may go on to develop secondary-progressive MS if they are untreated.
- **Primary-progressive MS**. This type of MS is less common and is characterized by progressively worsening symptoms from the beginning with no noticeable relapses or exacerbations of the disease although there may be temporary or minor relief from symptoms.
- **Progressive-relapsing MS**. The rarest form of MS is characterized by a steady worsening of symptoms from the beginning with acute relapses that can occur over time during the disease course.

The following are some rare and unusual variants of MS:

- **Marburg variant MS (also known as "malignant MS").** It causes swift and relentless symptoms and decline in function and may result in significant disability or even death shortly after disease onset.
- **Balo's concentric sclerosis.** It causes concentric rings of myelin destruction that can be seen on an MRI and is another variant type of MS that can progress rapidly.

Early MS symptoms often include the following:

- vision problems such as blurred or double vision, or optic neuritis, which causes pain with eye movement and rapid vision loss
- muscle weakness, often in the hands and legs, and muscle stiffness accompanied by painful muscle spasms
- tingling, numbness, or pain in the arms, legs, trunk, or face
- clumsiness, especially difficulty staying balanced when walking
- bladder control problems
- intermittent or constant dizziness

MS may also cause later symptoms, such as:

- mental or physical fatigue, which accompanies the early symptoms during an attack
- mood changes such as depression or difficulty with emotional expression or control
- cognitive dysfunction, such as problems concentrating, multitasking, thinking, learning, or difficulties with memory or judgment

Muscle weakness, stiffness, and spasms may be severe enough to affect walking or standing. In some cases, MS leads to partial or complete paralysis, and the use of a wheelchair is not uncommon, particularly in individuals who are untreated or have advanced disease. Many people with MS find that weakness and fatigue are worse when they have a fever or when they are exposed to heat. MS exacerbations may occur following common infections.

Pain is rarely the first sign of MS, but pain often occurs with optic neuritis and trigeminal neuralgia, a disorder that affects one of the nerves that provides sensation to different parts of the face. Painful limb spasms and sharp pain shooting down the legs or around the abdomen can also be symptoms of MS.

Conditions Associated with Multiple Sclerosis

- Transverse myelitis (inflammation of the spinal cord) may develop in those with MS. Transverse myelitis can affect spinal cord function over several hours to several weeks before partial or complete recovery. It usually begins as a sudden onset of lower back pain, muscle weakness, abnormal sensations in the toes and feet, or difficulties with bladder control or bowel movements. This can rapidly progress to more severe symptoms, including arm and/or leg paralysis. In most cases, people recover at least some function within the first 12 weeks after an attack begins.
- Neuromyelitis optica is a disorder associated with transverse myelitis as well as optic nerve inflammation (also known as "optic neuritis"). People with this disorder usually have abnormal antibodies (proteins that normally target viruses and bacteria) against a specific channel in optic nerves, the brain stem or spinal cord, called the "aquaporin-4 channel." These individuals respond to certain treatments, which are different from those commonly used to treat MS.
- Trigeminal neuralgia is a chronic pain condition that causes sporadic, sudden burning or shock-like facial pain. The condition is more common in young adults with MS and is caused by lesions in the brain stem, the part of the brain that controls facial sensation.

WHO IS MORE LIKELY TO GET MULTIPLE SCLEROSIS?

Females are more frequently affected than males. Researchers are looking at several possible explanations for why the immune system attacks CNS myelin, including:

- fighting an infectious agent (e.g., a virus) that has components that mimic components of the brain (molecular mimicry)
- destroying brain cells because they are unhealthy
- mistakenly identifying normal brain cells as foreign

There is also something known as the "blood-brain barrier," which separates the brain and spinal cord from the immune system. If there is a break in this barrier, it exposes the brain to the immune system. When this happens, the immune system may misinterpret structures in the brain, such as myelin, as "foreign."

Research shows that genetic vulnerabilities combined with environmental factors may cause MS.

Genetic Susceptibility

MS itself is not inherited, but susceptibility to MS may be inherited. Studies show that some individuals with MS have one or more family members or relatives who also have MS.

Current research suggests that dozens of genes and possibly hundreds of variations in the genetic code (gene variants) combine to create vulnerability to MS. Some of these genes have been identified, and most are associated with functions of the immune system. Many of the known genes are similar to those that have been identified in people with other autoimmune diseases such as type 1 diabetes, rheumatoid arthritis, or lupus.

Infectious Factors and Viruses

Several viruses have been found in people with MS, but the virus most consistently linked to the development of MS is the Epstein-Barr virus (EBV), which causes infectious mononucleosis.

Only about 5 percent of the population has not been infected by EBV. These individuals are at a lower risk for developing MS than those who have been infected. People who were infected with EBV in adolescence or adulthood and who therefore develop an exaggerated immune response to EBV are at a significantly higher risk for developing MS than those who were infected in early childhood. This suggests that it may be the type of immune response to EBV that may lead to MS rather than EBV infection itself. However, there is still no proof that EBV causes MS, and the mechanisms that underlie this process are poorly understood.

Environmental Factors

Several studies indicate that people who spend more time in the sun and those with relatively higher levels of vitamin D are less likely to develop MS or have a less severe course of disease and fewer relapses. Bright sunlight helps human skin produce vitamin D. Researchers believe that vitamin D may help regulate the immune system in ways that reduce the risk of MS or autoimmunity in general.

People from regions near the equator, where there is a great deal of bright sunlight, generally have a much lower risk of MS than people from temperate areas such as the United States and Canada. Studies have found that people who smoke are more likely to develop MS and have a more aggressive disease course. Indeed, people who smoke tend to have more brain lesions and brain shrinkage than nonsmokers.

DIAGNOSING MULTIPLE SCLEROSIS

There is no single test used to diagnose MS. The disease is confirmed when symptoms and signs develop and are related to different parts of the nervous system at more than one interval and after other alternative diagnoses have been excluded. Doctors use different tests to rule out or confirm the diagnosis. In addition to a complete medical history, physical examination, and a detailed neurological examination, a doctor may recommend the following:

- **MRI scans of the brain and spinal cord**. It is to look for the characteristic lesions of MS. A special dye or contrast agent may be injected into a vein to enhance brain images of the active MS lesions.

- **Lumbar puncture (sometimes called a "spinal tap").** This is done to obtain a sample of cerebrospinal fluid and examine it for proteins and inflammatory cells associated with the disease. Spinal tap analysis can also rule out diseases that may look like MS.
- **Evoked potential tests.** They use electrodes placed on the skin and painless electric signals to measure how quickly and accurately the nervous system responds to stimulation.

TREATING MULTIPLE SCLEROSIS

There is no cure for MS, but there are treatments that can reduce the number and severity of relapses and delay the long-term disability progression of the disease.

- **Corticosteroids.** Medicines, such as intravenous (infused into a vein) methylprednisolone, are prescribed over the course of three to five days. Intravenous steroids quickly and potently suppress the immune system and reduce inflammation. They may be followed by a tapered dose of oral corticosteroids. Clinical trials have shown that these drugs hasten recovery from MS attacks but do not alter the long-term outcome of the disease.
- **Plasma exchange (plasmapheresis).** This intervention can treat severe flare-ups in people with relapsing forms of MS who do not have a good response to methylprednisolone. Plasma exchange involves taking blood out of the body and removing components in the blood's plasma that are thought to be harmful. The rest of the blood, plus replacement plasma, is then transfused back into the body. This treatment has not been shown to be effective for secondary- or chronic-progressive MS.

MANAGING MULTIPLE SCLEROSIS SYMPTOMS

Multiple sclerosis causes a variety of symptoms that can interfere with daily activities but can usually be treated or managed. Many of these issues are best treated by neurologists who have advanced training in the treatment of MS and who can prescribe specific medications to treat these problems. Eye and vision problems are common in people with MS but rarely result in permanent blindness. Inflammation of the optic nerve (optic neuritis) or damage to the myelin that covers the nerve fibers in the visual system can cause blurred or grayed vision, temporary blindness in one eye, loss of normal color vision, depth perception, or loss of vision in parts of the visual field. Uncontrolled horizontal or vertical eye movements (nystagmus), "jumping vision" (opsoclonus), and double vision (diplopia) are common in people with MS. Intravenous steroid medications, special eyeglasses, and periodically resting the eyes may be helpful.

Muscle weakness and spasticity are common in MS. Mild spasticity can be managed by stretching and exercising muscles using water therapy, yoga, or physical therapy. Medications such as gabapentin or baclofen can reduce spasticity. It is very important that people with MS stay physically active because physical inactivity can contribute to worsening stiffness, weakness, pain, fatigue, and other symptoms. Tremor, or uncontrollable shaking, develops in some people with MS. Assistive devices and weights attached to utensils or even limbs are sometimes helpful for people with tremors. Deep brain stimulation and drugs, such as clonazepam, may also be useful.

Problems with walking and balance occur in many people with MS. The most common walking problem is ataxia—unsteady, uncoordinated movements—due to damage to the areas of the brain that coordinate muscle balance. People with severe ataxia generally benefit from the use of a cane, walker, or other assistive device. Physical therapy can also reduce walking problems. The FDA has approved the drug dalfampridine to improve walking speed in people with MS.

Fatigue is a common symptom of MS and may be both physical (tiredness in the arms or legs) and cognitive (slowed processing speed or mental exhaustion). Daily physical activity programs of mild-to-moderate intensity can significantly reduce fatigue although people should avoid excessive physical activity and minimize exposure to hot weather conditions or ambient temperature. Other drugs that may reduce fatigue include amantadine,

269

methylphenidate, and modafinil. Occupational therapy can help people learn how to walk using an assistive device or in a way that saves physical energy. Stress management programs, relaxation training, membership in an MS support group, or individual psychotherapy may help some people.

Pain from MS can be felt in different parts of the body. Trigeminal neuralgia (facial pain) is treated with anticonvulsants or antispasmodic drugs or, less commonly, painkillers. Central pain, a syndrome caused by damage to the brain and/or spinal cord, can be treated with gabapentin and nortriptyline. Treatments for chronic back or other musculoskeletal pain may include heat, massage, ultrasound, and physical therapy.

Problems with bladder control and constipation may include urinary frequency, urgency, or the loss of bladder control. A small number of individuals retain large amounts of urine. Medical treatments are available for bladder-related problems. Constipation is also common and can be treated with a high-fiber diet, laxatives, and stool softeners. Sexual dysfunction can result from damage to nerves running through the spinal cord. Sexual problems may also stem from MS symptoms such as fatigue, cramped or spastic muscles, and psychological factors. Some of these problems can be corrected with medications. Psychological counseling may be helpful.

Clinical depression is frequent among people with MS. MS may cause depression as part of the disease process and chemical imbalance in the brain. Depression can intensify symptoms of fatigue, pain, and sexual dysfunction. It is most often treated with cognitive-behavioral therapy and selective serotonin reuptake inhibitor (SSRI) antidepressant medications, which are less likely than other antidepressant medications to cause fatigue.

Inappropriate and involuntary expressions of laughter, crying, or anger—symptoms of a condition called "pseudobulbar affect"—sometimes are associated with MS. These expressions are often incongruent with mood; for example, people with MS may cry when they are actually happy or laugh when they are not especially happy. The combination treatment of the drugs dextromethorphan and quinidine can treat pseudobulbar affect, as can other drugs such as amitriptyline or citalopram.

Cognitive impairment—a decline in the ability to think quickly and clearly and to remember easily—affects up to 75 percent of people with MS. These cognitive changes may appear at the same time as the physical symptoms, or they may develop gradually over time. Drugs such as donepezil may be helpful in some cases.

Complementary and Alternative Therapies

Many people with MS benefit from complementary or alternative approaches such as acupuncture, aromatherapy, ayurvedic medicine, touch and energy therapies, physical movement disciplines such as yoga and tai chi, herbal supplements, and biofeedback.

Because of the risk of interactions between alternative and conventional therapies, people with MS should discuss all the therapies they are using with their doctor, especially herbal supplements. Herbal supplements have biologically active ingredients that could have harmful effects on their own or interact harmfully with other medications.[4]

Section 35.5 | Myasthenia Gravis

WHAT IS MYASTHENIA GRAVIS?

Myasthenia gravis (MG) is a chronic autoimmune, neuromuscular disease that causes weakness in the skeletal muscles (the muscles that connect to your bones and contract to allow body movement in the arms and legs and allow for breathing).

The hallmark of MG is muscle weakness that worsens after periods of activity and improves after periods of rest. Certain muscles are often (but not always) involved in the disorder such as those that control the following:
- eye and eyelid movement
- facial expressions

[4] "Multiple Sclerosis," National Institute of Neurological Disorders and Stroke (NINDS), January 23, 2023. Available online. URL: www.ninds.nih.gov/health-information/disorders/multiple-sclerosis. Accessed May 10, 2023.

- chewing
- talking
- swallowing

The onset of the disorder may be sudden, and symptoms may not be immediately recognized as MG. The degree of muscle weakness involved varies greatly among individuals.

SYMPTOMS OF MYASTHENIA GRAVIS

The following symptoms are commonly associated with MG:
- weakness of the eye muscles (ocular myasthenia)
- drooping of one or both eyelids (ptosis)
- blurred or double vision (diplopia)
- changes in facial expressions
- difficulty swallowing
- shortness of breath
- impaired speech (dysarthria)
- weakness in the arms, hands, fingers, legs, and neck

Sometimes, the severe weakness of MG may cause respiratory failure, which requires immediate emergency medical care.

WHO IS MORE LIKELY TO GET MYASTHENIA GRAVIS?

Myasthenia gravis affects both males and females and occurs across all racial and ethnic groups. It most commonly impacts young adult females (under 40) and older males (over 60), but it can occur at any age, including childhood. MG is not inherited, nor is it contagious. Occasionally, the disease may occur in more than one member of the same family.

Although MG is rarely seen in infants, the fetus may acquire antibodies from a female parent—a condition called "neonatal myasthenia." Neonatal MG is generally temporary, and the child's symptoms usually disappear within two to three months after birth. Rarely, children of a healthy female parent may develop congenital myasthenia. This is not an autoimmune disorder but is caused by defective genes that produce abnormal proteins in the connection between the end of a nerve that carries signals from the brain to a muscle (the neuromuscular junction) and can cause similar symptoms to MG.

CAUSES OF MYASTHENIA GRAVIS

- **Antibodies**. Myasthenia gravis is caused by an error in how nerve signals are transmitted to muscles. It occurs when communication between the nerve and muscle is interrupted at the neuromuscular junction—the place where nerve cells connect with the muscles they control. Neurotransmitters are chemicals that neurons, or brain cells, use to communicate information. When electrical signals or impulses travel down a motor nerve, the nerve endings release a neurotransmitter called "acetylcholine" that binds to sites called "acetylcholine receptors" on the muscle. The binding of acetylcholine to its receptor activates the muscle and causes muscle contraction. In MG, antibodies (immune proteins produced by the body's immune system) block, alter, or destroy the receptors for acetylcholine at the neuromuscular junction, which prevents the muscle from contracting. This is most often caused by antibodies to the acetylcholine receptor itself, but antibodies to other proteins, such as muscle-specific kinase (MuSK) protein, can also impair transmission at the neuromuscular junction.
- **Thymus gland**. The thymus gland controls immune function and may be associated with MG. It grows gradually until puberty and then gets smaller until it is replaced by fat. Throughout childhood, the thymus plays an important role in the development of the immune system because it is responsible for producing T lymphocytes (T cells), a specific type of white blood cell (WBC) that protects the body from viruses and infections. In many adults with MG, the thymus gland remains large. People with the disease typically have clusters of immune cells in their thymus gland and may develop thymomas (tumors of the thymus gland). Thymomas are most often harmless, but they can become cancerous. Scientists

273

believe the thymus gland may give incorrect instructions to developing immune cells, ultimately causing the immune system to attack its own cells and tissues and produce acetylcholine receptor antibodies—setting the stage for the attack on neuromuscular transmission.

- **Myasthenic crisis.** A myasthenic crisis is a medical emergency that occurs when the muscles that control breathing weaken to the point where a ventilator is required to breathe. It may be triggered by infection, stress, surgery, or an adverse reaction to medication. Approximately 15–20 percent of people with MG experience at least one myasthenic crisis, and up to 50 percent may have no obvious cause for their myasthenic crisis. Certain medications have been shown to cause MG; however, these medications may still be used if it is more important to treat an underlying condition.

DIAGNOSING MYASTHENIA GRAVIS

A doctor may perform or order several tests to confirm a diagnosis of MG:

- **Physical and neurological examination.** A doctor will review your medical history and conduct a physical examination. In a neurological examination, the physician will check:
  - muscle strength and tone
  - coordination
  - sense of touch
  - any impairment of eye movements
- **Edrophonium test.** This test is used to test eye muscle weakness and uses injections of edrophonium chloride to briefly relieve weakness. The drug blocks the breakdown of acetylcholine and temporarily increases the levels of acetylcholine at the neuromuscular junction.
- **Blood test.** People living with MG may have abnormally elevated levels of acetylcholine receptor

antibodies. A second antibody called the "anti-MuSK" antibody has been found in about half of the individuals with MG who do not have acetylcholine receptor antibodies. A blood test can also detect this antibody. However, in some individuals with MG, neither of these antibodies is present; this is called "seronegative (negative antibody) myasthenia."

- **Electrodiagnostics**. Diagnostic tests include repetitive nerve stimulation, which repeatedly stimulates your nerves with small pulses of electricity to tire specific muscles. Muscle fibers in MG, as well as other neuromuscular disorders, do not respond as well to repeated electrical stimulation. Single-fiber electromyography (EMG), which is considered the most sensitive test for MG, detects impaired nerve-to-muscle transmission. EMG can be very helpful in diagnosing mild cases of MG when other tests fail to demonstrate abnormalities.
- **Diagnostic imaging**. Diagnostic imaging of your chest using computed tomography (CT) or magnetic resonance imaging (MRI) may identify the presence of a thymoma.
- **Pulmonary function testing**. Measuring breathing strength can help predict if respiration may fail and lead to a myasthenic crisis.

Because weakness is a common symptom of many other disorders, the diagnosis of MG is often missed or delayed (sometimes up to two years) in people who have either mild weakness or in those individuals whose weakness is restricted to only a few muscles.

TREATING MYASTHENIA GRAVIS

Currently, there is no known cure. Available treatments can control symptoms and often allow you to have a relatively high quality of life (QOL). Most people with MG have an average life expectancy.

There are several therapies available to help reduce and improve muscle weakness, including the following:

- **Thymectomy.** An operation to remove the problematic thymus gland can reduce symptoms, possibly by rebalancing the immune system. A study of 126 people with MG with thymoma and those with no visible thymoma funded by the National Institute of Neurological Disorders and Stroke (NINDS) found the surgery reduced muscle weakness and the need for immunosuppressive drugs. Stable, long-lasting complete remissions are the goal of thymectomy and may occur in about 50 percent of individuals who undergo this procedure.
- **Monoclonal antibody**. This is a treatment that targets the process by which acetylcholine antibodies injure the neuromuscular junction. The U.S. Food and Drug Administration (FDA) has approved the use of the medication eculizumab for the treatment of generalized MG in adults who test positive for the antiacetylcholine receptor (AchR) antibody.
- **Anticholinesterase medications**. Medications to treat MG include anticholinesterase agents such as mestinon or pyridostigmine, which slow the breakdown of acetylcholine at the neuromuscular junction and improve neuromuscular transmission and increase muscle strength.
- **Immunosuppressive drugs**. These are a group of drugs that improve muscle strength by suppressing the production of abnormal antibodies, such as prednisone, azathioprine, mycophenolate mofetil (MMF), and tacrolimus. The drugs can cause significant side effects and must be carefully monitored by a physician.
- **Plasmapheresis and intravenous immunoglobulin**. These therapies are used in severe cases of MG to remove destructive antibodies that attack the neuromuscular junction although their effectiveness usually only lasts a few weeks or months.

- Plasmapheresis is a procedure using a machine to remove harmful antibodies in plasma and replace them with good plasma or a plasma substitute.
- Intravenous immunoglobulin is a highly concentrated injection of antibodies pooled from many healthy donors that temporarily changes the way the immune system operates. It works by binding to the antibodies that cause MG and removing them from circulation.

Some cases of MG may go into remission, either temporarily or permanently, and muscle weakness may disappear completely so that medications can be discontinued.

WHAT ARE THE LATEST UPDATES ON MYASTHENIA GRAVIS?

The NINDS is a component of the National Institutes of Health (NIH), a leading supporter of biomedical research in the world. Researchers continue to gain a better understanding of MG, its causes, and the structure and function of the neuromuscular junction. Technological advances have led to more timely and accurate diagnoses of MG, and new and enhanced therapies have improved treatment options. Researchers are working to develop better medications, identify new ways to diagnose and treat individuals, and improve treatment options.

Medication

Some people with MG do not respond well to available treatment options, which usually include long-term suppression of the immune system. New drugs are being tested, either alone or in combination with existing drug therapies, to see if they are more effective in targeting the causes of the disease.

Diagnostics and Biomarkers

The NINDS-funded researchers are exploring the assembly and function of connections between nerves and muscle fibers to understand the fundamental processes in neuromuscular development, which could reveal new therapies for neuromuscular diseases such as MG. Researchers are also exploring better ways to treat MG by developing new tools to diagnose people with undetectable antibodies and identify potential biomarkers (signs that can help diagnose or measure the progression of a disease) to predict an individual's response to immunosuppressive drugs.[5]

Section 35.6 | **Relapsing Polychondritis**

Relapsing polychondritis (RP) is a rare condition characterized by recurrent inflammation of the cartilage and other tissues throughout the body. Cartilage is a tough but flexible tissue that covers the ends of bones at a joint and gives shape and support to other parts of the body. It has been estimated that between 3 and 4 people per 1 million develop RP every year. Females are more likely to develop RP than males. The exact number of people with this condition is unknown.

SYMPTOMS OF RELAPSING POLYCHONDRITIS

The following list includes the most common signs and symptoms in people with RP. These features may be different from person to person. Some people may have more symptoms than others, and symptoms can range from mild to severe. This list does not include every symptom or feature that has been described in this condition.

The features of the condition and the severity of symptoms vary significantly from person to person but may include:
- pain and swelling of the ear
- damage to the outer part of the ear

---

[5] "Myasthenia Gravis," National Institute of Neurological Disorders and Stroke (NINDS), January 23, 2023. Available online. URL: www.ninds.nih.gov/health-information/disorders/myasthenia-gravis. Accessed May 10, 2023.

- swelling of the inner ear
- dizziness, hearing loss, and/or nausea
- joint pain
- swelling of the voice box (larynx)
- narrowing and blockage of the trachea (tracheal stenosis)
- coughing, wheezing, or hoarseness
- swelling of the outer parts of the eye (episcleritis, uveitis, and/or scleritis)
- nasal cartilage inflammation and damage

Less commonly, RP may affect the heart, kidneys, nervous system, gastrointestinal tract, and/or vascular (veins) system. Nonspecific symptoms such as fever, weight loss, malaise, and fatigue may also be present. Symptoms usually begin in adulthood between the ages of 20 and 60, but RP has been diagnosed in children as well.

In approximately one-third of affected people, RP is associated with other medical problems. Conditions reportedly associated with RP include hematological diseases (including Hodgkin lymphoma and myelodysplastic syndromes), gastrointestinal disorders (including Crohn's disease and ulcerative colitis), endocrine diseases (including diabetes mellitus type 1 and thyroid disorders), and others.

Episodes of RP may last a few days or weeks and typically resolve with or without treatment. However, it is generally progressive, and many people have persistent symptoms in between flares. The most serious symptoms involve the airways and heart.

CAUSES OF RELAPSING POLYCHONDRITIS

The exact underlying cause of RP is unknown. However, scientists suspect that it is an autoimmune condition. It is thought that RP occurs when the body's immune system mistakenly attacks its own cartilage and other tissues. In general, autoimmune conditions are complex traits that are associated with the effects of multiple genes in combination with lifestyle and environmental factors.

There is also evidence to suggest that some people may be born with a genetic susceptibility to RP. Studies have found that people with RP are roughly twice as likely as those without this condition to carry a certain genetic allele called "*HLA-DR4*." "HLA" stands for human leukocyte antigen, which is an important part of our immune system and plays a role in resistance and predisposition (risk) to disease. However, *HLA* genes are not solely responsible for specific diseases but instead may simply contribute along with other genetic or environmental factors to disease risk. Thus, many people with *HLA-DR4* will never develop RP.

DIAGNOSIS OF RELAPSING POLYCHONDRITIS

There are no tests available that are specific to RP. A diagnosis is, therefore, generally based on the presence of characteristic signs and symptoms. For example, people may be diagnosed as having RP if they have three or more of the following features:

- inflammation of the cartilage of both ears
- seronegative (negative for rheumatoid factor) polyarthritis (arthritis that involves five or more joints simultaneously)
- inflammation of the cartilage of the nose
- eye inflammation (conjunctivitis, episcleritis, scleritis, and/or uveitis)
- inflammation of the cartilage of the airway
- vestibular dysfunction (i.e., vertigo, hearing loss, tinnitus)

In some cases, a biopsy of affected tissue may be necessary to support the diagnosis.

TREATMENT FOR RELAPSING POLYCHONDRITIS

The primary goals of treatment for people with RP are to relieve present symptoms and preserve the structure of the affected cartilage. The main treatment for RP is corticosteroid therapy with prednisone to decrease the severity, frequency, and duration of relapses. Higher doses are generally given during flares, while lower doses can typically be prescribed during periods of remission. Other medications reported to control symptoms include dapsone, colchicine, azathioprine, methotrexate, cyclophosphamide, hydroxychloroquine, cyclosporine, and infliximab. People who develop severe heart or respiratory complications may require surgery.[6]

Section 35.7 | Rheumatoid Arthritis

WHAT IS RHEUMATOID ARTHRITIS?

Rheumatoid arthritis (RA) is a chronic (long-lasting) autoimmune disease that mostly affects joints. RA occurs when the immune system, which normally helps protect the body from infection and disease, attacks its own tissues. The disease causes pain, swelling, stiffness, and loss of function in joints.

Additional features of RA can include the following:

- It affects the lining of the joints, which damages the tissue that covers the ends of the bones in a joint.
- RA often occurs in a symmetrical pattern, meaning that if one knee or hand has the condition, the other hand or knee is often also affected.
- It can affect the joints in the wrists, hands, elbows, shoulders, feet, spine, knees, and jaw.
- RA may cause fatigue, occasional fevers, and a loss of appetite.
- RA may cause medical problems outside of the joints, in areas such as the heart, lungs, blood, nerves, eyes, and skin.

[6] Genetic and Rare Diseases Information Center (GARD), "Relapsing Polychondritis," National Center for Advancing Translational Sciences (NCATS), January 22, 2021. Available online. URL: https://rarediseases.info.nih.gov/diseases/7417/relapsing-polychondritis. Accessed May 25, 2023.

WHAT HAPPENS IN RHEUMATOID ARTHRITIS?

Doctors do not know why the immune system attacks joint tissues. However, they do know that when a series of events occurs, RA can develop. This series of events includes the following:

- A combination of genes and exposure to environmental factors starts the development of RA.
- The immune system may be activated years before symptoms appear.
- The start of the autoimmune process may happen in other areas of the body, but the impact of the immune malfunction typically settles in the joints.
- Immune cells cause inflammation in the inner lining of the joint, called the "synovium."
- This inflammation becomes chronic, and the synovium thickens due to an increase in cells, production of proteins, and other factors in the joint, which can lead to pain, redness, and warmth.
- As RA progresses, the thickened and inflamed synovium pushes further into the joint and destroys the cartilage and bone within the joint.
- As the joint capsule stretches, the forces cause changes within the joint structure.
- The surrounding muscles, ligaments, and tendons that support and stabilize the joint become weak over time and do not work as well. This can lead to more pain and joint damage and problems using the affected joint.

WHO GETS RHEUMATOID ARTHRITIS?

You are more likely to get RA if you have certain risk factors. These include the following:

- **Age**. The disease can happen at any age; however, the risk of developing RA increases with older age. Children and younger teenagers may be diagnosed with juvenile idiopathic arthritis, a condition related to RA.
- **Sex**. RA is more common among women than men. About two to three times as many women as men have

the disease. Researchers think that reproductive and hormonal factors may play a role in the development of the disease for some women.

- **Family history and genetics**. If a family member has RA, you may be more likely to develop the disease. There are several genetic factors that slightly increase the risk of getting RA.
- **Smoking**. Research shows that people who smoke over a long period of time are at an increased risk of getting RA. For people who continue to smoke, the disease may be more severe.
- **Obesity**. Some research shows that being obese may increase your risk for the disease as well as limit how much the disease can be improved.
- **Periodontitis**. Gum disease may be associated with developing RA.
- **Lung diseases**. Diseases of the lungs and airways may also be associated with developing RA.

SYMPTOMS OF RHEUMATOID ARTHRITIS

Common symptoms of RA include the following:

- RA affects people differently. In some people, RA starts with mild or moderate inflammation affecting just a few joints. However, if it is not treated or the treatments are not working, RA can worsen and affect more joints. This can lead to more damage and disability.
- RA can happen in any joint; however, it is more common in the wrists, hands, and feet. The symptoms often happen on both sides of the body in a symmetrical pattern. For example, if you have RA in the right hand, you may also have it in the left hand.
- At times, RA symptoms worsen in "flares" due to a trigger such as stress, environmental factors (such as cigarette smoke or viral infections), too much activity, or suddenly stopping medications. In some cases, there may be no clear cause.

RA can cause other medical problems, such as the following:

- joint pain at rest and when moving, along with tenderness, swelling, and warmth of the joint
- joint stiffness that lasts longer than 30 minutes, typically after waking in the morning or after resting for a long period of time
- joint swelling that may interfere with daily activities, such as difficulty making a fist, combing hair, buttoning clothes, or bending knees
- fatigue—feeling unusually tired or having low energy
- occasional low-grade fever
- loss of appetite
- rheumatoid nodules that are firm lumps just below the skin, typically on the hands and elbows
- anemia due to low red blood cell (RBC) counts
- dry eyes and mouth
- inflammation of the blood vessels, lung tissue, airways, the lining of the lungs, or the sac enclosing the heart
- lung disease, characterized by scarring and inflammation of the lungs that can be severe in some people with RA

CAUSES OF RHEUMATOID ARTHRITIS

Researchers do not know what causes the immune system to turn against the body's joints and other tissues. Studies show that a combination of the following factors may lead to the disease:

- **Genes**. Certain genes that affect how the immune system works may lead to RA. However, some people who have these genes never develop the disease. This suggests that genes are not the only factor in the development of RA. In addition, more than one gene may determine who gets the disease and how severe it will become.
- **Environment**. Researchers continue to study how environmental factors such as cigarette smoke may trigger RA in people who have specific genes that also increase their risk. In addition, some factors such as

inhalants, bacteria, viruses, gum disease, and lung disease may play a role in the development of RA.
- **Sex hormones**. Researchers think that sex hormones may play a role in the development of RA when genetic and environmental factors are also involved. Studies show:
  - women are more likely than men to develop RA
  - the disease may improve during pregnancy and flare after pregnancy

DIAGNOSIS OF RHEUMATOID ARTHRITIS

Doctors diagnose RA by:
- taking a medical history
- performing a physical exam
- ordering laboratory tests
- ordering imaging studies, such as x-rays or ultrasound

It can be difficult to diagnose RA when it is in the early stages because:
- the disease develops over time and only a few symptoms may be present in the early stages
- there is no single test for the disease
- symptoms differ from person to person
- symptoms can be similar to those of other types of arthritis and joint conditions

As a result, doctors use a variety of tools to diagnose the disease and to rule out other conditions.

Medical History

Remember to let your doctor know:
- about your symptoms, when and how they started, and how they have changed over time
- what limitations in activities you may have, such as difficulty with work, leisure, or activities around the house

- about your other medical problems
- if you have any family members with similar symptoms or if any family members have RA
- what medications you take

Answers to these questions can help your doctor make a diagnosis and understand the impact the disease has on your life.

Physical Examination

The doctor usually performs a physical exam that may include the following:

- Examine your joints.
- Watch how you walk, bend, and carry out activities of daily living.
- Look for a rash or nodules on your skin.
- Listen to your chest for signs of inflammation in the lungs.

Laboratory Tests

Lab tests may help diagnose RA. Some common tests are as follows:

- **Rheumatoid factor (RF).** This blood test checks for RF, an antibody that many people with RA can eventually have in their blood. An antibody is a special protein made by the immune system that normally helps fight invaders in the body. Not all people with RA test positive for RF; some people test positive for RF but never develop the disease; and some people test positive but have another disease. However, doctors can use this test, along with other test results and evaluations, to diagnose RA.
- **Anti-cyclic citrullinated peptide antibody (anti-CCP).** This blood test checks for anti-CCP antibodies, which appear in many people with RA. In addition, anti-CCP can appear before RA symptoms develop, which can help doctors diagnose the disease early. This test's results, along with the results from RF blood

tests, are very useful in confirming an RA diagnosis. However, it is important to know that some people can be diagnosed with RA even with normal blood tests.

- **Complete blood count**. This blood test measures different blood cell counts and can help diagnose anemia, which is common in people with RA.
- **Erythrocyte sedimentation rate (often called the "sed rate")**. This test measures inflammation in the body and monitors disease activity and response to treatments.
- **C-reactive protein**. This is another common test for inflammation that can help diagnose RA and monitor disease activity and response to treatments.
- **Other blood tests**. Your doctor may also use other tests to check your kidney function, electrolytes, liver function, thyroid function, muscle markers, other autoimmune markers, and markers of infection to evaluate your overall health and evaluate for other diagnoses. Other specific tests for RA are sometimes considered.

Imaging Tests

To check for joint damage, doctors may use imaging tests such as the following:

- X-rays help check for RA; however, they are not generally abnormal in the early stages of RA before joint damage occurs. Doctors may use x-rays to monitor the progression of the disease or to rule out other causes of joint pain.
- Magnetic resonance imaging (MRI) and ultrasound may help diagnose RA in the early stages of the disease. In addition, these imaging tests can help evaluate the amount of damage in the joints and the severity of the disease.
- Other imaging tests sometimes considered for RA include computed tomography (CT) scanning, positron emission tomography (PET) scan, bone scan, and dual-energy x-ray absorptiometry (DEXA).

TREATMENT FOR RHEUMATOID ARTHRITIS

Treatment for RA continues to improve, which can give many people relief from symptoms, improving their quality of life (QOL). Doctors may use the following options to treat RA:

- medications
- physical therapy and occupational therapy
- surgery
- routine monitoring and ongoing care
- complementary therapies

Your doctor may recommend a combination of treatments, which may change over time based on your symptoms and the severity of your disease. No matter which treatment plan your doctor recommends, the overall goals are to help:

- relieve pain
- decrease inflammation and swelling
- prevent, slow, or stop joint and organ damage
- improve your ability to participate in daily activities

RA may start causing joint damage in the first or second year that a person has the disease. Once joint damage occurs, it generally cannot be reversed, so early diagnosis and treatment are very important.[7]

Section 35.8 | Systemic Lupus Erythematosus

WHAT IS SYSTEMIC LUPUS ERYTHEMATOSUS?

Systemic lupus erythematosus (SLE) (lupus) is a chronic (long-lasting) autoimmune disease that can affect many parts of the body. Lupus occurs when the immune system, which normally helps protect the body from infection and disease, attacks its own tissues. This attack causes inflammation and, in some cases, permanent

---

[7] "Rheumatoid Arthritis," National Institute of Arthritis and Musculoskeletal and Skin Diseases (NIAMS), November 2022. Available online. URL: www.niams.nih.gov/health-topics/rheumatoid-arthritis. Accessed May 10, 2023.

tissue damage, which can be widespread—affecting the skin, joints, heart, lungs, kidneys, circulating blood cells, and brain.

If you have lupus, you may experience periods of illness (flares) and periods of wellness (remission). Lupus flares can be mild to serious, and they are unpredictable. However, with treatment, many people with lupus can manage the disease.

WHO GETS SYSTEMIC LUPUS ERYTHEMATOSUS?

Anyone can get lupus; however, women get the disease about nine times more often than men. Most often, it happens in people between ages 15 and 45, but lupus can occur in childhood or later in life as well.

Lupus is more common in African Americans than in White people and is also more common in people of American Indian and Asian descent. Men, African Americans, Chinese people, and Hispanic people are also more likely to have serious organ system involvement. If you have a family member with lupus or another autoimmune disease, you may be more likely to develop lupus.

SYMPTOMS OF SYSTEMIC LUPUS ERYTHEMATOSUS

The symptoms of lupus vary from person to person and can range from mild to severe. You may have just a few symptoms affecting just one area of your body, or you could have many symptoms throughout your body. Symptoms may come and go, and you may develop new symptoms over time. Some symptoms happen when the disease causes inflammation in organs, such as the joints, skin, kidneys, lining of the heart and lungs, brain, and blood cells. Symptoms of lupus can include the following:
- arthritis, causing painful and swollen joints and morning stiffness
- fevers
- fatigue, or feeling tired often
- a rash that appears on the face across the nose and cheeks, which is called a "malar" or "butterfly" rash
- round, scaly rashes that can appear anywhere on the body

- sensitivity to the sun that may cause a rash
- hair loss
- sores, which are usually painless, in the nose and mouth (most often on the roof of the mouth)
- change of color in the fingers and toes—blue-purplish, white, or red—from cold and stress (Raynaud phenomenon)
- swollen glands
- swelling in the legs or around the eyes
- pain when breathing deeply or lying down from inflammation of the lining around the lungs or heart
- headaches, dizziness, depression, confusion, or seizures
- abdominal pain

Lupus causes inflammation throughout the body, which can cause problems in organs, including the following:
- kidney damage that can lead to changes in kidney function, including kidney failure, which is called "lupus nephritis"
- seizures and memory problems due to changes in the brain and central nervous system
- heart problems:
  - heart valve damage due to inflammation that leads to scarring
  - inflammation of the lining around the heart muscle called "pericarditis"
  - inflammation of the heart muscle itself, called "myocarditis"
- inflammation of blood vessels called "vasculitis"
- blood clots due to high levels of certain autoantibodies referred to as antiphospholipid antibodies
- low blood cell counts, including red blood cells (RBCs), white blood cells (WBCs), and platelets
- inflammation of the tissue that surrounds the lungs, making it painful to breathe, which is called "pleurisy"

Some people with lupus may be more likely to develop other conditions, such as cardiovascular disease, due to inflammation of the heart and blood vessel tissues caused by lupus, which can lead to the following:

- **Atherosclerosis**. It happens when fat and other materials attach to the blood vessel wall and form plaque. This can happen in blood vessels throughout the body.
- **Coronary artery disease**. It happens when plaque builds up in the arteries that supply blood to the heart. This can interrupt blood flow when a blood clot forms or a piece of plaque breaks off, causing a heart attack.

CAUSES OF SYSTEMIC LUPUS ERYTHEMATOSUS

The cause of lupus is unknown, and researchers are still trying to learn what may trigger or lead to the disease. Doctors know that it is a complex autoimmune disease in which the body's immune system attacks the person's tissues and organs. Studies show that certain factors may trigger your immune system, causing the disease. These factors include the following:

- **Genes**. Research shows that certain genes play a role in the development of lupus. The different forms of these genes carry instructions for proteins that may affect the immune system. Researchers are studying how high or low levels of these proteins may be important in the development of the disease.
- **Environment**. Exposure to certain factors in the environment—such as viral infections, sunlight, certain medications, and smoking—may trigger lupus.
- **Immune and inflammatory influences**. Researchers think that if the body does not remove damaged or dead cells normally, this could trick the immune system into constantly fighting against itself. This process could cause an autoimmune response, which could lead to lupus. In addition, researchers are studying different cell types and how changes could lead to lupus.

DIAGNOSIS OF SYSTEMIC LUPUS ERYTHEMATOSUS

Lupus can be difficult to diagnose because it has many symptoms that come and go and can mimic symptoms of other disorders or diseases. When speaking to your doctor about your symptoms, be sure to include symptoms that may no longer be present. Your doctor may need to rule out other causes before diagnosing lupus. At this time, no single test diagnoses lupus. Doctors can diagnose the condition by:

- asking about your medical history and symptoms and, if necessary, reading your previous medical records
- asking if anyone in your family has lupus or other autoimmune diseases
- performing a complete physical exam
- taking samples of blood for laboratory tests, such as:
  - **Antinuclear antibodies (ANAs).** The ANA test is a sensitive test for lupus. Almost all people with lupus have a positive ANA test. However, having a positive ANA test does not mean you have lupus since totally healthy people can have a positive ANA test.
  - **Antiphospholipid antibodies, anti-Smith, and anti-double-strand deoxyribonucleic acid (DNA) antibodies**. Doctors order these when you have a positive ANA test and can help determine if you have lupus.
  - **Complete blood counts**. It is to check for low platelet counts, low RBC counts, and low WBC levels, which can happen if you have lupus.
  - **Metabolic panel**. It is to look for changes in kidney function.
- taking urine samples to check for abnormal levels of protein in the urine
- performing a biopsy of the skin or kidney (when labs indicate there may be a problem with the kidney) by taking a small sample of tissue to examine under a microscope

TREATMENT FOR SYSTEMIC LUPUS ERYTHEMATOSUS

Doctors treat lupus based on your symptoms. The goal of treatment is to:

- manage symptoms
- prevent, limit, and stop flares
- maintain the lowest level of disease activity and, if possible, achieve complete remission
- prevent or slow organ damage
- improve your quality of life (QOL)

Lupus is a chronic (long-lasting) disease, and there is no cure at the present time. However, treatments have improved dramatically, giving doctors more choices to manage the disease. Because symptoms can change and treatments can have side effects, your doctor may recommend a combination of treatments to manage lupus. Treatments for lupus may include the following.

Medications

- Anti-inflammatory drugs help treat pain or fever.
- Antimalarials, which are used to prevent and treat malaria, have been found to be useful for treating fatigue, joint pain, skin rashes, and inflammation of the lungs caused by lupus. These drugs may also prevent flares from recurring.
- Corticosteroids help lower inflammation in the body. Because they are potent drugs, your doctor will prescribe the lowest dose possible to achieve the desired benefit. Doctors prescribe these medicines in the following forms:
  - liquid or pills that you swallow
  - cream that you apply to the skin
  - injection
  - intravenous (IV) infusion that doctors give to you through a tube in your vein
- Immunosuppressants help suppress or curb the overactive immune system, and they may be given by mouth or by

IV infusion. The risk for side effects increases with the length of treatment.

- The B-lymphocyte stimulator (BlyS) protein inhibitor, a type of biologic medication, can help reduce the activation and life span of abnormal B cells in the body, which may help control lupus. Inhibitors to the type I interferon receptor, a type of biologic medication, may improve skin, joint, and overall lupus symptoms.

You may need to take medicines to treat or prevent complications related to lupus or side effects from the medicines that treat the disease, such as heart disease, high blood pressure, osteoporosis or other bone problems, or infection.

Alternative and Complementary Therapies
Some people may try alternative and complementary therapies to improve symptoms. However, research has not definitively shown whether they help or treat lupus, for example:
- special diets
- nutritional supplements
- fish oils
- ointments and creams
- acupuncture
- chiropractic treatment
- homeopathy

Some over-the-counter (OTC) medicines, herbs, and supplements can interfere with other medicines you are taking. Before beginning any new therapy, speak with your doctor. No matter what treatment you receive, it is important that you have regular visits with your doctor to monitor your disease and the potential side effects of prescribed therapies. Never stop your medicines or treatments without speaking to your doctor.

Who Treats Systemic Lupus Erythematosus?
Most people will see a rheumatologist for their lupus treatment. A rheumatologist is a doctor who specializes in rheumatic diseases,

such as arthritis and other inflammatory or autoimmune disorders. Clinical immunologists, doctors who specialize in immune system disorders, may also treat people with lupus. Other health-care providers may provide treatment, including:

- primary care providers, such as family physicians or internal medicine specialists
- mental health professionals, who provide counseling and treat mental health disorders such as depression and anxiety
- nephrologists, who treat kidney disease
- cardiologists, who specialize in treating diseases of the heart and blood vessels
- hematologists, who specialize in blood disorders
- endocrinologists, who treat problems related to the glands and hormones
- dermatologists, who specialize in conditions of the skin, hair, and nails
- pulmonologists, who treat lung problems
- neurologists, who treat disorders and diseases of the spine, brain, and nerves

LIVING WITH SYSTEMIC LUPUS ERYTHEMATOSUS

Living with lupus can be physically and emotionally hard. At times, you may think that your friends, family, and coworkers do not understand how you feel. You may experience sadness and anger. A good place to start managing the disease is working with your doctor to determine the best treatment plan and taking your medications as prescribed. But, keep in mind, many people with lupus live wonderfully happy lives, and therefore, a positive outlook is very important.

You can do several things to help you live with lupus:

- Learn to recognize the warning signs of a flare so that you and your doctor might reduce or prevent them. Warning signs include the following:
  - increased tiredness
  - joint swelling
  - pain
  - rash

- fever
- abdominal pain
- headache
- Eat a healthy, well-balanced diet rich in fruits, vegetables, and whole grains.
- Exercise to help keep your body strong; however, talk to your doctor before starting an exercise program.
- If you smoke, quit. This will help lower your risk for heart disease that can be a complication of lupus.
- Protect yourself from the sun—sometimes, exposure to the sun can cause a flare. Wear protective clothing, such as a hat or long-sleeved shirt, and use sunscreen any time you go outside.
- Reach out to online and community support groups.
- Keep the lines of communication open. Talk to your family and friends about your lupus to help them understand the disease.
- Ask for help when you need it.
- Take a break from focusing on the disease and spend some time doing activities you enjoy.
- Lower your stress—try meditating, reading, or deep breathing. Remember, stress can trigger a flare.

Most people with mild disease or who are in remission can usually participate in the same life activities they did before they were diagnosed.[8]

---

[8] "Systemic Lupus Erythematosus (Lupus)," National Institute of Arthritis and Musculoskeletal and Skin Diseases (NIAMS), October 2022. Available online. URL: www.niams.nih.gov/health-topics/lupus. Accessed May 10, 2023.

Chapter 36 | **Autoimmune Disorders of the Eyes**

Chapter Contents

WHAT IS KERATOCONUS?

Keratoconus is an eye condition that affects the shape of the cornea, which is the clear outer covering of the eye. In this condition, the cornea thins and bulges outward, eventually resembling a cone shape. These corneal abnormalities, which worsen over time, can lead to nearsightedness (myopia), blurred vision that cannot be improved with corrective lenses (irregular astigmatism), and vision loss.

Other corneal changes typical of keratoconus that can be seen during an eye exam include iron deposits in the cornea that form a yellow-to-brownish ring, called the "Fleischer ring," surrounding the colored part of the eye (iris). Affected individuals may also develop Vogt's striae, which are thin, vertical, white lines in the tissue at the back of the cornea.

Keratoconus may affect only one eye at first, but eventually, the corneas of both eyes become misshapen although they might not be affected with the same severity. As keratoconus worsens, people with this condition can develop corneal scarring, often caused by exposure of the abnormally thin cornea to prolonged contact lens use or excessive eye rubbing.

The eye changes characteristic of keratoconus typically begin in adolescence and slowly worsen until mid-adulthood at which point the shape of the cornea remains stable.

Other Names of Keratoconus
- bulging cornea
- conical cornea
- KC

FREQUENCY OF KERATOCONUS

Keratoconus is estimated to affect 1 in 500–2,000 individuals worldwide.

CAUSES OF KERATOCONUS

The cause of keratoconus is unknown. Researchers have studied many different factors, both genetic and environmental, that are thought to influence the risk of developing keratoconus.

The environmental factors that may contribute to keratoconus include excessive eye rubbing and the tendency to develop allergic disorders (atopy).

Excessive and vigorous eye rubbing can cause trauma to the cornea and may lead to its thinning. However, it is unclear whether eye rubbing leads to keratoconus or if eye rubbing is a response to eye discomfort in the early stages of the condition. If eye rubbing is not involved in the development of keratoconus, it likely contributes to the worsening of the condition.

Approximately one-third of individuals with keratoconus have an allergic disorder although it is unclear how allergic disorders are related to the development of keratoconus. Allergies might trigger eye rubbing, which can aggravate eye problems.

Changes in multiple genes have been associated with developing keratoconus. Many of these variants have been found only in small populations or single families. In most individuals with keratoconus, a combination of genetic and environmental factors is needed for the condition to develop. However, some affected individuals seem to have a largely environmental cause for the condition, while others seem to have a largely genetic cause. Individuals with a relative who has keratoconus have an increased risk of developing the condition compared to people without a family history.

More than a dozen genes have been associated with keratoconus. These genes have varied functions. The most frequently associated genes play roles in eye development, the formation and structure of the cornea, the intricate lattice of proteins and other molecules that form in the space between cells (extracellular matrix), an immune system response called "inflammation," and the regulation of cell growth. It is thought that a disruption in one of these processes, in combination with an environmental trigger, may lead to the development of keratoconus.

Keratoconus can be a feature of genetic syndromes, such as Leber congenital amaurosis and arterial tortuosity syndrome. When it is part of a syndrome, keratoconus is caused by the same genetic mutation that causes the syndrome. Mutations in the genes that cause syndromes with keratoconus have not been found to cause keratoconus without other features.

INHERITANCE OF KERATOCONUS

In most cases, keratoconus is not inherited and occurs in individuals with no family history of the disorder.

The condition can also occur in families. In some cases, keratoconus is inherited in an autosomal dominant pattern, which means one copy of the altered gene in each cell is sufficient to cause the disorder. An affected person often has one parent with the condition although some people who have a gene variant never develop the condition, a situation known as "reduced penetrance."

Keratoconus can also be inherited in an autosomal recessive pattern, which means variants occur in both copies of the gene in each cell. The parents of an individual with an autosomal recessive condition each carry one copy of the altered gene, but they typically do not show signs and symptoms of the condition.[1]

Section 36.2 | Neuromyelitis Optica

WHAT IS NEUROMYELITIS OPTICA?

Neuromyelitis optica (NMO) is an autoimmune disorder that affects the nerves of the eyes and the central nervous system (CNS), which includes the brain and spinal cord. Autoimmune disorders occur when the immune system malfunctions and attacks the body's own tissues and organs. In NMO, the autoimmune attack

---

[1] MedlinePlus, "Keratoconus," National Institutes of Health (NIH), July 1, 2017. Available online. URL: https://medlineplus.gov/genetics/condition/keratoconus. Accessed May 11, 2023.

causes inflammation of the nerves, and the resulting damage leads to the signs and symptoms of the condition. NMO is characterized by optic neuritis, which is inflammation of the nerve that carries information from the eye to the brain (optic nerve). Optic neuritis causes eye pain and vision loss, which can occur in one or both eyes.

NMO is also characterized by transverse myelitis, which is inflammation of the spinal cord. The inflammation associated with transverse myelitis damages the spinal cord, causing a lesion that often extends the length of three or more bones of the spine (vertebrae). In addition, myelin, which is the covering that protects nerves and promotes the efficient transmission of nerve impulses, can be damaged. Transverse myelitis causes weakness, numbness, and paralysis of the arms and legs. Other effects of spinal cord damage can include disturbances in sensations, loss of bladder and bowel control, uncontrollable hiccupping, and nausea. In addition, muscle weakness may make breathing difficult and can cause life-threatening respiratory failure in people with NMO.

There are two forms of NMO: the relapsing form and the monophasic form. The relapsing form is the most common. This form is characterized by recurrent episodes of optic neuritis and transverse myelitis. These episodes can be months or years apart, and there is usually partial recovery between episodes. However, most affected individuals eventually develop permanent muscle weakness and vision impairment that persist even between episodes. For unknown reasons, approximately nine times more women than men have the relapsing form. The monophasic form, which is less common, causes a single episode of NMO that can last several months. People with this form of the condition can also have lasting muscle weakness or paralysis and vision loss. This form affects men and women equally. The onset of either form of NMO can occur anytime from childhood to adulthood although the condition most frequently begins in a person's forties.

Approximately one-quarter of individuals with NMO have signs or symptoms of another autoimmune disorder, such as myasthenia gravis (MG), systemic lupus erythematosus (SLE), or Sjögren syndrome.

Other Names of Neuromyelitis Optica
- Devic disease
- Devic neuromyelitis optica
- Devic syndrome
- Devic's disease
- optic-spinal MS
- opticospinal MS

FREQUENCY OF NEUROMYELITIS OPTICA
Neuromyelitis optica affects approximately 1–2 per 100,000 people worldwide. Women are affected by this condition more frequently than men.

CAUSES OF NEUROMYELITIS OPTICA
No genes associated with NMO have been identified. However, a small percentage of people with this condition have a family member who is also affected, which indicates that there may be one or more genetic changes that increase susceptibility. It is thought that the inheritance of this condition is complex and that many environmental and genetic factors are involved in the development of the condition.

The aquaporin-4 protein (AQP4), a normal protein in the body, plays a role in NMO. The AQP4 is found in several body systems but is most abundant in tissues of the CNS. Approximately 70 percent of people with this disorder produce an immune protein called an "antibody" that attaches (binds) to the AQP4. Antibodies normally bind to specific foreign particles and germs, marking them for destruction, but the antibody in people with NMO attacks a normal human protein; this type of antibody is called an "autoantibody." The autoantibody in this condition is called "neuromyelitis optica immunoglobulin G" (NMO-IgG) or "anti-AQP4."

The binding of the NMO-IgG autoantibody to the AQP4 turns on (activates) the complement system, which is a group of immune system proteins that work together to destroy pathogens, trigger inflammation, and remove debris from cells and tissues. Complement activation leads to the inflammation of the optic nerve and spinal cord that is characteristic of NMO, resulting in the signs and symptoms of the condition.

The levels of the NMO-IgG autoantibody are high during episodes of NMO, and the levels decrease between episodes with the treatment for the disorder. However, it is unclear what triggers episodes to begin or end.

INHERITANCE OF NEUROMYELITIS OPTICA

Neuromyelitis optica is usually not inherited. Rarely, this condition is passed through generations in families, but the inheritance pattern is unknown.[2]

Section 36.3 | Uveitis

WHAT IS UVEITIS?

Uveitis is inflammation inside your eye. Inflammation usually happens when your immune system is fighting an infection. Sometimes, uveitis means your immune system is fighting an eye infection—but it can also happen when your immune system attacks healthy tissue in your eyes. Uveitis can cause problems such as pain, redness, and vision loss.

Uveitis damages the part of the eye called the "uvea"—but it often affects other parts of the eye, too. Sometimes, uveitis goes away quickly, but it can come back. And, sometimes, it is a chronic (long-term) condition. It can affect one eye or both eyes.

Uveitis can cause vision loss if it is not treated—so it is important to see your eye doctor right away if you have symptoms.

_____

[2] MedlinePlus, "Neuromyelitis Optica," National Institutes of Health (NIH), March 1, 2015. Available online. URL: https://medlineplus.gov/genetics/condition/neuromyelitis-optica. Accessed May 11, 2023.

WHAT IS THE UVEA?

The uvea is the middle layer of the eye between the sclera (white part of the eye) and the retina (light-sensitive layer at the back of the eye). It has three parts (refer to Figure 36.1):

- iris (the colored part of the eye)
- ciliary body (the part of the eye that helps the lens focus)
- choroid (the part of the eye that connects the retina to the sclera)

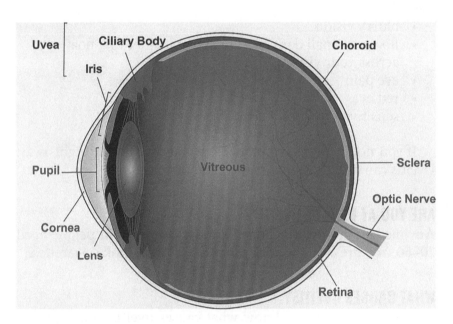

Figure 36.1. Parts of Eye

National Institutes of Health (NIH)

WHAT ARE THE TYPES OF UVEITIS?

The following are the different types of uveitis that affect different parts of the eye:

- **Anterior uveitis.** It affects the iris at the front of the eye. It is the most common type, and it is usually less serious.

- **Intermediate uveitis**. It affects the ciliary body and the vitreous (gel-like fluid that fills the eye).
- **Posterior uveitis**. It affects the retina and the choroid at the back of the eye.
- **Panuveitis**. It affects all parts of the uvea, from the front to the back of the eye.

WHAT ARE THE SYMPTOMS OF UVEITIS?

Early uveitis symptoms usually start suddenly. Symptoms include the following:
- blurry vision
- floaters (small dark spots or squiggly lines that float across your vision)
- eye pain
- red eyes
- sensitivity to light

If you notice these symptoms, see your eye doctor right away. Uveitis can cause vision loss if you do not treat it.

ARE YOU AT RISK OF UVEITIS?

Anyone can get uveitis, but it is most common in people aged 20–60. You are at higher risk for uveitis if you smoke cigarettes.

WHAT CAUSES UVEITIS?

Doctors do not always know what causes uveitis, but there are several known causes.

Sometimes, uveitis is caused by autoimmune diseases, such as the following:
- acquired immunodeficiency syndrome (AIDS)
- ankylosing spondylitis
- Behcet's disease
- lupus
- multiple sclerosis (MS)
- psoriasis

- rheumatoid arthritis (RA)
- sarcoidosis
- ulcerative colitis
- Vogt-Koyanagi-Harada (VKH) disease

Sometimes, it is caused by an infection or a condition related to an infection, such as the following:
- cytomegalovirus (CMV) retinitis
- histoplasmosis
- reactive arthritis
- shingles
- syphilis
- toxoplasmosis

Uveitis can also be caused by cancers that can affect the eye, like lymphoma.

HOW WILL YOUR EYE DOCTOR CHECK FOR UVEITIS?
Eye doctors can check for uveitis as part of a dilated eye exam. The exam is simple and painless—your doctor will give you some eye drops to dilate (widen) your pupil and then check your eyes for uveitis and other eye problems.

Your doctor will also ask about your medical history—and may recommend some tests to see if you have an infection or another disease that can cause uveitis.

WHAT IS THE TREATMENT FOR UVEITIS?
Medicines called "steroids" can reduce inflammation in your eye. This can ease symptoms and prevent vision loss. Your eye doctor may prescribe steroids in a few different ways:
- **Eye drops**. Prescription eye drops are the most common treatment.
- **Pills**. Your eye doctor may also prescribe steroids as a pill.
- **Injections**. In some cases, your eye doctor might put the steroid in or around your eye with a small needle.

- **Implants**. If other treatments do not work, your doctor might suggest surgery to put a small device called an "implant into your eye." The implant gives you regular small doses of the steroid over time.

Steroids can have side effects and can increase your risk for cataracts and glaucoma. If you take steroids for uveitis, it is important to get regular eye exams to check for signs of these problems.

Your treatment plan will depend on several factors—such as which part of your eye is affected and other health conditions you have. For example, your doctor may prescribe medicines to help control your immune system. You can work with your doctor to find the right treatments for you.[3]

[3] "Uveitis," National Eye Institute (NEI), November 16, 2021. Available online. URL: www.nei.nih.gov/learn-about-eye-health/eye-conditions-and-diseases/uveitis. Accessed May 11, 2023.

Chapter 37 | **Autoimmune Disorders of Glands**

Chapter Contents

Section 37.1 | Addison Disease

WHAT IS ADDISON DISEASE?

Autoimmune Addison disease affects the function of the adrenal glands, which are small hormone-producing glands located on top of each kidney. It is classified as an autoimmune disorder because it results from a malfunctioning immune system that attacks the adrenal glands. As a result, the production of several hormones is disrupted, which affects many body systems.

The signs and symptoms of autoimmune Addison disease can begin at any time although they most commonly begin between ages 30 and 50. Common features of this condition include extreme tiredness (fatigue), nausea, decreased appetite, and weight loss. In addition, many affected individuals have low blood pressure (hypotension), which can lead to dizziness when standing up quickly; muscle cramps; and a craving for salty foods. A characteristic feature of autoimmune Addison disease is abnormally dark areas of skin (hyperpigmentation), especially in regions that experience a lot of friction, such as the armpits, elbows, knuckles, and palm creases. The lips and the inside lining of the mouth can also be unusually dark. Because of an imbalance of hormones involved in the development of sexual characteristics, women with this condition may lose their underarm and pubic hair.

Other signs and symptoms of autoimmune Addison disease include low levels of sugar (hypoglycemia) and sodium (hyponatremia) and high levels of potassium (hyperkalemia) in the blood. Affected individuals may also have a shortage of red blood cells (anemia) and an increase in the number of white blood cells (WBCs; lymphocytosis), particularly those known as "eosinophils (eosinophilia)."

Autoimmune Addison disease can lead to a life-threatening adrenal crisis, characterized by vomiting, abdominal pain, back or leg cramps, and severe hypotension leading to shock. The adrenal crisis is often triggered by a stressor, such as surgery, trauma, or infection.

Individuals with autoimmune Addison disease or their family members can have another autoimmune disorder, most commonly autoimmune thyroid disease or type 1 diabetes.

Other Names of This Condition
- autoimmune Addison disease
- autoimmune adrenalitis
- classic Addison disease
- primary Addison disease

FREQUENCY OF ADDISON DISEASE
Addison disease affects approximately 11–14 in 100,000 people of European descent. The autoimmune form of the disorder is the most common form in developed countries, accounting for up to 90 percent of cases.

CAUSES OF ADDISON DISEASE
The cause of autoimmune Addison disease is complex and not completely understood. A combination of environmental and genetic factors plays a role in the disorder, and changes in multiple genes are thought to affect the risk of developing the condition.

The genes that have been associated with autoimmune Addison disease participate in the body's immune response. The most commonly associated genes belong to a family of genes called the "human leukocyte antigen (HLA) complex." The HLA complex helps the immune system distinguish the body's own proteins from proteins made by foreign invaders (such as viruses and bacteria). Each HLA gene has many different normal variations, allowing each person's immune system to react to a wide range of foreign proteins. The most well-known risk factor for autoimmune Addison disease is a variant of the *HLA-DRB1* gene called "*HLA-DRB1*04:04*." This and other disease-associated HLA gene variants likely contribute to an inappropriate immune response that leads to autoimmune Addison disease although the mechanism is unknown.

Normally, the immune system responds only to proteins made by foreign invaders, not to the body's own proteins. In autoimmune

Addison disease, however, an immune response is triggered by a normal adrenal gland protein, typically a protein called "21-hydroxylase." This protein plays a key role in producing certain hormones in the adrenal glands. The prolonged immune attack triggered by 21-hydroxylase damages the adrenal glands (specifically the outer layers of the glands known collectively as the adrenal cortex), preventing hormone production. A shortage of adrenal hormones (adrenal insufficiency) disrupts several normal functions in the body, leading to hypoglycemia, hyponatremia, hypotension, muscle cramps, skin hyperpigmentation, and other features of autoimmune Addison disease.

Rarely, Addison disease is not caused by an autoimmune reaction. Other causes include infections that damage the adrenal glands, such as tuberculosis, or tumors in the adrenal glands. Addison disease can also be one of several features of other genetic conditions, including X-linked adrenoleukodystrophy and autoimmune polyglandular syndrome type 1, which are caused by mutations in other genes.

INHERITANCE PATTERN OF ADDISON DISEASE

A predisposition to developing autoimmune Addison disease is passed through generations in families, but the inheritance pattern is unknown.[1]

Section 37.2 | Graves Disease

WHAT IS GRAVES DISEASE?

Graves disease is an autoimmune disorder that can cause hyperthyroidism, or overactive thyroid. The thyroid is a small, butterfly-shaped gland in the front of your neck. Thyroid hormones control the way your body uses energy, so they affect nearly every

---

[1] MedlinePlus, "Autoimmune Addison Disease," National Institutes of Health (NIH), January 1, 2017. Available online. URL: https://medlineplus.gov/genetics/condition/autoimmune-addison-disease. Accessed May 22, 2023.

organ in your body, even the way your heart beats. With Graves disease, your immune system attacks your thyroid gland, causing it to make more thyroid hormones than your body needs. As a result, many of your body's functions speed up.

HOW COMMON IS GRAVES DISEASE?
Graves disease affects nearly 1 in 100 Americans. About four out of five cases of hyperthyroidism in the United States are caused by Graves disease.

WHO IS MORE LIKELY TO HAVE GRAVES DISEASE?
Graves disease is more common in women and people older than age 30. You are more likely to develop the disease if you:
- have a family history of Graves disease or Hashimoto disease
- have other autoimmune disorders, such as:
  - vitiligo, which causes some parts of your skin to lose color
  - autoimmune gastritis, which attacks the cells in your stomach lining
  - type 1 diabetes, which occurs when your blood glucose, also called "blood sugar," is too high
  - rheumatoid arthritis, which affects your joints and sometimes other parts of your body
- use nicotine products

WHAT ARE THE COMPLICATIONS OF GRAVES DISEASE?
Untreated, Graves disease can cause serious health problems, including the following:
- a rapid and irregular heartbeat that can lead to blood clots, stroke, heart failure, and other heart-related problems
- thinning bones, osteoporosis, and muscle problems
- problems with the menstrual cycle, fertility, and pregnancy
- eye discomfort and changes in vision

WHAT ARE THE SYMPTOMS OF GRAVES DISEASE?

Graves disease often causes symptoms of hyperthyroidism. Graves disease can also affect your eyes and skin. Symptoms can come and go over time.

Hyperthyroidism

Symptoms of hyperthyroidism can vary from person to person and may include the following:

- weight loss, despite an increased appetite
- rapid or irregular heartbeat
- nervousness, irritability, trouble sleeping, or fatigue
- shaky hands or muscle weakness
- sweating or trouble tolerating heat
- frequent bowel movements
- an enlarged thyroid gland, called a "goiter"

Eye Problems

More than one in three people with Graves disease develop an eye disease called "Graves ophthalmopathy" (GO). GO occurs when your immune system attacks the muscles and other tissues around your eyes. Symptoms can include the following:

- bulging eyes
- gritty, irritated eyes
- puffy eyes
- light sensitivity
- pressure or pain in the eyes
- blurred or double vision

These symptoms can start before or at the same time as symptoms of hyperthyroidism. Rarely, GO can develop after Graves disease has been treated. You can develop GO even if your thyroid function is normal. Most people have mild symptoms.

Skin Problems

Rarely do people with Graves disease develop a condition that causes the skin to become reddish and thick, with a rough texture. Also called "Graves dermopathy" or "pretibial myxedema," the condition usually affects your shins but can also develop on the top of your feet and other parts of your body. Most cases are mild and painless.

WHAT CAUSES GRAVES DISEASE?

Researchers are not sure why some people develop autoimmune disorders, such as Graves disease. These disorders probably develop from a combination of genes and an outside trigger, such as a virus. With Graves disease, your immune system makes an antibody called "thyroid-stimulating immunoglobulin" (TSI) that attaches to your thyroid cells. TSI acts like thyroid-stimulating hormone (TSH), a hormone made in your pituitary gland that tells your thyroid how much thyroid hormone to make. TSI causes your thyroid to make too much thyroid hormone.

HOW DO DOCTORS DIAGNOSE GRAVES DISEASE?

Your doctor will take your medical history and perform a physical exam to look for signs of Graves disease. To confirm a diagnosis of Graves disease, your doctor may order one or more of these thyroid tests:

- **Blood tests**. These tests can measure the levels of your thyroid hormones and also check for TSI.
- **Radioactive iodine uptake test**. This test measures the amount of iodine your thyroid is taking up from your bloodstream to make thyroid hormones. If your thyroid is taking up large amounts of iodine, you may have Graves disease.
- **Thyroid scan**. This test, often done together with the radioactive iodine uptake test, shows how and where iodine is distributed in your thyroid. With Graves disease, the iodine shows up throughout the gland. With other causes of hyperthyroidism, such as nodules—small lumps in the gland—the iodine shows up in a different pattern.
- **Doppler blood flow measurement**. This test, also called "Doppler ultrasound," uses sound waves to detect increased blood flow in your thyroid due

to Graves disease. Your doctor may order this test if radioactive iodine uptake is not a good option for you, such as during pregnancy or breastfeeding.

HOW DO DOCTORS TREAT GRAVES DISEASE?
Treating Hyperthyroidism

Hyperthyroidism is usually treated with medicines, radioiodine therapy, or thyroid surgery. Your doctor can help you identify the best option based on your age, health, symptoms, and other factors.

Medicines

- **Beta-blockers**. These are the drugs that block the action of substances, such as adrenaline, on nerve cells. They cause blood vessels to relax and widen.
  - Pros:
    - They can reduce symptoms—such as tremors, rapid heartbeat, and nervousness—until other treatments start working.
    - They can make you feel better within hours.
  - Cons:
    - They do not stop thyroid hormone production.
- **Antithyroid medicines**. Antithyroid therapy is the simplest way to treat hyperthyroidism. Methimazole is used most often. Propylthiouracil is often used for women during the first three months of pregnancy because methimazole can, on rare occasions, harm the fetus.
  - Pros:
    - They cause the thyroid to make less thyroid hormone.
    - Some of your symptoms may go away temporarily after taking antithyroid drugs.
  - Cons:
    - Antithyroid medicines can cause side effects, including:
      - allergic reactions, such as rashes and itching

317

- a decrease in the number of white blood cells (WBCs) in your body, which can lower resistance to infection
- liver failure, in rare cases
- Antithyroid medicines may:
  - temporarily treat symptoms but are not a permanent cure for Graves disease
  - take several weeks or months for thyroid hormone levels to move into the normal range
  - take about one to two years total average treatment time but can continue for many years

SEEK CARE RIGHT AWAY
While taking antithyroid drugs, call your doctor right away if you have any of the following symptoms:
- fatigue or weakness
- dull pain in your abdomen
- loss of appetite
- skin rash, itching, or easy bruising
- yellowing of your skin or the whites of your eyes, called "jaundice"
- fever, chills, or constant sore throat

Radioiodine Therapy
Radioiodine therapy is a common and effective treatment. You can take radioactive iodine-131 by mouth as a capsule or liquid.
- Pros:
  - Radioiodine therapy slowly destroys the cells of the thyroid gland that produce the thyroid hormone.
  - In the doses prescribed, radioiodine therapy does not affect other body tissues.
- Cons:
  - You might need more than one treatment to bring thyroid hormone levels into the normal range, but beta-blockers can control symptoms between treatments.

- Radioiodine therapy is not used for women who are pregnant or breastfeeding. It can harm the fetus' thyroid and can be passed from the mother to the child in breastmilk.
- Radioiodine therapy may worsen symptoms of GO.

Almost everyone who gets radioiodine therapy later develops hypothyroidism. But hypothyroidism is easier to treat than hyperthyroidism by taking a daily thyroid hormone medicine, and it causes fewer long-term health problems.

Thyroid Surgery

Surgery to remove part or most of the thyroid gland is used less often to treat hyperthyroidism. Sometimes, doctors use surgery to treat people with large goiters or pregnant women who cannot take antithyroid medicines.

- Pros:
  - When part of the thyroid is removed, your thyroid hormone levels may return to normal.
- Cons:
  - Thyroid surgery requires general anesthesia, which can lead to a condition called "thyroid storm"—a sudden, severe worsening of symptoms if antithyroid medicines are not taken before surgery to prevent this problem.

When part of your thyroid is removed, you may develop hypothyroidism after surgery and need to take thyroid hormone medicine. If your whole thyroid is removed, you will need to take thyroid hormone medicine for life. After surgery, your doctor will continue to check your thyroid hormone levels and will adjust your thyroid medicine dosage as needed.

Treating Graves Ophthalmopathy

- Most cases of GO are mild. The following tips may help you control mild symptoms.

- Eye drops can help relieve dry, gritty, irritated eyes.
- If your eyelids do not fully close, taping them shut at night or wearing an eye mask can help prevent dry eyes.
- If you have puffy eyelids, sleeping with your head raised may reduce swelling.
- Sunglasses can help with light sensitivity.
- Special eyeglass lenses may help reduce double vision if you have it.

If you have severe GO, your doctor may recommend:
- steroids or other medicines that reduce your body's immune response
- surgery to improve bulging eyes or correct changes to your vision
- radiation therapy to the muscles and tissues around the eyes (used rarely)

GO often improves with treatment or even resolves on its own. But it can come back or get worse. Triggers include stressful life events and smoking. Smoking makes GO worse. If you smoke or use other tobacco products, stop. Ask for help, so you do not have to do it alone. You can start by calling the National Quitline at 800-QUITNOW or 800-784-8669. For tips on quitting, go to the Smokefree.gov web page. (https://smokefree.gov).

HOW DO EATING, DIET, AND NUTRITION AFFECT GRAVES DISEASE?

Your thyroid uses iodine to make thyroid hormones. If you have Graves disease or another autoimmune thyroid disorder, you may be sensitive to harmful side effects from too much iodine in your diet. Eating foods that have large amounts of iodine—such as kelp, dulse, or other kinds of seaweed—may cause or worsen hyperthyroidism. Taking iodine supplements can have the same effect. Talk with your health-care professional about:
- what foods to limit or avoid
- any iodine supplements you take

- any cough syrups or multivitamins you take because some may contain iodine[2]

Section 37.3 | Hashimoto Disease

WHAT IS HASHIMOTO DISEASE?

Hashimoto disease is an autoimmune disorder that can cause hypothyroidism, or underactive thyroid. Rarely, the disease can cause hyperthyroidism, or overactive thyroid.

The thyroid is a small, butterfly-shaped gland in the front of your neck. People with Hashimoto disease may have the following:

- The immune system makes antibodies that attack the thyroid gland.
- Large numbers of white blood cells (WBCs), which are part of the immune system, build up in the thyroid.
- The thyroid becomes damaged and cannot make enough thyroid hormones.

Thyroid hormones control how your body uses energy, so they affect nearly every organ in your body—even the way your heart beats.

Does Hashimoto Disease Have Another Name?

Hashimoto disease is also called "Hashimoto thyroiditis," "chronic lymphocytic thyroiditis," or "autoimmune thyroiditis."

HOW COMMON IS HASHIMOTO DISEASE?

The number of people who have Hashimoto disease in the United States is unknown. However, the disease is the most common cause of hypothyroidism, which affects about 5 in 100 Americans.

---

[2] "Graves' Disease," National Institute of Diabetes and Digestive and Kidney Diseases (NIDDK), November 2021. Available online. URL: www.niddk.nih.gov/health-information/endocrine-diseases/Graves-disease. Accessed May 10, 2023.

WHO IS MORE LIKELY TO HAVE HASHIMOTO DISEASE?

Hashimoto disease is 4–10 times more common in women than in men. Although the disease may occur in teens or young women, it more often develops in women aged 30–50. Your chance of developing Hashimoto disease increases if other family members have the disease.

You are more likely to develop Hashimoto disease if you have other autoimmune disorders, including the following:

- celiac disease, a digestive disorder that damages the small intestine
- lupus, a chronic, or long-term, disorder that can affect many parts of the body
- rheumatoid arthritis, a disorder that affects the joints
- Sjögren syndrome, a disease that causes dry eyes and mouth
- type 1 diabetes, a disease that occurs when your blood glucose, also called "blood sugar," is too high

WHAT ARE THE COMPLICATIONS OF HASHIMOTO DISEASE?

Many people with Hashimoto disease develop hypothyroidism. Untreated, hypothyroidism can lead to several health problems, including the following:

- high cholesterol
- heart disease and heart failure
- high blood pressure
- myxedema, a rare condition in which the body's functions slow down to the point that it can threaten your life

Left untreated, hypothyroidism can also cause problems during pregnancy.

WHAT ARE THE SYMPTOMS OF HASHIMOTO DISEASE?

Many people with Hashimoto disease have no symptoms at first. As the disease progresses, they may have one or more of the symptoms of hypothyroidism.

Some common symptoms of hypothyroidism include the following:
- fatigue
- weight gain
- trouble tolerating cold
- joint and muscle pain
- constipation
- dry skin or dry, thinning hair
- heavy or irregular menstrual periods or fertility problems
- slowed heart rate

Hashimoto disease causes your thyroid to become damaged. Most people with Hashimoto disease develop hypothyroidism. Rarely, early in the course of the disease, thyroid damage may lead to the release of too much thyroid hormone into your blood, causing symptoms of hyperthyroidism.

Your thyroid may get larger and cause the front of the neck to look swollen. The enlarged thyroid, called a "goiter," may create a feeling of fullness in your throat though it is usually not painful. After many years, or even decades, damage to the thyroid may cause the gland to shrink and the goiter to disappear.

WHAT CAUSES HASHIMOTO DISEASE?

Researchers do not know why some people develop Hashimoto disease, but a family history of thyroid disease is common. Several factors may play a role, including the following:
- genes
- viruses, such as hepatitis C

Hypothyroidism can also be caused by the following:
- some medicines used to treat bipolar disorder or other mental health problems
- iodine-containing medicines used to treat abnormal heart rhythm
- exposure to toxins, such as nuclear radiation

HOW DO DOCTORS DIAGNOSE HASHIMOTO DISEASE?

Doctors diagnose Hashimoto disease based on the following:

- **Medical history and physical exam**. Your doctor will start by taking a medical history and performing a physical exam. In addition to asking about symptoms, the doctor will check your neck for a goiter, which some people with Hashimoto disease can develop.
- **Blood tests**. Your doctor will order one or more blood tests to check for hypothyroidism and its causes. Examples include tests for:
  - the thyroid hormones T4 (thyroxine) and T3 (triiodothyronine)
  - thyroid-stimulating hormone (TSH)
  - thyroid peroxidase antibodies (TPO), a type of thyroid antibody that is present in most people with Hashimoto disease

You probably will not need other tests to confirm you have Hashimoto disease. However, if your doctor suspects Hashimoto disease but you do not have antithyroid antibodies in your blood, you may have an ultrasound of your thyroid. The ultrasound images can show the size of your thyroid and other features of Hashimoto disease. The ultrasound can also rule out other causes of an enlarged thyroid, such as thyroid nodules—small lumps in the thyroid gland.

HOW DO DOCTORS TREAT HASHIMOTO DISEASE?

How your doctors treat Hashimoto disease usually depends on whether the thyroid is damaged enough to cause hypothyroidism. If you do not have hypothyroidism, your doctor may choose to simply check your symptoms and thyroid hormone levels regularly.

The medicine levothyroxine, which is identical to the natural thyroid hormone thyroxine (T4), is the recommended way to treat hypothyroidism. Prescribed in pill form for many years, this medicine is now also available as a liquid and in a soft gel capsule. These newer formulas may be helpful to people with digestive problems that affect how the thyroid hormone pill is absorbed.

Some foods and supplements can affect how well your body absorbs levothyroxine. Examples include grapefruit juice, espresso coffee, soy, and multivitamins that contain iron or calcium. Taking the medicine on an empty stomach can prevent this from happening. Your doctor may ask you to take levothyroxine in the morning, 30–60 minutes before you eat your first meal.

Your doctor will give you a blood test about six to eight weeks after you begin taking the medicine and adjust your dose if needed. Each time you change your dose, you will have another blood test. Once you have reached a dose that is working for you, your doctor will likely repeat the blood test in six months and then once a year.

Never stop taking your medicine or take a higher dose without talking with your doctor first. Taking too much thyroid hormone medicine can cause serious problems, such as atrial fibrillation or osteoporosis. Your hypothyroidism can be well-controlled with thyroid hormone medicine, as long as you take the medicine as instructed by your doctor and have regular follow-up blood tests.

HOW DO EATING, DIET, AND NUTRITION AFFECT HASHIMOTO DISEASE?

The thyroid uses iodine, a mineral in some foods, to make thyroid hormones. However, if you have Hashimoto disease or other types of autoimmune thyroid disorders, you may be sensitive to harmful side effects from iodine. Eating foods that have large amounts of iodine—such as kelp, dulse, or other kinds of seaweed and certain iodine-rich medicines—may cause hypothyroidism or make it worse. Taking iodine supplements can have the same effect.

Talk with members of your health-care team about:
- what foods and beverages to limit or avoid
- whether you take iodine supplements
- any cough syrups you take that may contain iodine

However, if you are pregnant, you need to take enough iodine because the baby gets iodine from your diet. Too much iodine can cause problems as well, such as a goiter in the baby. If you are pregnant, talk with your doctor about how much iodine you need.

Researchers are looking at other ways in which diet and supplements—such as vitamin D and selenium—may affect Hashimoto disease. However, no specific guidance is currently available.[3]

Section 37.4 | Sjögren Syndrome

WHAT IS SJÖGREN SYNDROME?

Sjögren syndrome is a chronic (long-lasting) autoimmune disorder that happens when the immune system attacks the glands that make moisture in the eyes, mouth, and other parts of the body. The main symptoms are dry eyes and mouth, but other parts of the body may be affected as well, with many people reporting fatigue and joint and muscle pain. In addition, the disease can damage the lungs, kidneys, and nervous system. Sjögren syndrome predominantly affects women.

WHO GETS SJÖGREN SYNDROME?

Most people with Sjögren syndrome are women. People can get it at any age, but it is most common in people in their 40s and 50s. It occurs across all racial and ethnic backgrounds.

TYPES OF SJÖGREN SYNDROME

Doctors divide Sjögren syndrome into the following two categories:
- **Primary form**. You have this form if you do not have another rheumatic disease.
- **Secondary form**. You have this form if you also have another rheumatic disease, such as rheumatoid arthritis, systemic lupus erythematosus (SLE), scleroderma, or polymyositis.

---

[3] "Hashimoto's Disease," National Institute of Diabetes and Digestive and Kidney Diseases (NIDDK), June 2021. Available online. URL: www.niddk.nih.gov/health-information/endocrine-diseases/hashimotos-disease. Accessed May 10, 2023.

SYMPTOMS OF SJÖGREN SYNDROME

Sjögren syndrome may have different effects on the body, and the symptoms vary from person to person. In some people, symptoms cycle between mild and severe.

The classic symptoms are as follows:

- **Dry eyes**. Your eyes may burn or itch or feel like they have sand in them. Sometimes, the dryness causes blurry vision or sensitivity to bright light. You may get irritated, itchy eyelids due to inflammation.
- **Dry mouth**. Your mouth may feel chalky, and you may have trouble swallowing, speaking, and tasting. Because you lack the protective effects of saliva, you may develop more dental decay (cavities) and mouth infections, such as candidiasis (also called "thrush").

In some people, the main problem is dry mouth, while for others, it is dry eyes, and some people experience both problems equally. In some cases, Sjögren syndrome affects other tissues and organs and has more widespread effects on the body. These other effects may cause the following:

- acid reflux
- dry nasal passages and throat and a dry cough
- dry skin
- fatigue
- joint pain
- muscle aches
- muscle weakness
- numbness, tingling, and weakness, especially in the extremities
- poor concentration and memory problems
- shortness of breath or trouble breathing
- skin rashes
- swelling of the glands around the face and neck
- trouble sleeping
- vaginal dryness

The symptoms can be severe, with some people reporting debilitating pain and fatigue. People with Sjögren syndrome have a higher chance of developing a type of cancer called "lymphoma," but the risk of developing it is low.

CAUSES OF SJÖGREN SYNDROME

Sjögren syndrome is an autoimmune disorder that happens when the immune system attacks healthy tissues. Normally, the immune system protects the body from infection and disease.

Researchers do not know what causes the immune system to turn on the body, but they believe that both genetic and environmental factors are involved. Studies have linked Sjögren syndrome to variants (changes) in several genes, many of which are involved in immunity.

In Sjögren syndrome, the immune system attacks the glands that make tears and saliva. The resulting inflammation damages the glands, limiting their production of the fluids that normally keep the eyes and mouth moist. In some cases, the immune system attacks additional parts of the body, damaging other organs and tissues and causing a range of other symptoms.

DIAGNOSIS OF SJÖGREN SYNDROME

There is no single test for Sjögren syndrome, so doctors will typically ask about your symptoms and conduct a series of tests to diagnose the disorder. A rheumatologist (a specialist in autoimmune diseases) may diagnose the disease. However, an ophthalmologist (eye doctor) or a dentist may also perform certain tests to help make the diagnosis. The diagnosis is based on how well the tear and salivary glands are working and whether there is evidence of autoimmunity.

To diagnose Sjögren syndrome, your doctor may ask about your medical history, including about dryness in your eyes and mouth, such as when it started and whether you feel it every day. Your doctor may also order the following tests:

- **Eye test**. It is to see if you produce a normal amount of tears and to find out if there has been any damage to your eyes due to dryness.
- **Salivary gland test**. It can measure how much saliva your mouth produces. Ultrasound imaging and biopsy

can help determine if the salivary gland tissues are altered by inflammation.

- **Blood test**. It can identify antibodies that are typically present in people with Sjögren syndrome and other autoimmune disorders. While the presence of these antibodies can help doctors diagnose Sjögren syndrome, this alone cannot diagnose the disorder because these antibodies may be present in healthy individuals and people with other disorders as well.

Your doctor may order other laboratory or imaging tests to determine if another disease or problem is causing your symptoms.

TREATMENT FOR SJÖGREN SYNDROME

There is no cure for Sjögren syndrome, so treatment focuses on relieving symptoms and preventing complications. Treatments are different for each person and will depend on which parts of your body are affected. Your treatment plan will likely include a combination of self-management approaches and over-the-counter (OTC) and prescription medications. Be sure to tell your doctor which medications you are currently taking because some make eye and mouth dryness worse.

Eye Treatments

- **Eye drops (artificial tears)**. There are many different types of eye drops, and you may have to try a few to find the one that works best for you. Some people need prescription eye drops that contain medications to suppress the immune system and reduce inflammation in the eye.
- **Eye ointments**. These are thicker than eye drops and keep the eyes wet for several hours. They can blur your vision, so most people use them while they sleep.
- **Plugs to block the tear ducts**. Small plugs placed in the tear duct in the corners of the eyes block drainage and keep tears in the eyes longer. The procedure only takes a few minutes and is done in the office of an ophthalmologist (eye doctor).

Mouth Treatments

- **Artificial saliva.** Using a saliva substitute prescribed by a doctor helps make the mouth feel wet.
- **Saliva production stimulators.** These medications cause salivary glands to make more saliva. These medications also stimulate tear production.
- **Antifungal medications.** These medications treat fungal infections, such as candidiasis (also called "thrush"), which are more common in people with dry mouths.

Treatments for Other Problems Related to Sjögren Syndrome

- **OTC or prescribed pain relievers.** These medicines alleviate joint and muscle pain and discomfort from swollen glands.
- **Disease-modifying antirheumatic drugs (DMARDs) and antimalarial drugs.** These drugs are often prescribed to people with joint pain, rashes, and other serious effects of the disease. While these medicines have not specifically been approved for Sjögren syndrome, they may be helpful in some people with the disorder.
- **Corticosteroids.** These medications help control inflammation and pain. Because they are potent drugs, your doctor will prescribe the lowest dose possible to achieve the desired benefit. They are usually reserved for people with rare, serious effects of the disorder.
- **Acid reflux medications.** Reduced saliva production may raise the stomach's acidity in people with Sjögren syndrome. Some people may take these medicines to counteract this effect.

WHO TREATS SJÖGREN SYNDROME?

Sjögren syndrome is primarily treated by:

- **Rheumatologists.** These are doctors who treat diseases of the joints, muscles, and bones. Rheumatologists are also specialists in autoimmune diseases.

Other specialists who may be involved in your care include the following:

- dentists, who care for your gums and teeth
- mental health professionals, who can help people cope with difficulties in the home and workplace that may result from their medical conditions
- nephrologists, who treat kidney disease problems
- neurologists, who specialize in treating diseases of the nervous system, which includes the brain and spinal cord
- ophthalmologists, who specialize in the care of the eyes
- otolaryngologists, who specialize in caring for the ears, nose, and throat
- primary care doctors, such as family physicians or internal medicine specialists, who coordinate care between the different health-care providers and treat other problems as they arise
- pulmonologists, who specialize in treating diseases of the lungs

LIVING WITH SJÖGREN SYNDROME

The symptoms of Sjögren syndrome can largely be managed, and most people can expect to live a normal life. The following tips can make living with Sjögren syndrome easier.

Caring for Your Eyes

- Protect your eyes from drafts, breezes, and smoky rooms.
- Have your glasses fitted with shields on the sides or use wraparound glasses.
- Do not use eye drops that irritate your eyes. If one brand or prescription bothers you, try another. Eye drops that do not contain preservatives are usually essential if you use them four or more times per day on a regular basis.
- Put humidifiers in the rooms where you spend the most time, including the bedroom, or install a humidifier in your heating and air-conditioning unit.

331

- If you get blepharitis (eyelid inflammation), use warm compresses on your eyes to alleviate the discomfort. You may also gently wash the eyelids with a dilute solution of a mild detergent such as baby shampoo.

Caring for Your Mouth

- Brush and floss your teeth regularly. There are some toothpaste designed for people with dry mouths. Most people should use toothpaste with fluoride to help prevent cavities.
- Carry a water bottle and sip on it throughout the day to keep your mouth moist. Keeping hydrated will also help combat dry eyes.
- Chewing gum or sucking on hard candy helps your glands make more saliva. Try to use sugar-free gum and candy.
- Visit a dentist at least twice a year to have your teeth examined and cleaned. Ask your dentist about fluoride treatments.
- See your doctor or dentist if you have symptoms of candidiasis (also called "thrush"), such as burning, soreness, and white patches inside your mouth.

Managing Other Sjögren Syndrome-Related Symptoms

- Moisturize other dry areas.
- For dry skin, moisturize your skin regularly, especially with products made for extra dry skin.
- Use lip balms, such as those containing petroleum jelly, for dry lips.
- Use products such as vaginal moisturizers or estrogen creams for vaginal dryness.
- Use saline sprays to help with dry nose.
- Educate yourself and get support.
- Learn as much as you can about the syndrome and talk with others who are dealing with it by joining a support group. Having a support network can help you manage difficult times.

- Having a long-term condition can be challenging, so visit a mental health professional if emotional problems arise.
- Maintain a healthy weight and watch what you eat to help control acid reflux. Eat slowly and avoid common triggers such as fried and fatty foods, tomato sauce, and onions.
- Eat a healthy and balanced diet and exercise regularly to help combat fatigue and to help you sleep better. Check with your doctor before beginning an exercise routine.

Remember to visit your health-care providers regularly and follow their recommendations.[4]

Section 37.5 | Type 1 Diabetes

WHAT IS TYPE 1 DIABETES?

Diabetes occurs when your blood glucose, also called "blood sugar," is too high. Blood glucose is your main source of energy and comes mainly from the food you eat. Insulin, a hormone made by the pancreas, helps the glucose in your blood get into your cells to be used for energy. Another hormone, glucagon, works with insulin to control blood glucose levels.

In most people with type 1 diabetes, the body's immune system, which normally fights infection, attacks and destroys the cells in the pancreas that make insulin. As a result, your pancreas stops making insulin. Without insulin, glucose cannot get into your cells, and your blood glucose rises above normal. People with type 1 diabetes need to take insulin every day to stay alive.

WHO IS MORE LIKELY TO DEVELOP TYPE 1 DIABETES?

Type 1 diabetes typically occurs in children and young adults although it can appear at any age. Having a parent or sibling with

---

[4] "Sjögren's Syndrome," National Institute of Arthritis and Musculoskeletal and Skin Diseases (NIAMS), January 2021. Available online. URL: www.niams.nih.gov/health-topics/sjogrens-syndrome. Accessed May 10, 2023.

the disease may increase your chance of developing type 1 diabetes. In the United States, about 5 percent of people with diabetes have type 1.

WHAT ARE THE SYMPTOMS OF TYPE 1 DIABETES?

Symptoms of type 1 diabetes are serious and usually happen quickly, over a few days to weeks. Symptoms can include:

- increased thirst and urination
- increased hunger
- blurred vision
- fatigue
- unexplained weight loss

Sometimes, the first symptoms of type 1 diabetes are signs of a life-threatening condition called "diabetic ketoacidosis" (DKA). Some symptoms of DKA are as follows:

- breath that smells fruity
- dry or flushed skin
- nausea or vomiting
- stomach pain
- trouble breathing
- trouble paying attention or feeling confused

WHAT CAUSES TYPE 1 DIABETES?

Experts think type 1 diabetes is caused by genes and factors in the environment, such as viruses, that might trigger the disease.

HOW DO HEALTH-CARE PROFESSIONALS DIAGNOSE TYPE 1 DIABETES?

Health-care professionals usually test people for type 1 diabetes if they have clear-cut diabetes symptoms. Health-care professionals most often use the random plasma glucose (RPG) test to diagnose type 1 diabetes. This blood test measures your blood glucose level at a single point in time. Sometimes, health professionals also use the A1C blood test to find out how long someone has had high blood glucose.

Even though these tests can confirm that you have diabetes, they cannot identify what type you have. Treatment depends on the type of diabetes, so knowing whether you have type 1 or type 2 is important.

To find out if your diabetes is type 1, your health-care professional may test your blood for certain autoantibodies. Autoantibodies are antibodies that attack your healthy tissues and cells by mistake. The presence of certain types of autoantibodies is common in type 1 but not in type 2 diabetes.

Because type 1 diabetes can run in families, your health-care professional can test your family members for autoantibodies. The presence of autoantibodies, even without diabetes symptoms, means the family member is more likely to develop type 1 diabetes. If you have a brother or sister, child, or parent with type 1 diabetes, you may want to get an autoantibody test. People aged 20 or younger who have a cousin, aunt, uncle, niece, nephew, grandparent, or half-sibling with type 1 diabetes may also want to get tested.

WHAT MEDICINES DO YOU NEED TO TREAT YOUR TYPE 1 DIABETES?

If you have type 1 diabetes, you must take insulin because your body no longer makes this hormone. Different types of insulin start to work at different speeds, and the effects of each last a different length of time. You may need to use more than one type. You can take insulin in a number of ways. Common options include a needle and syringe, insulin pen, or insulin pump.

Some people who have trouble reaching their blood glucose targets with insulin alone might also need to take another type of diabetes medicine that works with insulin, such as pramlintide. Pramlintide, given by injection, helps keep blood glucose levels from going too high after eating. Few people with type 1 diabetes take pramlintide, however.

Hypoglycemia, or low blood sugar, can occur if you take insulin but do not match your dose with your food or physical activity. Severe hypoglycemia can be dangerous and needs to be treated right away.

HOW ELSE CAN YOU MANAGE TYPE 1 DIABETES?

Along with insulin and any other medicines you use, you can manage your diabetes by taking care of yourself each day. Following your diabetes meal plan, being physically active, and checking your blood glucose often are some of the ways you can take care of yourself. Work with your health-care team to come up with a diabetes care plan that works for you. If you are planning a pregnancy with diabetes, try to get your blood glucose levels in your target range before you get pregnant.

DO YOU HAVE OTHER TREATMENT OPTIONS FOR YOUR TYPE 1 DIABETES?

The National Institute of Diabetes and Digestive and Kidney Diseases (NIDDK) has played an important role in developing "artificial pancreas" technology. An artificial pancreas replaces manual blood glucose testing and the use of insulin shots. A single system monitors blood glucose levels around the clock and provides insulin or a combination of insulin and glucagon automatically. The system can also be monitored remotely, for example, by parents or medical staff.

In 2016, the U.S. Food and Drug Administration (FDA) approved a type of artificial pancreas system called a "hybrid closed-loop system." This system tests your glucose level every five minutes throughout the day and night through a continuous glucose monitor and automatically gives you the right amount of basal insulin, long-acting insulin, through a separate insulin pump. You still need to manually adjust the amount of insulin the pump delivers at mealtimes and when you need a correction dose. You will also need to test your blood with a glucose meter several times a day. Talk with your health-care provider about whether this system might be right for you.

An artificial pancreas system uses a continuous glucose monitor, an insulin pump, and a control algorithm to give you the right amount of basal insulin.

The continuous glucose monitor sends information through a software program called "control algorithm." Based on your glucose level, the algorithm tells the insulin pump how much insulin to deliver. The software program could be installed on the pump or another device such as a cell phone or computer.

Pancreatic islets are clusters of cells in the pancreas that make insulin. Type 1 diabetes attacks these cells. A pancreatic islet transplant replaces destroyed islets with ones that make and release insulin. This procedure takes islets from the pancreas of an organ donor and transfers them to a person with type 1 diabetes.

WHAT HEALTH PROBLEMS CAN PEOPLE WITH TYPE 1 DIABETES DEVELOP?

Over time, high blood glucose leads to problems such as:
- dental disease
- depression
- eye problems
- foot problems
- heart disease
- kidney disease
- nerve damage
- sleep apnea
- stroke

If you have type 1 diabetes, you can help prevent or delay the health problems of diabetes by managing your blood glucose, blood pressure, and cholesterol and following your self-care plan.

CAN YOU LOWER YOUR CHANCE OF DEVELOPING TYPE 1 DIABETES?

At this time, type 1 diabetes cannot be prevented. However, through studies such as TrialNet, researchers are working to identify possible ways to prevent or slow down the disease.[5]

---

[5] "Type 1 Diabetes," National Institute of Diabetes and Digestive and Kidney Diseases (NIDDK), July 2017. Available online. URL: www.niddk.nih.gov/health-information/diabetes/overview/what-is-diabetes/type-1-diabetes. Accessed May 22, 2023.

Chapter 38 | Guillain-Barré Syndrome

WHAT IS GUILLAIN-BARRÉ SYNDROME?

Guillain-Barré syndrome (GBS) is a rare neurological disorder in which your immune system mistakenly attacks part of the peripheral nervous system (PNS)—the network of nerves located outside of the brain and spinal cord. GBS can range from a very mild case with brief weakness to nearly devastating paralysis, leaving you unable to breathe independently. Fortunately, most people eventually recover from even the most severe cases of GBS. After recovery, some people will continue to have some degree of weakness.

GBS can increase in intensity over a period of hours, days, or weeks until certain muscles cannot be used at all, and when severe, the person is almost totally paralyzed. In these cases, the disorder is life-threatening—potentially interfering with breathing and, at times, with blood pressure or heart rate.

SYMPTOMS OF GUILLAIN-BARRÉ SYNDROME

- **Weakness.** The weakness seen in GBS usually comes on quickly and worsens over hours or days. Symptoms are usually equal on both sides of the body (called "symmetric"). You may first notice weakness as difficulty climbing stairs or with walking. Symptoms often affect the arms, breathing muscles, and even the face, reflecting more widespread nerve damage. Occasionally symptoms start in the upper body and move down to the legs and feet. Muscles controlling breathing can weaken to the point that you might need a machine to help you breathe. Most people reach the greatest stage of weakness within the first two weeks after symptoms appear; by the third

339

week, 90 percent of affected individuals are at their weakest.

- **Sensation changes**. Since nerves are damaged in GBS, your brain may receive abnormal sensory signals from the rest of your body. This results in unexplained, spontaneous sensations, called "paresthesias," that you may feel as tingling, a sense of insects crawling under the skin (called "formications"), and pain. Deep muscular pain may be experienced in the back and/or legs. Unexplained sensations often occur first, such as tingling in the feet or hands, or even pain (especially in children), often starting in the legs or back. Children will also show symptoms of difficulty walking and may refuse to walk. These sensations tend to disappear before the major, longer-term symptoms appear.

Other symptoms may include the following:

- difficulty with eye muscles and vision
- difficulty swallowing, speaking, or chewing
- pricking or pins and needles sensations in the hands and feet
- pain that can be severe, particularly at night
- coordination problems and unsteadiness
- abnormal heartbeat/rate or blood pressure
- problems with digestion and/or bladder control

WHO IS MORE LIKELY TO GET GUILLAIN-BARRÉ SYNDROME?

Guillain-Barré syndrome can affect anyone. It can strike at any age (although it is more frequent in adults and older people), and both sexes are equally prone to the disorder. GBS is estimated to affect about one person in 100,000 each year. It is not contagious or inherited.

The exact cause of GBS is not known. Researchers do not know why it strikes some people and not others.

What they do know is that the affected person's immune system begins to attack the body itself. It may be this immune attack starts as a fight against an infection and that some chemicals on infecting bacteria and viruses resemble those on nerve cells, which, in turn, also become targets of attack. Since the body's own immune system does the damage, GBS is called an "autoimmune disease" ("auto" meaning "self"). Normally the immune system uses antibodies (molecules produced in an immune response) and special white blood cells (WBCs) to protect us by attacking infecting micro-organisms (bacteria and viruses). In GBS, however, the immune system mistakenly attacks the healthy nerves.

Many of the body's nerves are like household wires. There is a central conducting core in the nerves called the "axon" that carries an electric signal. The axon (an extension of a nerve cell) is sur-rounded by a covering, like insulation, called "myelin." The myelin sheath surrounding the axon speeds up the transmission of nerve signals and allows the transmission of signals over long distances.

In most cases of GBS, the immune system damages the myelin sheath that surrounds the axons of many peripheral nerves; how-ever, it may also damage the axons themselves. As a result, the nerves cannot transmit signals efficiently, and the muscles begin to lose their ability to respond to the brain's commands. This causes weakness.

Most GBS cases usually start a few days or weeks following a respiratory or gastrointestinal viral infection. Occasionally sur-gery will trigger the syndrome. In rare cases, vaccinations may increase the risk of GBS (there have been reports of a few people who received a vaccine for the severe acute respiratory syndrome coronavirus 2 (SARS-CoV-2) developing GBS, but the chance of this occurring is very low). Some countries worldwide reported an increased incidence of GBS following infection with the Zika virus.

DIAGNOSING GUILLAIN-BARRÉ SYNDROME

The initial signs and symptoms of GBS are varied, and there are several disorders with similar symptoms. Therefore, doctors may find it difficult to diagnose GBS in its earliest stages and may per-form the following tests:

- **Physical exam.** Your physician will look at your physical symptoms, ask about your medical history, and conduct exams to assess how your muscles and nerves are functioning. Your physician or a specialist will note whether your symptoms appear on both sides of the body (the typical finding in GBS) and the speed with which the symptoms appear (in other disorders, muscle weakness may progress over months rather than days or weeks). Your reflexes will also be checked: In GBS, deep tendon reflexes in the legs, such as knee jerks, are usually lost. Reflexes may also be absent in the arms.

- **Nerve conduction velocity (NCV) test**. This test measures the nerve's ability to send a signal. In GBS, the signals traveling along the damaged nerves are slow, and this can provide clues to aid the diagnosis.
- **Cerebrospinal fluid analysis**. Your doctor may also remove and have analyzed a small sample of the cerebrospinal fluid that bathes the spinal cord since the fluid in people with GBS contains more protein than usual but very few immune cells (measured by WBCs).

Key diagnostic findings include the following:
- recent onset, within days to at most four weeks of symmetric weakness, usually starting in the legs
- abnormal sensations such as pain, numbness, and tingling in the feet that accompany or even occur before weakness
- absent or diminished deep tendon reflexes in weak limbs
- elevated cerebrospinal fluid protein without elevated cell count (This may take up to 10 days from the onset of symptoms to develop.)
- abnormal nerve conduction velocity findings, such as slow signal conduction
- sometimes, a recent viral infection or diarrhea

TREATING GUILLAIN-BARRÉ SYNDROME

There is no known cure for GBS. However, some therapies can lessen the severity of the illness and shorten your recovery time. There are also several ways to treat the complications of the disease.

If you have GBS, you are usually admitted to and treated in the hospital's intensive care unit due to possible complications of muscle weakness, problems that can affect any paralyzed person (such as pneumonia or bed sores), and the need for sophisticated medical equipment.

Acute Care

There are currently two treatments commonly used to interrupt immune-related nerve damage. Both are equally effective if started within two weeks of GBS symptoms:

- Plasma exchange (PE), also called "plasmapheresis," involves removing some of your blood through a catheter. The blood cells from the liquid part of the blood (plasma) are extracted and treated and returned to your body. Plasma contains antibodies, and PE removes some plasma; PE may work by removing the antibodies that have been damaging the nerves.
- Intravenous immunoglobulin (IVIg) therapy involves intravenous injections of immunoglobulins— proteins that your immune system naturally makes to attack infecting organisms. The immunoglobulins are developed from a pool of thousands of healthy donors. IVIg therapy can lessen the immune attack on the nervous system and shorten recovery time. Investigators believe this treatment also lowers the levels or effectiveness of antibodies that attack the nerves by both "diluting" them with nonspecific antibodies and providing antibodies that bind to the harmful antibodies and take them out of commission.

Anti-inflammatory steroid hormones called "corticosteroids" have also been tried to reduce the severity of GBS, but controlled clinical trials showed this treatment is not effective.

Supportive care is very important to address the many complications of paralysis as your body recovers and damaged nerves begin to heal. Since respiratory failure can occur in GBS, your breathing should be closely monitored. Sometimes, a mechanical ventilator is used to help support or control breathing. The autonomic nervous system (that regulates the functions of internal organs and some of the muscles in your body) can also be disturbed, causing changes in heart rate, blood pressure, toileting, or sweating, so you should be put on a heart monitor or equipment that measures and tracks body function. You may also need help with any difficulty from secretions in the mouth and throat. In addition to choking and/or drooling, secretions can fall into your airway and cause pneumonia.

Rehabilitative Care

As you begin to improve, you may be transferred from the acute care hospital to a rehabilitation setting. Here, you can regain strength, receive physical rehabilitation and other therapy to resume activities of daily living, and prepare to return to pre-illness life.

Because GBS can affect several parts of your body, you may need different methods and approaches to prevent or treat complications. For example, you may need a physical therapist to manually move and position your limbs to help keep the muscles flexible and prevent muscle shortening. Injections of blood thinners can help prevent dangerous blood clots from forming in leg veins. Inflatable cuffs may also be placed around your legs to provide intermittent compression. All or any of these methods helps prevent blood stagnation and sludging (the buildup of red blood cells (RBCs) in veins), which could lead to reduced blood flow in the leg veins. Muscle strength may not return uniformly; some muscles that get stronger faster may tend to take over a function that weaker muscles normally perform—called "substitution." A physical therapist can select specific exercises to improve the strength of weaker muscles, so their original function can be regained.

Occupational and vocational therapy helps you learn new ways to handle everyday functions that may be affected by the disease, as well as work demands and the need for assistive devices and other adaptive equipment and technology.[1]

---

[1] "Guillain-Barré Syndrome," National Institute of Neurological Disorders and Stroke (NINDS), March 8, 2023. Available online. URL: www.ninds.nih.gov/health-information/disorders/guillain-barre-syndrome. Accessed May 12, 2023.

Chapter 39 | **Inflammatory Myopathies**

Chapter Contents

Section 39.1 | Inflammatory Myopathies: An Overview

WHAT ARE INFLAMMATORY MYOPATHIES?

Inflammatory myopathies are a group of diseases, with no known cause, that involve chronic muscle inflammation accompanied by muscle weakness. The majority of these disorders are considered to be autoimmune disorders, in which the body's immune response system that normally defends against infection and disease attacks its own muscle fibers, blood vessels, connective tissue, organs, or joints. These rare disorders may affect both adults and children.

The four main types of chronic, or long-term, inflammatory myopathies are:

- polymyositis, which affects skeletal muscles (involved with making movement)
- dermatomyositis, which includes a skin rash and progressive muscle weakness
- inclusion body myositis (IBM), which is characterized by progressive muscle weakness and shrinkage
- necrotizing autoimmune myopathy, with weakness in the upper and lower body, difficulty rising from low chairs or climbing stairs, fatigue, and muscle pain

SYMPTOMS OF INFLAMMATORY MYOPATHIES

The general symptoms of chronic inflammatory myopathy include progressive muscle weakness that starts in the proximal muscles, those muscles closest to the trunk of the body. Other symptoms include fatigue after walking or standing, tripping or falling, and difficulty swallowing or breathing. Polymyositis and dermato-myositis are more common in women than in men. IBM is most common after the age of 50. Dermatomyositis is more common in children.

TREATMENT FOR INFLAMMATORY MYOPATHIES

Chronic inflammatory myopathies cannot be cured in most adults, but many of the symptoms can be treated. Options include medication, physical therapy, and rest. Polymyositis, dermato-myositis, and necrotizing autoimmune myopathy are first treated with high doses of corticosteroid drugs such as prednisone. Immunosuppressant drugs may reduce inflammation in individuals who do not respond well to prednisone. Injections of adrenocorticotropic hormone gel may be another option for people who do not respond to or cannot tolerate other drug treatment options. Physical therapy is usually recommended to prevent muscle atrophy as well as to maintain muscle strength and range of motion. Some individuals may use a topical cream to treat skin problems associated with the disorder. IBM has no standard course of treatment.

PROGNOSIS OF INFLAMMATORY MYOPATHIES

Most cases of dermatomyositis respond to therapy. Approximately one-third of individuals with juvenile-onset dermatomyositis recover from their illness; one-third have a relapsing-remitting course of disease; and the other third have a more chronic course of illness. The prognosis for polymyositis varies. Most individuals respond fairly well to therapy, but some people have a more severe disease that does not respond adequately to therapies and may have a significant disability. IBM is generally resistant to all therapies, and its rate of progression appears to be unaffected by currently available treatments. Necrotizing autoimmune myopathy generally responds well to long-term combination immunosuppressive therapies.[1]

[1] "Inflammatory Myopathies," National Institute of Neurological Disorders and Stroke (NINDS), April 25, 2022. Available online. URL: www.ninds.nih.gov/health-information/disorders/inflammatory-myopathies. Accessed June 14, 2023.

Section 39.2 | **Dermatomyositis**

Dermatomyositis is one of a group of acquired muscle diseases called "inflammatory myopathies" (a disorder of muscle tissue or muscles), which are characterized by chronic muscle inflammation accompanied by muscle weakness. The cardinal symptom is a skin rash that precedes or accompanies progressive muscle weakness. Dermatomyositis may occur at any age, but it is most common in adults in their late 40s to early 60s or children between 5 and 15 years of age. There is no cure for dermatomyositis, but the symptoms can be treated. The options include medication, physical therapy, exercise, heat therapy (including microwave and ultrasound), orthotics and assistive devices, and rest.

SYMPTOMS OF DERMATOMYOSITIS

The signs and symptoms of dermatomyositis may appear suddenly or develop gradually, over weeks or months. The cardinal symptom of dermatomyositis is a skin rash that precedes or accompanies progressive muscle weakness. The rash looks patchy, with bluish-purple or red discolorations, and characteristically develops on the eyelids and on muscles used to extend or straighten joints, including knuckles, elbows, heels, and toes. Red rashes may also occur on the face, neck, shoulders, upper chest, back, and other locations, and there may be swelling in the affected areas. The rash sometimes occurs without obvious muscle involvement.

Adults with dermatomyositis may experience weight loss or a low-grade fever, have inflamed lungs, and be sensitive to light. Children and adults with dermatomyositis may develop calcium deposits, which appear as hard bumps under the skin or in the muscle (called "calcinosis"). Calcinosis most often occurs one to three years after the disease begins. These deposits are seen more often in children with dermatomyositis than in adults. In some cases of dermatomyositis, distal muscles (muscles located away from the trunk of the body, such as those in the forearms and around the ankles and wrists) may be affected as the disease progresses. Dermatomyositis may be associated with collagen vascular or autoimmune diseases, such as lupus.

CAUSES OF DERMATOMYOSITIS

The cause of this disorder is unknown. It is theorized that an auto-immune reaction (reactions caused by an immune response against the body's own tissues) or a viral infection of the skeletal muscle may cause the disease. In addition, some doctors think certain people may have a genetic susceptibility to the disease.

TREATMENT FOR DERMATOMYOSITIS

While there is no cure for dermatomyositis, the symptoms can be treated. The options include medication, physical therapy, exercise, heat therapy (including microwave and ultrasound), orthotics and assistive devices, and rest. The standard treatment for dermatomyositis is a corticosteroid drug, given either in pill form or intravenously. Immunosuppressant drugs, such as azathioprine and methotrexate, may reduce inflammation in people who do not respond well to prednisone. Periodic treatment using intravenous immunoglobulin can also improve recovery. Other immunosuppressive agents used to treat the inflammation associated with dermatomyositis include cyclosporine A, cyclophosphamide, and tacrolimus. Physical therapy is usually recommended to prevent muscle atrophy and to regain muscle strength and range of motion. Many individuals with dermatomyositis may need a topical ointment, such as topical corticosteroids, for their skin disorder. They should wear a high-protection sunscreen and protective clothing. Surgery may be required to remove calcium deposits that cause nerve pain and recurrent infections.

PROGNOSIS OF DERMATOMYOSITIS

Most cases of dermatomyositis respond to therapy. Some people may recover and have symptoms completely disappear. This is more common in children. In adults, death may result from severe and prolonged muscle weakness, malnutrition, pneumonia, or lung failure. The outcome is usually worse if the heart or lungs are involved.[2]

[2] Genetic and Rare Diseases Information Center (GARD), "Dermatomyositis," National Center for Advancing Translational Sciences (NCATS), August 26, 2013. Available online. URL: https://rarediseases.info.nih.gov/diseases/6263/dermatomyositis. Accessed May 23, 2022.

Section 39.3 | Inclusion Body Myositis

WHAT IS INCLUSION BODY MYOSITIS?

Inclusion body myositis (IBM) is one of a group of muscle diseases known as the "inflammatory myopathies," which are characterized by chronic, progressive muscle inflammation accompanied by muscle weakness. The onset of muscle weakness in IBM is generally gradual (over months or years) and affects both proximal (close to the trunk of the body) and distal (further away from the trunk) muscles. Muscle weakness may affect only one side of the body. Falling and tripping are usually the first noticeable symptoms of IBM. For some individuals, the disorder begins with weakness in the wrists and fingers that causes difficulty with pinching, buttoning, and gripping objects. There may be a weakness of the wrist and finger muscles and atrophy (thinning or loss of muscle bulk) of the forearm muscles and quadriceps in the legs. Difficulty swallowing occurs in approximately half of IBM cases. Symptoms of the disease usually begin after the age of 50 although the disease can occur earlier. IBM occurs more frequently in men than in women.

TREATMENT FOR INCLUSION BODY MYOSITIS

There is no cure for IBM, nor is there a standard course of treatment. The disease is generally unresponsive to corticosteroids and immunosuppressive drugs. Some evidence suggests that intravenous immunoglobulin may have a slight, but short-lasting, beneficial effect in a small number of cases. Physical therapy may be helpful in maintaining mobility.

PROGNOSIS OF INCLUSION BODY MYOSITIS

Inclusion body myositis is generally resistant to all therapies, and its rate of progression appears to be unaffected by currently available treatments.[3]

---

[3] "Inclusion Body Myositis," National Institute of Neurological Disorders and Stroke (NINDS), July 25, 2022. Available online. URL: www.ninds.nih.gov/health-information/disorders/inclusion-body-myositis. Accessed May 23, 2023.

Section 39.4 | **Myocarditis**

Myocarditis is a condition where the muscles in your heart, which help it pump blood, become swollen and inflamed, causing your heart to not work as efficiently as it should. It is estimated to affect thousands of Americans each year, and it is caused by a wide variety of factors, including viral infections, environmental toxins, autoimmune diseases, bacterial infections, and allergic reactions to certain toxins and medications. Myocarditis often produces no symptoms, and because it is relatively uncommon, the best ways to diagnose and treat the condition are still being studied. It usually affects people who are otherwise healthy, including a significant number of young adults. The best way to prevent myocarditis is by seeking immediate medical attention for infections or inflammatory conditions.

CAUSES OF MYOCARDITIS

Myocarditis is primarily caused by viral infections, the most common among them being those that affect the upper respiratory tract. Other less common causes include contagious infections, such as Lyme disease.

Viral infections, such as cold, flu, or COVID-19, are a major reason people get myocarditis. Most of the time, even after the infection is gone, the heart can still be stressed and swollen. Other things that can cause myocarditis are cancer, bacterial infections, fungi, parasites, or other contagious diseases such as hepatitis C, herpes, and human immunodeficiency virus (HIV). Additionally, allergic reactions to certain medicines and toxins such as drugs, alcohol, spider or snake bites, wasp stings, lead, radiation, and chemotherapy can also cause myocarditis.

Myocarditis can also be caused by autoimmune diseases, such as lupus or rheumatoid arthritis (RA).

SIGNS AND SYMPTOMS OF MYOCARDITIS

Some of the symptoms of myocarditis include the following:
- shortness of breath during exercise, which may lead to breathing troubles at night

- irregular heartbeat and, in some cases, fainting
- heart palpitations
- light-headedness
- sharp or stabbing chest pain or pressure
- fatigue
- swelling in the joints, legs, or neck veins
- indications of infection, such as fever, sore throat, muscle aches, headache, or diarrhea

These symptoms often follow a respiratory infection, and if they occur, it is important to seek medical attention promptly.

DIAGNOSIS OF MYOCARDITIS

In many cases, myocarditis has no symptoms and is not diagnosed. However, when there are symptoms, the doctor will conduct a physical exam to check for an abnormal heartbeat, fluid in the lungs, or swelling in the legs. Some of the following tests may also be conducted:

- blood test to analyze blood cell count and check for infection or antibodies
- an electrocardiogram to evaluate the electrical activity of the heart
- a chest x-ray to study the shape and size of the heart
- an echocardiogram to inspect the structure of the heart and measure blood flow
- occasionally, a cardiac magnetic resonance imaging (MRI) scan or a heart biopsy to confirm the diagnosis

TREATMENT FOR MYOCARDITIS

The first step for an individual affected with myocarditis is to treat the underlying root cause. The treatment typically includes medication to take the load off the heart, improve heart function, and prevent or control further complications.

In the presence of an abnormal heart rhythm, additional treatment, such as a pacemaker or defibrillator, could be required. Hospitalization may be necessary in case of serious complications, such as a blood clot or a weakened heart. Angiotensin-converting enzyme (ACE) inhibitors, angiotensin receptor blockers (ARBs), and beta-blockers help heal the heart after inflammation; diuretics reduce fluid buildup; and corticosteroids are used selectively to reduce inflammation in myocarditis and help the heart function better. Often, reduced physical activity for at least six months, rest, and a low-salt diet are recommended.

The cause of myocarditis, the overall health of the person, and complications, if any, determine the outlook. The infected person could either recover completely or develop a chronic condition. There is a slight possibility that myocarditis may recur and could, in rare cases, lead to dilated cardiomyopathy, where the ventricles enlarge by thinning and stretching and weaken the heart's pumping chambers.

COMPLICATIONS OF MYOCARDITIS

Not treating myocarditis can cause the heart to work harder to pump blood. This can lead to symptoms of heart failure and, in severe cases, may be fatal. Cardiomyopathy and pericarditis are other possible complications of this infection, both of which are leading causes of heart transplants in the United States. Cardiomyopathy is an increase in the size, thickness, or rigidity of the heart muscle, and pericarditis is the inflammation of the pericardium or the sac covering the heart.

PREVENTION OF MYOCARDITIS

While there is no specified prevention for myocarditis, a few steps can be taken to prevent infections that lead to the disease.
- practicing good personal hygiene by washing and sanitizing hands frequently
- staying away from those people with infections
- ensuring to stay up-to-date with vaccines which include those that protect against the flu and rubella and diseases that can lead to myocarditis
- practicing safe sex and getting tested for sexually transmitted infections (STIs)
- avoiding using illicit drugs

References

"About Myocarditis," Myocarditis Foundation, January 18, 2023. Available online. URL: www.myocarditisfoundation. org/about-myocarditis. Accessed April 20, 2023.

Dunkin, Mary Anne. "What You Should Know: Myocarditis," WebMD, November 1, 2022. Available online. URL: www. webmd.com/heart-disease/myocarditis. Accessed April 20, 2023.

Gilotra, Nisha Aggarwal. "Myocarditis," The Johns Hopkins University, June 25, 2021. Available online. URL: www. hopkinsmedicine.org/health/conditions-and-diseases/ myocarditis. Accessed April 20, 2023.

"Myocarditis," Mayo Foundation for Medical Education and Research (MFMER), May 20, 2022. Available online. URL: www.mayoclinic.org/diseases-conditions/ myocarditis/symptoms-causes/syc-20352539. Accessed April 20, 2023.

Section 39.5 | Polymyositis

WHAT IS POLYMYOSITIS?

Polymyositis is a type of inflammatory myopathy, which refers to a group of muscle diseases characterized by chronic muscle inflammation and weakness. It involves skeletal muscles (those involved with making movement) on both sides of the body. Although it can affect people of all ages, most cases are seen in adults between the ages of 31 and 60. The exact cause of polymyositis is unknown; however, the disease shares many characteristics with autoimmune disorders which occur when the immune system mistakenly attacks healthy body tissues. In some cases, the condition may be associated with viral infections, malignancies, or connective tissue disorders. Although there is no cure for polymyositis, treatment can improve muscle strength and function.

SYMPTOMS OF POLYMYOSITIS

Polymyositis is characterized by chronic muscle inflammation and weakness involving the skeletal muscles (those involved with making movement) on both sides of the body. Weakness generally starts in the proximal muscles which can eventually cause difficulties climbing stairs, rising from a sitting position, lifting objects, or reaching overhead. In some cases, distal muscles may also be affected as the disease progresses.

Other symptoms may include:
- arthritis
- shortness of breath
- difficulty swallowing and speaking
- mild joint or muscle tenderness
- fatigue
- heart arrhythmias

DIAGNOSIS OF POLYMYOSITIS

A diagnosis of polymyositis is often suspected in people with proximal muscle weakness and other signs and symptoms associated with the disease. Additional testing can then be ordered to confirm the diagnosis and rule out other diseases that may cause similar features. The testing may include:
- blood tests to measure the levels of certain muscle enzymes, such as creatine kinase and aldolase
- blood tests to detect specific autoantibodies that cause the autoimmune response associated with polymyositis
- electromyography to check the health of the muscles and the nerves that control them
- imaging studies such as magnetic resonance imaging (MRI) scan or muscle ultrasound to detect muscle inflammation
- a muscle biopsy to diagnose muscle abnormalities such as inflammation, damage, or infection

TREATMENT FOR POLYMYOSITIS

The treatment for polymyositis is based on the signs and symptoms present in each person. Although there is currently no cure, symptoms of the disease may be managed with the following:

- medications such as corticosteroids, corticosteroid-sparing agents, or immunosuppressive drugs
- physical therapy to improve muscle strength and flexibility
- speech therapy to address difficulties with swallowing and speech
- intravenous immunoglobulin: an infusion of healthy antibodies that are given to block damaging autoantibodies that attack the muscle

PROGNOSIS OF POLYMYOSITIS

The long-term outlook (prognosis) for people with polymyositis varies. Most affected people respond well to treatment and regain muscle strength, although a certain degree of muscle weakness may persist in some cases. If the treatment is not effective, people may develop significant disability.

In rare cases, people with severe and progressive muscle weakness will develop respiratory failure or pneumonia. Difficulty swallowing may cause weight loss and malnutrition.[4]

---

[4] Genetic and Rare Diseases Information Center (GARD), "Polymyositis," National Center for Advancing Translational Sciences (NCATS), September 9, 2015. Available online. URL: https://rarediseases.info.nih.gov/diseases/7425/polymyositis. Accessed May 23, 2023.

Chapter 40 | **Interrelated Autoimmune Inflammatory Disorders: Polymyalgia Rheumatica and Giant Cell Arteritis**

WHAT ARE POLYMYALGIA RHEUMATICA AND GIANT CELL ARTERITIS?

Polymyalgia rheumatica and giant cell arteritis are closely linked inflammatory disorders that almost always occur in people older than the age of 50. Polymyalgia rheumatica causes muscle pain and stiffness in the shoulders, upper arms, hip area, and, sometimes, the neck. The ache and stiffness are usually worse in the morning or when you have not been moving for a while. They can sometimes be very debilitating and tend to improve with activity.

People with polymyalgia rheumatica sometimes have another disorder called "giant cell arteritis," which is associated with inflammation of arteries, especially those located on each side of the head, scalp, and aorta (the large artery that carries blood from the heart) and its main branches. Headaches, scalp tenderness, and jaw pain are common features of giant cell arteritis. If the blood vessels that nourish the eyes are affected, there may be visual problems such as fleeting or permanent vision loss or double vision. It is important to seek treatment right away if you have visual symptoms because if left untreated they may potentially lead to permanent blindness.

Giant cell arteritis is also known as "temporal arteritis" and "Horton disease."

Both disorders generally respond well to treatment although it is common for symptoms to recur after decreasing or stopping therapy.

WHO GETS POLYMYALGIA RHEUMATICA AND GIANT CELL ARTERITIS?

You are more likely to get polymyalgia rheumatica and giant cell arteritis if you have certain risk factors. These include the following:

- **Age**. They occur almost exclusively in people older than the age of 50, typically in people in their late 60s and in their 70s.
- **Sex**. Women get these disorders more frequently than men.
- **Ethnic and racial background**. They are more common in Caucasians, especially people of Northern European ancestry, but are also observed in patients of other ethnic and racial backgrounds.

SYMPTOMS OF POLYMYALGIA RHEUMATICA AND GIANT CELL ARTERITIS

Polymyalgia rheumatica and giant cell arteritis are related conditions, with some people having symptoms of both. About 10 percent of people with polymyalgia rheumatica have giant cell arteritis, and about 50 percent of those with giant cell arteritis have polymyalgia rheumatica.

The symptoms of polymyalgia rheumatica include the following:

- pain and stiffness in the shoulders, neck, upper arms, and hip area (The pain and stiffness are usually worse upon waking in the morning or after resting and usually last an hour or more. You may have difficulty with activities such as getting up from a bed or chair and dressing and brushing your hair. It is also typical to have difficulty raising your arms above the shoulders.)

- flu-like symptoms, including low-grade fever, weakness, loss of appetite, and weight loss
- occasional swelling of the wrists or joints in the hands

The symptoms of polymyalgia rheumatica can come on quickly, usually in a matter of a few days and in some cases even overnight. The symptoms of giant cell arteritis include the following:

- **Headaches and scalp tenderness**. These are the most common symptoms. The headache pain may be severe and is usually located in the temple areas. Some people notice tenderness of the scalp, often prior to the onset of headaches.
- **Jaw pain**. People sometimes experience jaw pain, especially when chewing.
- **Visual disturbances**. Many people have episodes of double vision or vision loss in one or both eyes. At first, the visual disturbances may last only a few minutes and resolve on their own. It is important to see a health-care provider right away if you develop visual symptoms because if left untreated, they can lead to permanent vision loss within hours or days.
- **Flu-like symptoms**. These include low-grade fever, weakness, loss of appetite, and weight loss.
- **Large artery involvement**. This, including inflammation of the aorta and its major branches, can lead to bulging of the artery (aneurysms) or, due to blockages in the arteries, cause cramping or aching pain in the arms or legs with activity. At times, inflammation of the aorta does not cause any symptoms but is detected by chance in imaging studies (such as computed tomography (CT) or magnetic resonance imaging (MRI)).

In most people, symptoms of giant cell arteritis develop over the course of weeks or months, but in some cases, the onset is more abrupt. Some people may have only large artery involvement (such as the aorta) and not have any symptoms in the head or scalp; these people may experience flu-like symptoms or no symptoms at all.

CAUSES OF POLYMYALGIA RHEUMATICA AND GIANT CELL ARTERITIS

Inflammation causes polymyalgia rheumatica and giant cell arteritis, but scientists do not know what triggers it. Some studies have linked certain gene variants with the disorders, but these genetic links have not been consistent across different populations. Because the disorders occur in older people, the aging process may contribute to the disease onset.

DIAGNOSIS OF POLYMYALGIA RHEUMATICA AND GIANT CELL ARTERITIS

There is no single test to tell if you have polymyalgia rheumatica or giant cell arteritis. The doctor usually does the following:

- Takes your medical history and performs a physical exam. He or she will likely examine the temporal arteries for evidence of swelling or tenderness, signs of giant cell arteritis.
- Orders blood tests, such as the erythrocyte sedimentation rate (ESR or "sed" rate) and C-reactive protein (CRP) test. These tests are measures of inflammation, but they are not specific for polymyalgia rheumatica or giant cell arteritis. They can indicate any inflammatory disorder.

The doctor may also do the following:

- Obtain a biopsy of the temporal artery if giant cell arteritis is suspected. The procedure is performed using a local anesthetic. A pathologist will examine the sample under a microscope and look for signs of inflammation.
- Order imaging tests. An ultrasound, positron emission tomography (PET), CT, or MRI scan can reveal changes consistent with the disorders, such as swelling and inflammation in large vessels, or may help rule out other diseases and conditions.

- Request consultation from specialists such as an ophthalmologist if concerning visual symptoms are occurring.

TREATMENT FOR POLYMYALGIA RHEUMATICA AND GIANT CELL ARTERITIS

The primary goal of treatment for polymyalgia rheumatica is relief of symptoms. For giant cell arteritis, the aim is to alleviate symptoms and to prevent vision loss and other potential complications. Polymyalgia rheumatica and giant cell arteritis are primarily treated with the following:

- **Corticosteroids**. These anti-inflammatory medications are a mainstay of treatment for both disorders. Doctors usually prescribe low-to-moderate doses, taken orally, for polymyalgia rheumatica and higher doses for giant cell arteritis. Most people respond to these medications within days to weeks, and once symptoms resolve, the dosage is usually gradually decreased. You may remain on a maintenance dose for a year or possibly longer. Because these are potent drugs, your doctor will prescribe the lowest dose possible to achieve the desired benefit.

Osteoporosis, a condition characterized by weak and brittle bones, can be a complication of taking corticosteroids, so your doctor may also prescribe medications to strengthen the bones.

Other medications your doctor may prescribe include the following:

- **Disease-modifying antirheumatic drugs (DMARDs)**. These medications, approved for other conditions, are small molecules that act on inflammation at the cellular level. Doctors may prescribe them in combination with corticosteroids, especially in people who experience side effects from these medications or to quell a flare of symptoms.
- **Biologic response modifiers**. These medications, which are also DMARDs, target specific immune messages and interrupt the signal, helping to decrease

or stop inflammation. They are sometimes prescribed in combination with corticosteroids, in people with giant cell arteritis.

Who Treats Polymyalgia Rheumatica and Giant Cell Arteritis?

Polymyalgia rheumatica and giant cell arteritis are primarily treated by:

- rheumatologists, who specialize in treating arthritis and other diseases that affect the joints, bones, muscles, and immune system
- primary care doctors, such as family physicians or internal medicine specialists

Other health-care providers who may be involved in your care include the following:

- **Ophthalmologists.** In cases of giant cell arteritis in which the eyes are affected, they treat the patients. Ophthalmologists specialize in treating disorders and diseases of the eye.
- **Cardiologists or vascular surgeons.** In cases of giant cell arteritis affecting the aorta and its main branches, they treat the patients. These specialists focus on treating blood vessel problems.
- **Mental health professionals**. They help people cope with difficulties in the home and workplace that may result from their medical conditions.
- **Physical therapists and movement specialists**. They improve the quality of life (QOL) through prescribed exercise, hands-on care, and patient education.

LIVING WITH POLYMYALGIA RHEUMATICA AND GIANT CELL ARTERITIS

Corticosteroids can cause side effects, even at low doses, and it is important to let your doctor know if you experience any of them. The side effects include the following:

- heightened risk of infections
- mood swings

- insomnia
- high blood pressure
- vision problems (such as cataracts or glaucoma)
- diabetes
- osteoporosis (thinning, weakened bones)
- weight gain
- swelling of the face, legs, or other parts of the body
- loss of muscles

If you notice signs of any of these adverse effects, your doctor may need to adjust the corticosteroid dose. Below are some tips to help you avoid side effects:

- To protect your bones, make sure you get enough calcium and vitamin D and do weight-bearing exercises, such as walking.
- To avoid weight gain and lower the risk of diabetes and high blood pressure, eat a healthy balanced diet and exercise regularly.
- If you smoke, see your doctor about making a plan to quit. Smoking can affect bone and heart health.

It is also important to do the following:

- Visit your health-care providers regularly and follow their recommendations.
- Talk to your doctor before beginning an exercise program. He or she may refer you to a physical therapist, who can develop a plan to help you be more active and manage pain.
- Talk to a mental health professional or join a support group if you develop anxiety or depression. Living with polymyalgia rheumatica or giant cell arteritis may be challenging at times, and sharing your experiences with others may help.

RESEARCH PROGRESS RELATED TO POLYMYALGIA RHEUMATICA AND GIANT CELL ARTERITIS

Investigators at the National Institutes of Health (NIH) and at other research centers across the country, many supported by the NIH, are working to understand what causes polymyalgia rheumatica and giant cell arteritis and to develop new treatment strategies. Current research efforts include the following:

- More effective and safer therapies are being studied throughout the world. Several large clinical trials are currently underway to find steroid-sparing immunosuppressives that block inflammation caused by giant cell arteritis or polymyalgia rheumatica.

- Researchers are working to evaluate how long patients need to stay on medications for polymyalgia rheumatica and giant cell arteritis.

- By comparing the deoxyribonucleic acid (DNA) of people with the disorders to healthy controls, investigators are searching for gene variants that may raise the risk of polymyalgia rheumatica and giant cell arteritis.

- Polymyalgia rheumatica and giant cell arteritis can be difficult to diagnose because there is no specific test for them. Scientists are analyzing the patterns of inflammatory molecules in blood samples from people with the disorders in an effort to find biomarkers that help detect disease or predict outcomes.

- Researchers are working on optimizing visualization techniques, such as ultrasound, PET/CT, and MRI, for diagnosing polymyalgia rheumatica and giant cell arteritis.[1]

---

[1] "Polymyalgia Rheumatica and Giant Cell Arteritis," National Institute of Arthritis and Musculoskeletal and Skin Diseases (NIAMS), February 2022. Available online. URL: www.niams.nih.gov/health-topics/polymyalgia-rheumatica-giant-cell-arteritis. Accessed May 12, 2023.

Chapter 41 | Autoimmune Diseases of the Intestine

Section 41.1 | Celiac Disease

WHAT IS CELIAC DISEASE?

Celiac disease is a chronic digestive and immune disorder that damages the small intestine. The disease is triggered by eating foods containing gluten. Gluten is a protein found naturally in wheat, barley, and rye and is common in foods such as bread, pasta, cookies, and cakes. Many products contain gluten, such as prepackaged foods, lip balms and lipsticks, toothpaste, vitamin and nutrient supplements, and, rarely, medicines.

Celiac disease can be serious. The disease can cause long-lasting digestive problems and keep your body from getting all the nutrients it needs. Celiac disease can also affect the body outside the small intestine. Celiac disease is different from gluten sensitivity or wheat intolerance. If you have gluten sensitivity, you may have symptoms like those of celiac disease, such as abdominal pain and tiredness. Unlike celiac disease, gluten sensitivity does not damage the small intestine.

Celiac disease is also different from a wheat allergy, a type of food allergy. In both cases, your body's immune system reacts to wheat. However, some symptoms of wheat allergies, such as having itchy eyes or a hard time breathing, are different from celiac disease. Wheat allergies also do not cause long-term damage to the small intestine.

DOES CELIAC DISEASE HAVE OTHER NAMES?

Celiac disease is also called "celiac sprue," "nontropical sprue," and "gluten-sensitive enteropathy."

HOW COMMON IS CELIAC DISEASE?

Many people who have celiac disease have not been diagnosed. However, experts estimate about 2 million people in the United States have celiac disease and about 1 percent of people around the world have celiac disease.

WHO IS MORE LIKELY TO DEVELOP CELIAC DISEASE?

Celiac disease can only occur in people who have certain genes. You are more likely to develop celiac disease if someone in your family has the disease.

Celiac disease affects children and adults in all parts of the world. In the United States, celiac disease is more common among White Americans than among other racial or ethnic groups. A celiac disease diagnosis is more common in females than in males. Celiac disease is also more common in people who have certain chromosomal disorders, such as Down syndrome, Turner syndrome, and Williams syndrome.

WHAT OTHER HEALTH PROBLEMS DO PEOPLE WITH CELIAC DISEASE HAVE?

Experts have found that some people have both celiac disease and other disorders related to the immune system. These disorders include the following:

- type 1 diabetes
- thyroid diseases, such as Hashimoto disease, Graves disease, Addison disease, and primary hyperparathyroidism
- selective immunoglobulin A (IgA) deficiency, a condition in which your body makes little or no IgA, an antibody that fights infections
- rheumatic diseases, such as Sjögren syndrome
- liver diseases, such as autoimmune hepatitis, primary sclerosing cholangitis, and primary biliary cholangitis

WHAT ARE THE COMPLICATIONS OF CELIAC DISEASE?

Long-term complications of celiac disease include the following:

- accelerated osteoporosis or bone softening, known as "osteomalacia"
- anemia
- malnutrition, a condition in which you do not get enough vitamins, minerals, and other nutrients you need to be healthy

- nervous system problems
- problems related to the reproductive system

Rare complications can include the following:
- adenocarcinoma, a type of cancer of the small intestine
- liver damage, which may lead to cirrhosis or liver failure
- non-Hodgkin lymphoma (NHL)

In rare cases, you may continue to have trouble absorbing nutrients even though you have been following a strict gluten-free diet. If you have this condition, called "refractory celiac disease," your small intestine is severely damaged and cannot heal. You may need to receive intravenous (IV) nutrients and specialized treatment.

WHAT ARE THE SYMPTOMS OF CELIAC DISEASE?

Symptoms of celiac disease vary widely, and a person may have multiple symptoms that come and go. If you have celiac disease, you may have digestive problems or other symptoms. Digestive symptoms are more common in children than in adults. Digestive symptoms of celiac disease may include the following:
- bloating
- chronic diarrhea
- constipation
- gas
- lactose intolerance due to damage to the small intestine
- loose, greasy, bulky, and bad-smelling stools
- nausea or vomiting
- pain in the abdomen

For children with celiac disease, being unable to absorb nutrients at a time when they are so important to normal growth and development can lead to:
- damage to the permanent teeth enamel
- delayed puberty
- failure to thrive, meaning that an infant or a child weighs less or is gaining less weight than expected for his or her age

371

- mood changes or feeling annoyed or impatient
- slowed growth and short height
- weight loss

Some people with celiac disease have symptoms that affect other parts of the body. These symptoms may include the following:
- dermatitis herpetiformis
- fatigue or feeling tired
- joint or bone pain
- mental health problems, such as depression or anxiety
- nervous system symptoms, such as headaches, balance problems, seizures, or peripheral neuropathy
- reproductive problems in women and girls—which may include infertility, delayed start of menstrual periods, missed menstrual periods, or repeated miscarriages—and male infertility
- symptoms involving the mouth, such as canker sores; a dry mouth; or a red, smooth, shiny tongue

Most people with celiac disease have one or more symptoms before they are diagnosed and begin treatment. Symptoms typically improve and may go away after a person begins eating a gluten-free diet. Symptoms may return if a person consumes small amounts of gluten.

Depending on how old you are when a doctor diagnoses your celiac disease, some symptoms, such as short height and tooth defects, may not improve. People with celiac disease who have no symptoms can still develop complications over time if they do not get treatment.

Dermatitis Herpetiformis

Dermatitis herpetiformis is an itchy, blistering skin rash that usually appears on the elbows, knees, buttocks, back, or scalp. Among people with untreated celiac disease, about 2–3 percent of children and 10–20 percent of adults have dermatitis herpetiformis. Some people with celiac disease may have the rash and no other symptoms. After a person starts a gluten-free diet, the rash may take some time to heal and may return if a person consumes small amounts of gluten.

WHAT CAUSES CELIAC DISEASE?

Research suggests that celiac disease only occurs in people who have certain genes and eat food that contains gluten. Experts are studying other factors that may play a role in causing the disease.

Genes

Celiac disease almost always occurs in people who have one of two groups of normal gene variants, called "DQ2" and "DQ8." People who do not have these gene variants are very unlikely to develop celiac disease. About 30 percent of people have DQ2 or DQ8. However, only about 3 percent of people with DQ2 or DQ8 develop celiac disease.

Researchers are studying other genes that may increase the chance of developing celiac disease in people who have DQ2 or DQ8.

Gluten

Consuming gluten triggers the abnormal immune system response that causes celiac disease. However, not all people who have the gene variant DQ2 or DQ8 and eat gluten develop the disease. Research suggests that among children with a genetic predisposition for celiac disease, those who eat more gluten in early childhood may have a greater risk for celiac disease.

Other Factors

Researchers are studying other factors that may increase a person's chances of developing celiac disease. For example, research suggests that a higher number of infections in early life and certain digestive tract infections may increase the risk. Experts also think changes in the microbiome—the bacteria in the digestive tract that help with digestion—could play a role in the development of celiac disease.

HOW DO DOCTORS DIAGNOSE CELIAC DISEASE?

Doctors use information from your medical and family history, a physical exam, a dental exam, and medical test results to look for signs that you might have celiac disease. Doctors typically diagnose celiac disease with blood tests and biopsies of the small intestine.

Medical and Family History

Your doctor will ask about your symptoms. Celiac disease is not diagnosed based on symptoms alone because some of the symptoms are like the symptoms of other digestive disorders, such as irritable bowel syndrome (IBS) or lactose intolerance. Some people with celiac disease have symptoms that affect parts of the body outside the digestive tract.

The doctor will review your medical history, including your history of conditions that are more common in people who have celiac disease. Your doctor will also ask about your family's medical history and whether anyone in your family has been diagnosed with celiac disease.

Physical Exam

During a physical exam, a doctor may:
- check for signs of weight loss or growth problems
- examine your skin for rashes, such as dermatitis herpetiformis
- listen to sounds in the abdomen using a stethoscope
- tap on the abdomen to check for pain or swelling

In some cases, a dentist may notice signs of celiac disease during an exam. Celiac disease may cause problems with the teeth and mouth, such as defects in tooth enamel or canker sores.

WHAT TESTS DO DOCTORS USE TO DIAGNOSE CELIAC DISEASE?

Doctors most often use blood tests and biopsies of the small intestine to diagnose or rule out celiac disease. Doctors do not recommend starting a gluten-free diet before diagnostic testing because a gluten-free diet can affect test results.

In some cases, doctors may order additional tests, such as skin biopsies and genetic tests, to help diagnose or rule out celiac disease.

Blood Tests

A health-care professional will take a blood sample from you and send the sample to a lab. Blood tests can show levels of certain antibodies that are often higher than normal in people who have untreated celiac disease. Blood tests may also show signs of health problems that could be related to celiac disease, such as anemia.

Biopsies of the Small Intestine

A doctor obtains biopsies of the small intestine during an upper gastrointestinal (GI) endoscopy. For an upper GI endoscopy, a doctor uses an endoscope—a flexible tube with a camera—to see the lining of your upper GI tract, including the first part of your small intestine. The doctor passes an instrument through the endoscope to take small pieces of tissue from your small intestine. A pathologist will examine the tissue under a microscope to look for signs of celiac disease.

Skin Biopsies

A doctor may order skin biopsies if you have a rash that could be dermatitis herpetiformis. For skin biopsies, a doctor removes small pieces of skin tissue on and next to the rash. A pathologist will examine the tissue under a microscope to look for signs of dermatitis herpetiformis.

Genetic Testing

In some cases, a health-care professional may take a blood sample or use a swab to collect cells from the inside of your cheek. The sample will be tested for groups of gene variants called "*DQ2*" and "*DQ8*." If you do not have these gene variants, you are very unlikely to have celiac disease.

Having *DQ2* or *DQ8* alone does not mean you have celiac disease. Most people with these gene variants do not develop celiac disease. If you do have *DQ2* or *DQ8*, your doctor may recommend additional tests to check for or rule out celiac disease.

DO DOCTORS SCREEN FOR CELIAC DISEASE?

Screening is testing for diseases when you have no symptoms. Doctors in the United States do not routinely screen people for celiac disease. However, blood relatives of people with celiac disease and those with type 1 diabetes should talk with their doctor about their chances of getting the disease to see if they should be tested.

HOW DO DOCTORS TREAT CELIAC DISEASE?
Gluten-Free Diet

Doctors treat celiac disease by helping people follow a gluten-free diet. Gluten is a protein found naturally in certain grains, including wheat, barley, and rye. Gluten is also added to many other foods and products. In people who have celiac disease, consuming gluten triggers an abnormal immune system reaction that damages the small intestine.

Symptoms greatly improve for most people with celiac disease who stick to a gluten-free diet. For most people, following a gluten-free diet will heal damage in the small intestine and prevent more damage. Many people see symptoms improve within days to weeks of starting the diet. Your doctor will explain the gluten-free diet and may refer you to a registered dietitian who specializes in treating people who have celiac disease. The dietitian will teach you how to avoid gluten while following a healthy diet and recommend substitutes for foods that contain gluten. He or she will help you:

- check food and product labels for gluten
- design everyday meal plans
- make healthy choices about foods and drinks

Avoiding Medicines and Other Products That May Contain Gluten

In addition to prescribing a gluten-free diet, your doctor will want you to avoid all hidden sources of gluten. If you have celiac disease, ask a pharmacist about ingredients in:

- herbal and nutritional supplements
- prescription and over-the-counter medicines
- vitamin and mineral supplements

Medicines are rare sources of gluten. Even if gluten is present in a medicine, it is likely to be in such small quantities that it would not cause any symptoms.

Other products can be hidden sources of gluten. You may take in small amounts of gluten if you consume these products, use them around your mouth, or transfer them from your hands to your mouth by accident. Products that may contain gluten include the following:

- children's modeling dough, such as Play-Doh
- cosmetics
- lipstick, lip gloss, and lip balm
- skin and hair products
- toothpaste and mouthwash
- communion wafers

Reading product labels can sometimes help you avoid gluten. Some companies label their products as being gluten-free. In the United States, products labeled gluten-free must have less than 20 parts per million of gluten, which should not be a problem for the vast majority of people. If a label does not tell you what is in a product, ask the company that makes the product for an ingredients list. You cannot assume that the product is gluten-free.

TREATMENTS FOR SYMPTOMS OR COMPLICATIONS

A gluten-free diet will treat or prevent many of the symptoms and complications of celiac disease. Some symptoms may take longer to get better than others, and some symptoms may need additional help. Dermatitis herpetiformis may not go away until a person has been following a gluten-free diet for six months to two years. In some cases, doctors may prescribe a medicine, such as dapsone, to help treat dermatitis herpetiformis until the rash is under control with a gluten-free diet alone.

In untreated celiac disease, damage to the small intestine can lead to malabsorption and malnutrition. When you are diagnosed with celiac disease, your doctor may test you for low levels of certain vitamins and minerals and may recommend or prescribe supplements if you need them. For safety reasons, talk with your doctor before using dietary supplements, such as vitamins, or any complementary or alternative medicines or medical practices.

Follow-Up

Your doctor may recommend regular follow-up visits to make sure symptoms and health problems related to celiac disease are improving on a gluten-free diet. Follow-up may include blood tests to check levels of certain antibodies, which are higher in untreated celiac disease but typically return to normal after treatment. In some cases, doctors may recommend additional biopsies to find out if the small intestine has healed.

HOW CAN YOU IDENTIFY AND AVOID FOODS AND DRINKS THAT CONTAIN GLUTEN?

A registered dietitian can help you learn to identify and avoid foods and drinks that contain gluten when you shop, prepare foods at home, or eat out.

For example, when you shop and eat at home, do the following:
- Carefully read food labels to check for grains that contain gluten—such as wheat, barley, and rye—and ingredients or additives made from those grains.
- Check for gluten-free food labeling.
- Do not eat foods if you are not sure whether they contain gluten. If possible, contact the company that makes the food or visit the company's website for more information.

- Store and prepare your gluten-free foods separately from other family members' foods that contain gluten to prevent cross-contact.

When you eat out at restaurants or social gatherings, do the following:

- Before you go out to eat, search online for restaurants that offer a gluten-free menu.
- Review restaurant menus online or call ahead to make sure a restaurant can accommodate you safely.
- At the restaurant, let the server know that you have celiac disease. Ask about food ingredients, how food is prepared, and whether a gluten-free menu is available. Ask to talk with the chef if you would like more details about the menu.
- When attending social gatherings, let the host know you have celiac disease and find out if gluten-free foods will be available. If not or if you are unsure, bring gluten-free foods that are safe for you to eat.[1]

Section 41.2 | Crohn's Disease

WHAT IS CROHN'S DISEASE?

Crohn's disease is a chronic disease that causes inflammation and irritation in your digestive tract. Most commonly, Crohn's disease affects your small intestine and the beginning of your large intestine. However, the disease can affect any part of your digestive tract, from your mouth to your anus.

Crohn's disease is an inflammatory bowel disease (IBD). Crohn's disease most often begins gradually and can become worse over time. You may have periods of remission that can last for weeks or years.

---

[1] "Definition and Facts for Celiac Disease," National Institute of Diabetes and Digestive and Kidney Diseases (NIDDK), October 2020. Available online. URL: www.niddk.nih.gov/health-information/digestive-diseases/celiac-disease/definition-facts. Accessed May 8, 2023.

HOW COMMON IS CROHN'S DISEASE?

Researchers estimate that more than half a million people in the United States have Crohn's disease. Studies show that over time, Crohn's disease has become more common in the United States and other parts of the world. Experts do not know the reason for this increase.

WHO IS MORE LIKELY TO DEVELOP CROHN'S DISEASE?

Crohn's disease can develop in people of any age and is more likely to develop in people:

- between the ages of 20 and 29
- who have a family member, most often a sibling or parent, with IBD
- who smoke cigarettes

WHAT ARE THE COMPLICATIONS OF CROHN'S DISEASE?

Complications of Crohn's disease can include the following:

- **Intestinal obstruction**. Crohn's disease can thicken the wall of your intestines. Over time, the thickened areas of your intestines can narrow, which can block your intestines. A partial or complete intestinal obstruction, also called a "bowel blockage," can block the movement of food or stool through your intestines.
- **Fistulas**. In Crohn's disease, inflammation can go through the wall of your intestines and create tunnels or fistulas. Fistulas are abnormal passages between two organs or between an organ and the outside of your body. Fistulas may become infected.
- **Abscesses**. Inflammation that goes through the wall of your intestines can also lead to abscesses. Abscesses are painful, swollen, pus-filled pockets of infection.
- **Anal fissures**. Anal fissures are small tears in your anus that may cause itching, pain, or bleeding.
- **Ulcers**. Inflammation anywhere along your digestive tract can lead to ulcers or open sores in your mouth, intestines, anus, or perineum.

- **Malnutrition**. Malnutrition develops when your body does not get the right amount of vitamins, minerals, and nutrients it needs to maintain healthy tissues and organ function.
- **Inflammation in other areas of your body**. You may have inflammation in your joints, eyes, and skin.

WHAT OTHER HEALTH PROBLEMS DO PEOPLE WITH CROHN'S DISEASE HAVE?

If you have Crohn's disease in your large intestine, you may be more likely to develop colon cancer. If you receive ongoing treatment for Crohn's disease and stay in remission, you may reduce your chances of developing colon cancer.

Talk with your doctor about how often you should get screened for colon cancer. Screening is testing for diseases when you have no symptoms. Screening for colon cancer can include a colonoscopy with biopsies. Although screening does not reduce your chances of developing colon cancer, it may help find cancer at an early stage and improve the chance of curing the cancer.

WHAT ARE THE SYMPTOMS OF CROHN'S DISEASE?

The most common symptoms of Crohn's disease are:
- diarrhea
- cramping and pain in your abdomen
- weight loss

Other symptoms include:
- anemia
- eye redness or pain
- feeling tired
- fever
- joint pain or soreness
- nausea or loss of appetite
- skin changes that involve red, tender bumps under the skin

Your symptoms may vary depending on the location and severity of your inflammation.

Some research suggests that stress, including the stress of living with Crohn's disease, can make symptoms worse. Also, some people may find that certain foods can trigger or worsen their symptoms.

WHAT CAUSES CROHN'S DISEASE?

Doctors are not sure what causes Crohn's disease. Experts think the following factors may play a role in causing Crohn's disease.

Autoimmune Reaction

One cause of Crohn's disease may be an autoimmune reaction—when your immune system attacks healthy cells in your body. Experts think bacteria in your digestive tract can mistakenly trigger your immune system. This immune system response causes inflammation, leading to symptoms of Crohn's disease.

Genes

Crohn's disease sometimes runs in families. Research has shown that if you have a parent or sibling with Crohn's disease, you may be more likely to develop the disease. Experts continue to study the link between genes and Crohn's disease.

Other Factors

Some studies suggest that other factors may increase your chance of developing Crohn's disease:

- Smoking may double your chance of developing Crohn's disease.
- Nonsteroidal anti-inflammatory drugs (NSAIDs) such as aspirin or ibuprofen, antibiotics, and birth control pills may slightly increase the chance of developing Crohn's disease.
- A high-fat diet may also slightly increase your chance of getting Crohn' disease.

Stress and eating certain foods do not cause Crohn's disease.

DIAGNOSIS OF CROHN'S DISEASE
How Do Doctors Diagnose Crohn's Disease?

Doctors typically use a combination of tests to diagnose Crohn's disease. Your doctor will also ask you about your medical history—including medicines you are taking—and your family history and will perform a physical exam.

PHYSICAL EXAM

During a physical exam, a doctor most often:
- checks for bloating in your abdomen
- listens to sounds within your abdomen using a stethoscope
- taps on your abdomen to check for tenderness and pain and to see if your liver or spleen is abnormal or enlarged

DIAGNOSTIC TESTS

Your doctor may use the following tests to help diagnose Crohn's disease:
- lab tests
- intestinal endoscopy
- upper gastrointestinal (GI) series
- computed tomography (CT) scan

Your doctor may also perform tests to rule out other diseases, such as ulcerative colitis, diverticular disease, or cancer, that cause symptoms similar to those of Crohn's disease.

What Tests Do Doctors Use to Diagnose Crohn's Disease?

Your doctor may perform the following tests to help diagnose Crohn's disease.

LAB TESTS

Lab tests to help diagnose Crohn's disease include the following:
- **Blood tests**. A health-care professional may take a blood sample from you and send the sample to a lab to test for changes in the following:

- **Red blood cells (RBCs).** If your RBCs are fewer or smaller than normal, you may have anemia.
- **White blood cells (WBCs).** When your WBC count is higher than normal, you may have inflammation or infection somewhere in your body.
- **Stool tests**. A stool test is the analysis of a sample of stool. Your doctor will give you a container for catching and storing the stool. You will receive instructions on where to send or take the kit for analysis. Doctors use stool tests to rule out other causes of digestive diseases.

Intestinal Endoscopy

Intestinal endoscopies are the most accurate methods for diagnosing Crohn's disease and ruling out other possible conditions, such as ulcerative colitis, diverticular disease, or cancer. Intestinal endoscopies include the following:

- **Colonoscopy.** Colonoscopy is a procedure in which a doctor uses a long, flexible, narrow tube with a light and tiny camera on one end, called a colonoscope or endoscope, to look inside your rectum and colon. The doctor may also examine your ileum to look for signs of Crohn's disease.

A trained specialist performs a colonoscopy in a hospital or an outpatient center. A health-care professional will give you written bowel prep instructions to follow at home before the procedure. You will receive sedatives, anesthesia, or pain medicine during the procedure.

During a colonoscopy, you will be asked to lie on a table while the doctor inserts a colonoscope into your anus and slowly guides it through your rectum and colon and into the lower part of your ileum. If your doctor suspects that you have Crohn's disease, the colonoscopy will include biopsies of your ileum, colon, and rectum. You will not feel the biopsies.

- **Upper GI endoscopy and enteroscopy**. In an upper GI endoscopy, your doctor uses an endoscope to see inside your upper digestive tract, also called your upper GI tract.

A trained specialist performs the procedure at a hospital or an outpatient center. You should not eat or drink before the procedure. A health-care professional will tell you how to prepare for an upper GI endoscopy. You most often receive a liquid anesthetic to numb your throat and a light sedative to help you stay relaxed and comfortable during the procedure.

During the procedure, the doctor carefully feeds the endoscope down your esophagus and into your stomach and duodenum.

During an enteroscopy, a doctor examines your small intestine with a special, longer endoscope using one of the following procedures:

- **Push enteroscopy**. It uses a long endoscope to examine the upper portion of your small intestine.
- **Single- or double-balloon enteroscopy**. It uses small balloons to help move the endoscope into your small intestine.
- **Spiral enteroscopy**. It uses a tube attached to an endoscope that acts as a corkscrew to move the instrument into your small intestine.
- **Capsule endoscopy**. In capsule endoscopy, you swallow a capsule containing a tiny camera that allows your doctor to see inside your digestive tract. You should not eat or drink before the procedure. A health-care professional will tell you how to prepare for a capsule endoscopy. You do not need anesthesia for this procedure.

The test begins in a doctor's office where you swallow the capsule. You can leave the doctor's office during the test. As the capsule passes through your digestive tract, the camera will record and transmit images to a small receiver device that you wear. When the recording is done, your doctor downloads and reviews the images. The camera capsule leaves your body during a bowel movement, and you can safely flush it down the toilet.

Upper Gastrointestinal Series

An upper GI series is a procedure in which a doctor uses x-rays, fluoroscopy, and a chalky liquid called barium to view your upper GI tract.

An x-ray technician and a radiologist perform this test at a hospital or an outpatient center. You should not eat or drink before the procedure. A health-care professional will tell you how to prepare for an upper GI series. You do not need anesthesia for this procedure.

For the procedure, you will be asked to stand or sit in front of an x-ray machine and drink barium. The barium will make your upper GI tract more visible on an x-ray. You will then lie on the x-ray table, and the radiologist will watch the barium move through your upper GI tract on the x-ray and fluoroscopy.

Computed Tomography Scan

A CT scan uses a combination of x-rays and computer technology to create images of your digestive tract.

For a CT scan, a health-care professional may give you a solution to drink and an injection of a special dye called contrast medium. The contrast medium makes the structures inside your body easier to see during the procedure. You will lie on a table that slides into a tunnel-shaped device that takes the x-rays. CT scans can diagnose both Crohn's disease and the complications of the disease.

TREATMENT FOR CROHN'S DISEASE
How Do Doctors Treat Crohn's Disease?

Doctors treat Crohn's disease with medicines, bowel rest, and surgery.

No single treatment works for everyone with Crohn's disease. The goals of treatment are to decrease the inflammation in your intestines, prevent flare-ups of your symptoms, and keep you in remission.

MEDICINES

Many people with Crohn's disease need medicines. Which medicines your doctor prescribes will depend on your symptoms. Although no medicine cures Crohn's disease, many can reduce symptoms.

Aminosalicylates

These medicines contain 5-aminosalicylic acid (5-ASA), which helps control inflammation. Doctors use aminosalicylates to treat people newly diagnosed with Crohn's disease who have mild symptoms. Aminosalicylates include:

- balsalazide
- mesalamine
- olsalazine
- sulfasalazine

Some of the common side effects of aminosalicylates include:

- diarrhea
- headaches
- heartburn
- nausea and vomiting
- pain in your abdomen

Corticosteroids

Corticosteroids, also known as steroids, help reduce the activity of your immune system and decrease inflammation. Doctors prescribe corticosteroids for people with moderate-to-severe symptoms. Corticosteroids include:

- budesonide
- hydrocortisone
- methylprednisolone
- prednisone

Side effects of corticosteroids include:

- acne
- bone mass loss
- high blood glucose

- high blood pressure
- a higher chance of developing infections
- mood swings
- weight gain

In most cases, doctors do not prescribe corticosteroids for long-term use.

Immunomodulators

These medicines reduce immune system activity, resulting in less inflammation in your digestive tract. Immunomodulators can take several weeks to three months to start working. Immunomodulators include:

- 6-mercaptopurine (6-MP)
- azathioprine
- cyclosporine
- methotrexate

Doctors prescribe these medicines to help you go into remission or help you if you do not respond to other treatments. You may have the following side effects:

- a low WBC count, which can lead to a higher chance of infection
- feeling tired
- nausea and vomiting
- pancreatitis

Doctors most often prescribe cyclosporine only if you have severe Crohn's disease because of the medicine's serious side effects. Talk with your doctor about the risks and benefits of cyclosporine.

Biologic Therapies

These medicines target proteins made by the immune system. Neutralizing these proteins decreases inflammation in the intestines. Biologic therapies work to help you go into remission, especially if you do not respond to other medicines. Biologic therapies include:

- anti-tumor necrosis factor-alpha therapies, such as adalimumab, certolizumab, and infliximab
- anti-integrin therapies, such as natalizumab and vedolizumab
- anti-interleukin-12 and anti-interleukin-23 therapy, such as ustekinumab

Doctors most often give patients infliximab every six to eight weeks at a hospital or an outpatient center. Side effects may include a toxic reaction to the medicine and a higher chance of developing infections, particularly tuberculosis.

Other Medicines

Other medicines doctors prescribe for symptoms or complications may include the following:

- **Acetaminophen for mild pain**. You should avoid using ibuprofen, naproxen, and aspirin because these medicines can make your symptoms worse.
- **Antibiotics**. They help prevent or treat complications that involve infection, such as abscesses and fistulas.
- **Loperamide**. It helps slow or stop severe diarrhea. In most cases, people only take this medicine for short periods of time because it can increase the chance of developing a megacolon.

BOWEL REST

If your Crohn's disease symptoms are severe, you may need to rest your bowel for a few days to several weeks. Bowel rest involves drinking only certain liquids or not eating or drinking anything. During bowel rest, your doctor may:

- ask you to drink a liquid that contains nutrients
- give you a liquid that contains nutrients through a feeding tube inserted into your stomach or small intestine
- give you intravenous (IV) nutrition through a special tube inserted into a vein in your arm

You may stay in the hospital, or you may be able to receive the treatment at home. In most cases, your intestines will heal during bowel rest.

SURGERY

Even with medicines, many people will need surgery to treat their Crohn's disease. One study found that nearly 60 percent of people had surgery within 20 years of having Crohn's disease. Although surgery will not cure Crohn's disease, it can treat complications and improve symptoms. Doctors most often recommend surgery to treat:

- fistulas
- bleeding that is life-threatening
- intestinal obstructions
- side effects from medicines when they threaten your health
- symptoms when medicines do not improve your condition

A surgeon can perform different types of operations to treat Crohn's disease.

For any surgery, you will receive general anesthesia. You will most likely stay in the hospital for three to seven days following the surgery. Full recovery may take four to six weeks.

- **Small bowel resection**. Small bowel resection is surgery to remove part of your small intestine. When you have an intestinal obstruction or severe Crohn's disease in your small intestine, a surgeon may need to remove that section of your intestine. The two types of small bowel resection are as follows:
  - **Laparoscopic**. It is when a surgeon makes several small, half-inch incisions in your abdomen. The surgeon inserts a laparoscope—a thin tube with a tiny light and video camera on the end—through the small incisions. The camera sends a magnified image from inside your body to a video monitor, giving

the surgeon a close-up view of your small intestine. While watching the monitor, the surgeon inserts tools through the small incisions and removes the diseased or blocked section of the small intestine. The surgeon will reconnect the ends of your intestine.

- **Open surgery**. It is when a surgeon makes one incision about six inches long in your abdomen. The surgeon will locate the diseased or blocked section of the small intestine and remove or repair that section. The surgeon will reconnect the ends of your intestine.

- **Subtotal colectomy**. A subtotal colectomy, also called a large bowel resection, is surgery to remove part of your large intestine. When you have an intestinal obstruction, a fistula, or severe Crohn's disease in your large intestine, a surgeon may need to remove that section of the intestine. A surgeon can perform a subtotal colectomy by the following:

  - **Laparoscopic colectomy**. It is when a surgeon makes several small, half-inch incisions in your abdomen. While watching the monitor, the surgeon removes the diseased or blocked section of your large intestine. The surgeon will reconnect the ends of your intestine.

  - **Open surgery**. It is when a surgeon makes one incision about six to eight inches long in your abdomen. The surgeon will locate the diseased or blocked section of the large intestine and remove that section. The surgeon will reconnect the ends of your intestine.

- **Proctocolectomy and ileostomy**. A proctocolectomy is a surgery to remove your entire colon and rectum. An ileostomy is a stoma, or opening in your abdomen, that a surgeon creates from a part of your ileum. The surgeon brings the end of your ileum through an opening in your abdomen and attaches it to your skin, creating an opening outside your body. The stoma is about three-quarters of an inch to a little less than two inches wide and is most often located in the lower part of your abdomen, just below the beltline.

A removable external collection pouch, called an ostomy pouch or ostomy appliance, connects to the stoma and collects stool outside your body. The stool passes through the stoma instead of passing through your anus. The stoma has no muscle, so it cannot control the flow of stool, causing a continuous flow. If you have this type of surgery, you will have the ileostomy for the rest of your life.

How Do Doctors Treat the Complications of Crohn's Disease?

Your doctor may recommend treatments for the following complications of Crohn's disease:

- **Intestinal obstruction**. A complete intestinal obstruction is life-threatening. If you have a complete obstruction, you will need medical attention right away. Doctors often treat complete intestinal obstruction with surgery.
- **Fistulas**. How your doctor treats fistulas will depend on what type of fistulas you have and how severe they are. For some people, fistulas heal with medicine and diet changes, whereas other people will need to have surgery.
- **Abscesses**. Doctors prescribe antibiotics and drain abscesses. A doctor may drain an abscess with a needle inserted through your skin or with surgery.
- **Anal fissures**. Most anal fissures heal with medical treatment, including ointments, warm baths, and diet changes.
- **Ulcers**. In most cases, the treatment for Crohn's disease will also treat your ulcers.
- **Malnutrition**. You may need IV fluids or feeding tubes to replace lost nutrients and fluids.

- **Inflammation in other areas of your body**. Your doctor can treat inflammation by changing your medicines or prescribing new medicines.

EATING, DIET, AND NUTRITION FOR CROHN'S DISEASE
How Can Your Diet Help the Symptoms of Crohn's Disease?

Changing your diet can help reduce symptoms. Your doctor may recommend that you make changes to your diet such as:
- avoiding carbonated, or "fizzy," drinks
- avoiding popcorn, vegetable skins, nuts, and other high-fiber foods
- drinking more liquids
- eating smaller meals more often
- keeping a food diary to help identify foods that cause problems

Depending on your symptoms or medicines, your doctor may recommend a specific diet, such as a diet that is:
- high in calorie
- lactose-free
- low in fat
- low in fiber
- low in salt

Talk with your doctor about specific dietary recommendations and changes.

Your doctor may recommend nutritional supplements and vitamins if you do not absorb enough nutrients. For safety reasons, talk with your doctor before using dietary supplements, such as vitamins, or any complementary or alternative medicines or medical practices.[2]

---

[2] "Definition and Facts for Crohn's Disease," National Institute of Diabetes and Digestive and Kidney Diseases (NIDDK), September 2017. Available online. URL: www.niddk.nih.gov/health-information/digestive-diseases/crohns-disease/definition-facts. Accessed May 18, 2023.

Section 41.3 | Ulcerative Colitis

WHAT IS ULCERATIVE COLITIS?

Ulcerative colitis is a chronic inflammatory bowel disease (IBD) in which abnormal reactions of the immune system cause inflammation and ulcers on the inner lining of your large intestine.

Ulcerative colitis can begin gradually and become worse over time. However, it can also start suddenly. Symptoms can range from mild to severe. In between periods of flares—times when people have symptoms—most people have periods of remission—times when symptoms disappear. Periods of remission can last for weeks or years. The goal of treatment is to keep people in remission long-term.

FREQUENCY OF ULCERATIVE COLITIS

Research estimates that about 600,000–900,000 people in the United States have ulcerative colitis.

WHO IS MORE LIKELY TO HAVE ULCERATIVE COLITIS?

Ulcerative colitis is more likely to develop in people:
- between the ages of 15 and 30 although the disease may develop in people of any age
- who have a first-degree relative—a parent, sibling, or child—with IBD
- of Jewish descent

WHAT ARE THE COMPLICATIONS OF ULCERATIVE COLITIS?

Ulcerative colitis may lead to complications that develop over time, including the following:
- **Anemia.** It is a condition in which you have fewer red blood cells (RBCs) than normal. Ulcerative colitis may lead to more than one type of anemia, including iron deficiency anemia and anemia of inflammation or chronic disease.

- **Bone problems**. Ulcerative colitis and corticosteroids used to treat the disease can affect the bones. Bone problems include low bone mass, such as osteopenia or osteoporosis.
- **Problems with growth and development in children**. They include gaining less weight than normal, slowed growth, short stature, or delayed puberty.
- **Colorectal cancer**. Patients with long-standing ulcerative colitis that involves a third or more of the colon are at increased risk and require closer screening.

In some cases, ulcerative colitis may lead to serious complications that develop quickly and can be life-threatening. These complications require treatment at a hospital or emergency surgery. Serious complications include the following:

- **Fulminant ulcerative colitis**. It causes extremely severe symptoms, such as more than 10 bloody bowel movements in a day, often with fever, rapid heart rate, and severe anemia. People with fulminant ulcerative colitis have a higher chance of developing other complications, such as toxic megacolon and perforation.
- **Toxic megacolon**. It occurs when inflammation spreads to the deep tissue layers of the large intestine, and the large intestine swells and stops working.
- **Perforation**. It is otherwise known as "a hole in the wall of the large intestine."
- **Severe rectal bleeding, or passing a lot of blood from the rectum**. In some cases, people with ulcerative colitis may have severe or heavy rectal bleeding that may require emergency surgery.

Severe ulcerative colitis or serious complications may lead to additional problems, such as severe anemia and dehydration. These problems may require treatment at a hospital with blood transfusions or intravenous (IV) fluids and electrolytes.

Health Problems Affecting Other Parts of the Body

Some people with ulcerative colitis also have inflammation in parts of the body other than the large intestine, including the following:

- joints, causing certain types of arthritis
- skin
- eyes
- liver and bile ducts, causing conditions such as primary sclerosing cholangitis

People with ulcerative colitis also have a higher risk of blood clots in their blood vessels.

COLORECTAL CANCER

Ulcerative colitis increases the chance of getting colorectal cancer. People have a higher risk for developing colorectal cancer if ulcerative colitis affects more of their large intestine, is more severe, has started at a younger age, or has been present for a longer time. People with ulcerative colitis also have a higher risk of developing colorectal cancer if they have primary sclerosing cholangitis or have a family history of colorectal cancer.

If you have ulcerative colitis, your doctor may recommend a colonoscopy to screen for colorectal cancer. Screening is testing for diseases when you have no symptoms. Screening can check for dysplasia—precancerous cells—or colorectal cancer. Diagnosing cancer early can improve chances for recovery.

For people with ulcerative colitis, doctors typically recommend colonoscopies every one to three years, starting eight years after ulcerative colitis started. For people with ulcerative colitis and primary biliary cholangitis, doctors typically recommend colonoscopies every year, starting at diagnosis.

WHAT ARE THE SYMPTOMS OF ULCERATIVE COLITIS?

Symptoms of ulcerative colitis vary from person to person. Common symptoms of ulcerative colitis include the following:

- diarrhea
- passing blood with your stool or rectal bleeding

- cramping and pain in the abdomen
- passing mucus or pus with your stool
- tenesmus, which means feeling a constant urge to have a bowel movement even though your bowel may be empty
- an urgent need to have a bowel movement

Symptoms of ulcerative colitis may vary in severity. For example, mild symptoms may include having fewer than four bowel movements a day and sometimes passing blood with stool. Severe symptoms may include having more than six bowel movements a day and passing blood with stool most of the time. In extremely severe—or fulminant—ulcerative colitis, you may have more than 10 bloody bowel movements in a day.

Some symptoms are more likely to occur if ulcerative colitis is more severe or affects more of the large intestine. These symptoms include the following:

- fatigue, or feeling tired
- fever
- nausea or vomiting
- weight loss

You may have periods of remission—times when symptoms disappear—that can last for weeks or years. After a period of remission, you may have a relapse, or a return of symptoms.

WHAT CAUSES ULCERATIVE COLITIS?

Doctors are not sure what causes ulcerative colitis. Experts think that the following factors may play a role in causing ulcerative colitis.

- **Genes**. Ulcerative colitis sometimes runs in families. Research suggests that certain genes increase the chance that a person will develop ulcerative colitis.
- **Abnormal immune reactions**. Abnormal reactions of the immune system may play a role in causing ulcerative colitis. Abnormal immune reactions lead to inflammation in the large intestine.
- **Microbiome**. The microbes in your digestive tract— including bacteria, viruses, and fungi—that help with

digestion are called the "microbiome." Studies have found differences between the microbiomes of people who have IBD and those who do not. Researchers are still studying the relationship between the microbiome and IBD.

- **Environment.** Experts think a person's environment— one's surroundings and factors outside the body—may play a role in causing ulcerative colitis. Researchers are still studying how people's environments interact with genes, the immune system, and the microbiome to affect the chance of developing ulcerative colitis.

HOW DO DOCTORS DIAGNOSE ULCERATIVE COLITIS?

To diagnose ulcerative colitis, doctors review medical and family history, perform a physical exam, and order medical tests. Doctors order tests to:

- confirm the diagnosis of ulcerative colitis
- find out how severe ulcerative colitis is and how much of the large intestine is affected
- rule out other health problems—such as infections, irritable bowel syndrome, or Crohn's disease—that may cause symptoms similar to those of ulcerative colitis

Medical and Family History

To help diagnose ulcerative colitis, your doctor will ask about your symptoms, your medical history, and any medicines you take. Your doctor will also ask about lifestyle factors, such as smoking, and about your family medical history.

Physical Exam

During a physical exam, your doctor may:

- check your blood pressure, heart rate, and temperature (If you have ulcerative colitis, doctors may use these measures, along with information about your symptoms and test results, to find out how severe the disease is.)

- use a stethoscope to listen to sounds within your abdomen
- press on your abdomen to feel for tenderness or masses

The physical exam may also include a digital rectal exam to check for blood in your stool.

WHAT TESTS DO DOCTORS USE TO DIAGNOSE ULCERATIVE COLITIS?

Doctors may use blood tests, stool tests, and endoscopy of the large intestine to diagnose ulcerative colitis.

Blood Tests

A health-care professional will take a blood sample from you and send the sample to a lab. Doctors use blood tests to check for signs of ulcerative colitis and complications, such as anemia. Blood tests can also show signs of infection or other digestive diseases.

Stool Tests

A health-care professional will give you a container for catching and storing the stool. You will receive instructions on where to send or take the container for analysis. Doctors may use stool tests to check for conditions other than ulcerative colitis, such as infections that could be causing your symptoms. Doctors may also use stool tests to check for signs of inflammation in the intestines.

Endoscopy of the Large Intestine

Doctors order an endoscopy of the large intestine with biopsies to diagnose ulcerative colitis and rule out other digestive conditions. Doctors also use endoscopy to find out how severe ulcerative colitis is affected and how much of the large intestine is affected.

During an endoscopy, doctors use an endoscope—a long, flexible, narrow tube with a light and a tiny camera on one end—to view the lining of the large intestine. Doctors obtain biopsies by passing an instrument through the endoscope to take small pieces of tissue from the lining of your rectum and colon. A pathologist will examine the tissue under a microscope. The following are the two types of endoscopy used to diagnose ulcerative colitis:

- **Colonoscopy.** During this endoscopy, a doctor uses a type of endoscope called a "colonoscope" to view the lining of your rectum and your entire colon.
- **Flexible sigmoidoscopy.** During this endoscopy, a doctor uses a type of endoscope called a "sigmoidoscope" to view the lining of your rectum and lower colon.

HOW DO DOCTORS TREAT ULCERATIVE COLITIS?

Doctors treat ulcerative colitis with medicines and surgery. Each person experiences ulcerative colitis differently, and doctors recommend treatments based on how severe ulcerative colitis is and how much of the large intestine is affected. Doctors most often treat severe and fulminant ulcerative colitis in a hospital.

Medicines

Doctors prescribe medicines to reduce inflammation in the large intestine and to help bring on and maintain remission—a time when your symptoms disappear. People with ulcerative colitis typically need lifelong treatment with medicines unless they have surgery to remove the colon and rectum.

Which medicines your doctor prescribes will depend on how severe ulcerative colitis is. Ulcerative colitis medicines that reduce inflammation in the large intestine include the following:

- **Aminosalicylates.** Doctors prescribe these medicines to treat mild or moderate ulcerative colitis or to help people stay in remission.
- **Corticosteroids.** These are also called "steroids." Doctors prescribe these medicines to treat moderate-to-severe ulcerative colitis and to treat mild-to-moderate ulcerative colitis in people who do not respond to aminosalicylates. Doctors typically do not prescribe

corticosteroids for long-term use or to maintain remission. Long-term use may cause serious side effects.
- **Immunosuppressants**. Doctors may prescribe these medicines to treat people with moderate-to-severe ulcerative colitis and help them stay in remission. Doctors may also prescribe immunosuppressants to treat severe ulcerative colitis in people who are hospitalized and do not respond to other medicines.
- **Biologics**. Doctors prescribe these medicines to treat people with moderate-to-severe ulcerative colitis and help them stay in remission.
- **A novel small molecule medicine**. Doctors may prescribe this medicine for adults with moderate-to-severe ulcerative colitis who do not respond to other medicines or who have severe side effects with other medicines.

Surgery
Your doctor may recommend surgery if you have:
- colorectal cancer
- dysplasia, or precancerous cells that increase the risk of developing colorectal cancer
- complications that are life-threatening, such as severe rectal bleeding, toxic megacolon, or perforation of the large intestine
- symptoms that do not improve or stop after treatment with medicines
- symptoms that only improve with continuous treatment with corticosteroids, which may cause serious side effects when used for a long time

To treat ulcerative colitis, surgeons typically remove the colon and rectum and change how your body stores and passes stool. The most common types of surgery for ulcerative colitis are as follows:
- **Ileoanal reservoir surgery**. Surgeons create an internal reservoir, or pouch, from the end part of the small intestine, called the "ileum." Surgeons attach the pouch

to the anus. Ileoanal reservoir surgery most often requires two or three operations. After the operations, the stool will collect in the internal pouch and pass through the anus during bowel movements.

- **Ileostomy**. Surgeons attach the end of your ileum to an opening in your abdomen called a "stoma." After an ileostomy, the stool will pass through the stoma. You will use an ostomy pouch—a bag attached to the stoma and worn outside the body—to collect stool.

Surgery may be laparoscopic or open. In laparoscopic surgery, surgeons make small cuts in your abdomen and insert special tools to view, remove, or repair organs and tissues. In open surgery, surgeons make a larger cut to open your abdomen.

If you are considering surgery to treat ulcerative colitis, talk with your doctor or surgeon about what type of surgery might be right for you and the possible risks and benefits.

HOW DO DOCTORS TREAT SYMPTOMS AND COMPLICATIONS OF ULCERATIVE COLITIS?

Doctors may recommend or prescribe other treatments for symptoms or complications of ulcerative colitis. Talk with your doctor before taking any over-the-counter (OTC) medicines.

To treat mild pain, doctors may recommend acetaminophen instead of nonsteroidal anti-inflammatory drugs (NSAIDs). People with ulcerative colitis should avoid taking NSAIDs for pain because these medicines can make symptoms worse.

To prevent or slow the loss of bone mass and osteoporosis, doctors may recommend calcium and vitamin D supplements or medicines, if needed. For safety reasons, talk with your doctor before using dietary supplements or any other complementary or alternative medicines or practices.

Doctors most often treat severe complications in a hospital. Doctors may give:
- antibiotics, if severe ulcerative colitis or complications lead to infection
- blood transfusions to treat severe anemia

- IV fluids and electrolytes to prevent and treat dehydration

Doctors may treat life-threatening complications with surgery.

WHAT SHOULD YOU EAT IF YOU HAVE ULCERATIVE COLITIS?

If you have ulcerative colitis, you should eat a healthy, well-balanced diet. Talk with your doctor about a healthy eating plan.

Ulcerative colitis symptoms may cause some people to lose their appetite and eat less, and they may not get enough nutrients. In children, a lack of nutrients may play a role in problems with growth and development.

Researchers have not found that specific foods cause ulcerative colitis symptoms although healthier diets appear to be associated with less risk of developing IBD. Researchers have not found that specific foods worsen ulcerative colitis. Talk with your doctor about any foods that seem to be related to your symptoms. Your doctor may suggest keeping a food diary to help identify foods that seem to make your symptoms worse.

Depending on your symptoms and the medicines you take, your doctor may recommend changes to your diet. Your doctor may also recommend dietary supplements.[3]

[3] "Definition and Facts of Ulcerative Colitis," National Institute of Diabetes and Digestive and Kidney Diseases (NIDDK), September 2020. Available online. URL: www.niddk.nih.gov/health-information/digestive-diseases/ulcerative-colitis/definition-facts. Accessed May 10, 2023.

Chapter 42 | **Autoimmune Liver Disorders**

Chapter Contents

WHAT IS AUTOIMMUNE HEPATITIS?

Autoimmune hepatitis is a chronic disease in which your body's immune system attacks the liver and causes inflammation and liver damage. Without treatment, autoimmune hepatitis may get worse and lead to complications such as cirrhosis and liver failure.

Autoimmune hepatitis is an autoimmune disease. Your immune system normally makes large numbers of antibodies and lymphocytes that help fight off infections. The normal immune system does not attack healthy cells in a person's body. In autoimmune diseases, your immune system makes certain types of antibodies—called "autoantibodies"—and lymphocytes that attack your body's own cells and organs.

WHAT ARE THE TYPES OF AUTOIMMUNE HEPATITIS?

Experts have identified two types of autoimmune hepatitis: type 1 and type 2. The immune system makes different autoantibodies in each type. Type 1 autoimmune hepatitis is much more common than type 2, in both adults and children. Only about 5–10 percent of people with autoimmune hepatitis have type 2, and type 2 most often develops during childhood.

HOW COMMON IS AUTOIMMUNE HEPATITIS?

Rates of autoimmune hepatitis vary in different parts of the world and in different age groups. Studies have found that about 4–43 out of 100,000 adults and about 2–10 out of 100,000 children have autoimmune hepatitis.

WHO IS MORE LIKELY TO HAVE AUTOIMMUNE HEPATITIS?

Autoimmune hepatitis can occur at any age and affects people of all racial and ethnic groups. The disease is more common in females and women than in males. Studies have found that 71–95 percent of adults with autoimmune hepatitis are women and 60–76 percent of children with the disease are girls.

WHAT OTHER CONDITIONS DO PEOPLE WITH AUTOIMMUNE HEPATITIS HAVE?

Some people who have autoimmune hepatitis may also have features of liver diseases that affect their bile ducts—the tubes that carry bile out of the liver—such as:

- primary biliary cholangitis (PBC)
- primary sclerosing cholangitis (PSC)
- bile duct problems that cannot be classified as PBC or PSC

People with autoimmune hepatitis are at risk of having other autoimmune diseases, for example:

- celiac disease
- thyroid conditions, such as Graves disease and Hashimoto disease
- rheumatoid arthritis (RA)
- type 1 diabetes
- inflammatory bowel disease (IBD), such as ulcerative colitis
- vitiligo
- lupus

WHAT ARE THE COMPLICATIONS OF AUTOIMMUNE HEPATITIS?

Autoimmune hepatitis may lead to complications, but early diagnosis and treatment can lower your chances of developing them.

Acute Liver Failure

Very rarely, autoimmune hepatitis can cause acute liver failure, a condition in which your liver fails rapidly without warning.

Cirrhosis

Many people have cirrhosis when they are first diagnosed with autoimmune hepatitis. In cirrhosis, scar tissue replaces healthy liver tissue and prevents your liver from working normally. Scar tissue also partly blocks the flow of blood through the liver. As cirrhosis gets worse, the liver begins to fail.

Liver Failure

Cirrhosis may eventually lead to liver failure, also called "end-stage liver disease." With liver failure, your liver is badly damaged and stops working. People with liver failure may require a liver transplant.

Liver Cancer

Cirrhosis increases your chance of getting liver cancer. Your doctor may suggest blood tests and an ultrasound or another type of imaging test to check for liver cancer. Finding cancer at an early stage improves the chance of curing the cancer.

SYMPTOMS OF AUTOIMMUNE HEPATITIS

People with autoimmune hepatitis may have some of the following symptoms:

- feeling tired
- joint pain
- nausea
- poor appetite
- pain over the liver, in the upper part of the abdomen
- yellowish color of the whites of the eyes and skin, called "jaundice"
- darkening of the color of urine
- lightening of the color of stools
- skin conditions, such as rash, psoriasis, vitiligo, or acne

If you have symptoms of autoimmune hepatitis, they can range from mild to severe.

Many people with autoimmune hepatitis have no symptoms. In such cases, doctors may find you have signs of liver problems during routine blood tests, and this may lead to a diagnosis of autoimmune hepatitis. People without symptoms at diagnosis may develop symptoms later.

Some people with autoimmune hepatitis do not have symptoms until they develop complications due to cirrhosis. These symptoms include the following:

- feeling tired or weak
- losing weight without trying
- swelling of the abdomen from a buildup of fluid, called "ascites"
- swelling of the lower legs, ankles, or feet, called "edema"
- itchy skin
- jaundice
- vomiting blood if cirrhosis leads to enlarged veins in the esophagus, called "esophageal varices," and those varices burst
- confusion or difficulty thinking if cirrhosis leads to a buildup of toxins in the brain, called "hepatic encephalopathy"

CAUSES OF AUTOIMMUNE HEPATITIS

Experts are not sure what causes autoimmune hepatitis. Studies suggest that certain genes make some people more likely to develop autoimmune diseases. In people with these genes, factors in the environment may trigger an autoimmune reaction that causes their immune system to attack the liver.

Researchers are still studying the environmental triggers that play a role in autoimmune hepatitis. These triggers may include certain viruses and medicines.

Some medicines can cause liver injury that resembles autoimmune hepatitis. In most cases, the liver injury goes away when the medicine is stopped. Telling your doctor the names of all the medicines you take, even over-the-counter (OTC) medicines or herbal or botanical products, is important.

HOW DO DOCTORS DIAGNOSE AUTOIMMUNE HEPATITIS?

Doctors diagnose autoimmune hepatitis based on a combination of information from your medical history, a physical exam, and tests.

Medical History

Your doctor will ask about your symptoms and other factors that could be damaging your liver. For example, your doctor may ask about any medicines and herbal or botanical products you take and how much alcohol you drink. Your doctor will ask you about other autoimmune diseases that you might have, such as IBD or thyroid conditions.

Physical Exam

During a physical exam, your doctor will check for signs of liver damage such as:

- yellowish color of the whites of the eyes
- changes in the skin
- enlargement of the liver or spleen
- tenderness or swelling in the abdomen
- swelling in the lower legs, feet, or ankles, called "edema"

WHAT TESTS DO DOCTORS USE TO DIAGNOSE AUTOIMMUNE HEPATITIS?

Your doctor may order blood tests, imaging tests, and a liver biopsy to diagnose autoimmune hepatitis. No single test can diagnose autoimmune hepatitis. In most cases, doctors order a combination of tests, including a liver biopsy, to make a diagnosis.

Blood Tests

Your doctor may order one or more blood tests to look for signs of autoimmune hepatitis or other liver diseases. A health-care professional will take a blood sample from you and send the sample to a lab.

Liver Tests

Liver tests can check levels of the liver enzymes alanine amino-transferase (ALT) and aspartate aminotransferase (AST). ALT and AST are particularly important because these liver enzymes are highly elevated in people with autoimmune hepatitis. Doctors check ALT and AST levels to follow the progress of the disease and how it responds to treatment.

Antibody Tests

Doctors order antibody tests to check for autoantibodies—antibodies that attack your healthy tissues and cells by mistake—such as antinuclear antibody (ANA) and anti-smooth muscle antibody (anti-SMA). Doctors may also order blood tests to check levels of a type of protein called "immunoglobulin G" (IgG).

Other Blood Tests

Doctors order additional blood tests to look for other liver diseases that have symptoms similar to autoimmune hepatitis, such as viral hepatitis, PBC, PSC, nonalcoholic steatohepatitis (NASH), or Wilson disease.

Imaging Tests

Your doctor may order imaging tests of your abdomen and liver.

Ultrasound

Ultrasound uses a hand-held device, called a "transducer," that bounces safe, painless sound waves off organs to create images of their structure. An ultrasound can show whether the liver is enlarged, has an abnormal shape or texture, or has blocked bile ducts.

Computed Tomography

Computed tomography (CT) uses a combination of x-rays and computer technology to create images. A CT scan can show the size and shape of the liver and spleen and whether there are signs of cirrhosis.

Magnetic Resonance Imaging

Magnetic resonance imaging (MRI) uses radio waves and magnets to produce detailed images of organs and soft tissues without using x-rays. An MRI scan can show the shape and size of the liver and detect evidence of cirrhosis. Special MRI scans can estimate the amount of fat and scarring in the liver.

Liver Biopsy

During a liver biopsy, a doctor will take a piece of tissue from your liver. A pathologist will examine the tissue under a microscope to look for the amount of damage and features of specific liver diseases. A doctor can use a liver biopsy to look for the features of autoimmune hepatitis and to check the amount of scarring to find out if you have cirrhosis.

HOW DO DOCTORS TREAT AUTOIMMUNE HEPATITIS?

Doctors treat autoimmune hepatitis with medicines that suppress—or decrease the activity of—your immune system, reducing your immune system's attack on your liver. The medicines doctors most often prescribe are as follows:

- corticosteroids, also called "steroids"
- immunosuppressants

Doctors typically start with a relatively high dose of corticosteroids and then gradually lower the dose. The medicines used to treat autoimmune hepatitis can cause side effects, so your doctor will try to find the lowest dose that works for you.

Your doctor will use blood tests to check levels of the liver enzymes ALT and AST. If your ALT and AST levels drop, it means you are responding to the medicines.

Treatment can relieve symptoms and prevent or reverse liver damage in many people with autoimmune hepatitis. Early treatment of autoimmune hepatitis can lower the chances of developing cirrhosis and other complications. A minority of people with autoimmune hepatitis, including some people who have a mild form of the disease or increased risks related to the treatment, may not need medicines.

Remission

With treatment, you may experience remission. Remission is a period when you do not have any symptoms and your test results show that your liver is working better and is no longer being damaged. Many people with autoimmune hepatitis go into remission.

If the first medicines doctors prescribe do not bring on remission, doctors may prescribe other medicines.

ALT and AST levels falling to normal is a sign of remission. If you are in remission, your doctor may gradually lower the dose of medicines again to help reduce the medicines' side effects. After you stay in remission for at least two years, your doctor may try to stop your medicines to see if you remain in remission without them.

Your doctor will continue to perform routine blood tests for ALT and AST and monitor your symptoms while you are in remission to check for relapse. Your doctor may suggest a repeat liver biopsy to monitor liver damage and guide management.

Autoimmune hepatitis is often a long-term, if not lifelong, condition. Your doctor will need to watch your condition carefully, particularly when treatment is stopped because the liver damage may return quickly and may be severe. Stopping treatment without your doctor's guidance and monitoring may be very dangerous.

Relapse

Some people with autoimmune hepatitis stay in remission without medicines. However, most people relapse after stopping medicines and need to start taking medicines again. When you relapse, blood tests show a rise in ALT and AST levels, and autoimmune hepatitis begins causing symptoms or damaging your liver again.

If you relapse, your doctor will restart or adjust your medicines to treat autoimmune hepatitis.

Incomplete or Failed Response to Treatment

Some people with autoimmune hepatitis have:
- an incomplete response to treatment, meaning that treatment helps but does not lead to remission
- a failed response to treatment, meaning the inflammation and liver damage of autoimmune hepatitis keep getting worse despite treatment

If you have an incomplete response to treatment, your doctor may change the medicines you take to treat autoimmune hepatitis.

If the disease continues to damage your liver, you may develop complications and need additional treatments.

Do Medicines Used to Treat Autoimmune Hepatitis Have Side Effects?

Medicines for autoimmune hepatitis can cause side effects. Your doctor will monitor any side effects and help you manage them while you take these medicines. Your doctor may also adjust the doses or change the medicines you take. You may need to stop taking medicines if you have severe side effects.

Side effects of corticosteroids may include the following:
- changes in how you look, which may include weight gain, a fuller face, acne, or more facial hair
- diabetes
- eye problems, such as cataracts or glaucoma
- high blood pressure
- loss of bone density, called "osteopenia"
- mental health problems, such as extreme changes in mood or psychosis
- pancreatitis

Side effects of azathioprine may include the following:
- low white blood cell (WBC) count
- nausea or vomiting
- skin rash
- liver damage
- pancreatitis

Corticosteroids and azathioprine suppress, or decrease, the activity of your immune system, which increases your risk for infections. These medicines can also increase your risk of developing cancers, especially skin cancers.

Before you start taking medicines to treat autoimmune hepatitis, your doctor may do the following:
- Make sure you have had recommended vaccines, including vaccines for hepatitis A and hepatitis B.
- Order tests to check for hepatitis B infection. In people with a current or past hepatitis B infection, medicines

used to treat autoimmune hepatitis may cause hepatitis B reactivation. In some cases, doctors may recommend medicines to prevent hepatitis B reactivation.

- Order a genetic test for thiopurine S-methyltransferase (TPMT) deficiency. When the TPMT enzyme does not work the way it should, people have a higher risk for serious side effects from certain immunosuppressants.

How Do Doctors Treat the Complications of Autoimmune Hepatitis?

If autoimmune hepatitis leads to cirrhosis, doctors can treat the related health problems and complications with medicines, medical procedures, or surgery.

If you have cirrhosis, you have a greater chance of developing liver cancer. Your doctor may suggest blood tests and an ultrasound or another type of imaging test to check for liver cancer. Finding cancer at an early stage improves the chance of curing the cancer.

If autoimmune hepatitis causes acute liver failure or if cirrhosis leads to liver cancer or liver failure, you may need a liver transplant.

WHAT SHOULD YOU EAT IF YOU HAVE AUTOIMMUNE HEPATITIS?

Researchers have not found that eating, diet, and nutrition play a role in causing or preventing autoimmune hepatitis.

If you have autoimmune hepatitis, you should eat a healthy, well-balanced diet. A healthy diet is also important if autoimmune hepatitis leads to cirrhosis.

Using corticosteroids for a long time to treat autoimmune hepatitis can lead to a loss of bone density, called "osteopenia," which can lead to osteoporosis. Doctors may recommend that people who take corticosteroids also take dietary supplements of calcium and vitamin D to help prevent osteoporosis. Follow your doctor's instructions on the type and dose of supplements you should take.[1]

---

[1] "Autoimmune Hepatitis," National Institute of Diabetes and Digestive and Kidney Diseases (NIDDK), March 2023. Available online. URL: www.niddk.nih.gov/health-information/liver-disease/autoimmune-hepatitis. Accessed May 11, 2023.

Section 42.2 | Primary Biliary Cholangitis

WHAT IS PRIMARY BILIARY CHOLANGITIS?

Primary biliary cholangitis (PBC) is a chronic disease in which the small bile ducts in the liver become inflamed and are eventually destroyed. When there are no bile ducts, bile builds up and causes liver damage. Over time, this damage can lead to liver scarring, cirrhosis, and eventually liver failure. PBC is believed to be an autoimmune disease in which a person's own immune system becomes overactive and attacks normal, healthy bile duct cells.

Does Primary Biliary Cholangitis Have Another Name?

Doctors and patients often use the abbreviation PBC for primary biliary cholangitis. The disease used to be called "primary biliary cirrhosis."

HOW COMMON IS PRIMARY BILIARY CHOLANGITIS?

Researchers estimated that in 2014, about 58 out of every 100,000 U.S. women and about 15 out of every 100,000 U.S. men had PBC.

WHO IS MORE LIKELY TO GET PRIMARY BILIARY CHOLANGITIS?

Primary biliary cholangitis is more common in:
- women than in men
- people who are middle-aged (The average age at diagnosis is 60.)
- people who are White compared with other racial or ethnic groups
- people who have a parent or sibling—particularly an identical twin—with PBC

WHAT OTHER HEALTH PROBLEMS DO PEOPLE WITH PRIMARY BILIARY CHOLANGITIS HAVE?

People with PBC may have other autoimmune diseases, including the following:
- autoimmune thyroid diseases—conditions in which the immune system attacks the thyroid gland

- Raynaud disease
- Sjögren syndrome
- scleroderma
- autoimmune hepatitis

Women with PBC may also have frequent urinary tract infections (UTIs).

WHAT ARE THE COMPLICATIONS OF PRIMARY BILIARY CHOLANGITIS?

Common complications of PBC include the following:
- high blood cholesterol levels
- osteoporosis, or loss of calcium from the bones
- low levels of fat-soluble vitamins A, D, E, and K

These common complications can be prevented and treated.

Liver Complications

Primary biliary cholangitis can also damage the liver, leading to liver complications.
- **Cirrhosis**. In cirrhosis, scar tissue replaces healthy liver tissue and prevents your liver from working normally. As cirrhosis gets worse, the liver begins to fail.
- **Portal hypertension**. Portal hypertension most often occurs when scar tissue in a liver with cirrhosis partly blocks and slows the normal flow of blood, which causes high blood pressure in the portal vein. However, people with PBC may develop portal hypertension before they develop cirrhosis. When portal hypertension reaches a certain level, it can cause additional complications, such as:
  - swelling in your legs, ankles, or feet, called "edema"
  - buildup of fluid in your abdomen, called "ascites"
  - enlarged veins—called "varices"—in your esophagus, stomach, or intestines, which can lead to internal bleeding if the veins burst

- confusion or difficulty thinking caused by the buildup of toxins in your brain, called "hepatic encephalopathy"
- **Liver failure.** Cirrhosis may eventually lead to liver failure, also called "end-stage liver disease." With liver failure, your liver is badly damaged and stops working. People with liver failure may require a liver transplant.
- **Liver cancer.** Research suggests that people with cirrhosis caused by PBC and men with PBC have an increased risk for liver cancer.

WHAT ARE THE SYMPTOMS OF PRIMARY BILIARY CHOLANGITIS?

The most common symptoms of PBC are the following:
- feeling tired
- itchy skin

Other symptoms may include the following:
- discomfort or pain in the upper right side of your abdomen
- joint pain or arthritis
- symptoms of other health problems that may occur along with PBC, such as dry eyes and dry mouth due to Sjögren syndrome

As the disease gets worse, symptoms may include the following:
- darkening of skin color
- fatty deposits that appear as yellow bumps on the skin, called "xanthomas"
- symptoms of cirrhosis, such as edema, jaundice, and weight loss

Many people have no symptoms when they are first diagnosed with PBC. Doctors diagnose about 60 percent of people with PBC before symptoms begin. People with PBC and no symptoms are identified through blood tests. Some people do not have symptoms for years after they have been diagnosed with PBC.

WHAT CAUSES PRIMARY BILIARY CHOLANGITIS?

Experts are not sure what causes PBC. Studies suggest that certain genes make some people more likely to develop the disease. In people with these genes, factors in the environment may trigger an autoimmune reaction that causes their immune system to attack the small bile ducts in the liver, causing PBC.

Possible environmental triggers include the following:
- infections
- cigarette smoking
- exposure to certain chemicals

HOW DO DOCTORS DIAGNOSE PRIMARY BILIARY CHOLANGITIS?

Doctors diagnose PBC based on your medical and family history, a physical exam, and the results of medical tests.

Medical and Family History

Your doctor will ask you about your symptoms. He or she will also ask whether:
- you have a history of certain autoimmune diseases
- one of your parents or siblings has been diagnosed with PBC
- you have a history of infections and exposure to certain chemicals

Physical Exam

Your doctor will examine your body, use a stethoscope to listen to sounds in your abdomen, and tap or press on specific areas of your abdomen. He or she will:
- look for yellowing of the whites of your eyes and your skin
- check to see if your liver and spleen are larger than they should be
- check for abdominal tenderness or pain, particularly in the upper right side of your abdomen

WHAT TESTS DO DOCTORS USE TO DIAGNOSE PRIMARY BILIARY CHOLANGITIS?
Blood Tests
For a blood test, a health-care professional will take a blood sample from you and send the sample to a lab. Your doctor may recommend the following blood tests.

- **Antimitochondrial antibodies (AMAs).** AMAs are found in the blood of about 95 percent of people with PBC.
- **Liver tests.** Liver tests can show abnormal liver enzyme levels, which may be a sign of damage in your liver or biliary tract. Higher-than-normal levels of the liver enzyme alkaline phosphatase occur in people with diseases that destroy or block the bile ducts, such as PBC.
- Your doctor may diagnose PBC if you have AMAs and higher-than-normal levels of alkaline phosphatase in your blood, even if you have no other signs or symptoms of the disease.
- **Cholesterol.** People with PBC may have higher-than-normal cholesterol levels.

Imaging Tests
Your doctor may use imaging tests such as x-rays and ultrasounds to help diagnose PBC by ruling out other causes of bile duct damage, such as gallstones, bile duct strictures, and tumors.

Liver Biopsy
During a liver biopsy, a doctor will take small pieces of tissue from the liver. A pathologist will examine the tissue with a microscope. Your doctor may perform a liver biopsy to:
- rule out other diseases that may be causing your symptoms
- confirm the diagnosis of PBC
- determine whether the disease is advanced—as shown by the amount of liver scarring or cirrhosis—or is very active

HOW DO DOCTORS TREAT PRIMARY BILIARY CHOLANGITIS?

Doctors treat PBC with medicines. Your doctor may prescribe ursodiol. Although ursodiol does not cure PBC, it can slow the progression of liver damage. People who respond to ursodiol early in the course of PBC can live longer without needing a liver transplant.

If you do not respond to ursodiol, your doctor may prescribe obeticholic acid. Although obeticholic acid may improve blood test results, it may worsen symptoms. Obeticholic acid has not been shown to improve the course of illness or prevent cirrhosis. People with cirrhosis should not use obeticholic acid because it can cause worsening of the disease.

How Do Doctors Treat the Symptoms of Primary Biliary Cholangitis?

Your doctor may recommend over-the-counter (OTC) medicines or prescribe medicines to treat symptoms of PBC, such as itchy skin.

How Do Doctors Treat the Complications of Primary Biliary Cholangitis?

Doctors may treat common complications of PBC with medicines, dietary supplements, or changes in your diet and lifestyle.

- If you have higher-than-normal blood cholesterol levels, your doctor may prescribe medicines called "statins" and recommend lifestyle changes.
- For osteoporosis, your doctor may prescribe medicines that slow or stop bone loss and improve bone density. Your doctor may recommend dietary supplements of calcium and vitamin D.
- For low levels of fat-soluble vitamins, your doctor may recommend dietary supplements of vitamins A, D, E, and K. Follow your doctor's instructions on the type and amount of vitamins you should take.
- If you have dry eyes and dry mouth due to Sjögren syndrome, you should have regular eye and dental examinations.

Liver Complications

Doctors may recommend additional treatments for liver complications of PBC.

- **Cirrhosis or portal hypertension**. If PBC leads to cirrhosis or portal hypertension, doctors can treat the health problems related to these conditions with medicines, minor medical procedures, and surgery.
- **Liver failure**. If cirrhosis leads to liver failure, you may need a liver transplant.
- **Liver cancer**. If you have cirrhosis or other risk factors, your doctor may suggest blood tests and an ultrasound or another type of imaging test to check for liver cancer. Finding cancer at an early stage improves the chance of curing the cancer.

When Do Doctors Consider a Liver Transplant for Primary Biliary Cholangitis?

Your doctor will consider a liver transplant when your PBC leads to liver failure. Doctors consider liver transplants only after they have ruled out all other treatment options. Talk with your doctor to find out whether a liver transplant is right for you.

What Can You Do to Help Prevent Further Liver Damage?

If you have PBC, you can take the following steps to help prevent further liver damage:

- Carefully follow your doctor's instructions and take your medicines and dietary supplements as directed.
- Quit smoking.
- Avoid drinking alcohol. If you have cirrhosis, completely stop drinking alcohol.
- Have regular checkups, as recommended by your doctor.
- Talk with your doctor before taking:
  - prescription medicines
  - OTC medicines

- dietary supplements
- complementary and alternative medicines
- Try to reach and stay at a healthy body weight.

WHAT SHOULD YOU EAT IF YOU HAVE PRIMARY BILIARY CHOLANGITIS?

You should eat a healthy, well-balanced diet. Good nutrition is important in all stages of PBC to help your liver work properly and manage complications.

Your doctor can recommend a healthy eating plan that is well-balanced and provides enough calories and nutrients. Your doctor may recommend that you eat foods high in calcium and vitamin D or take dietary supplements of these nutrients to help prevent osteoporosis. If you have low levels of fat-soluble vitamins A, D, E, or K, your doctor may also recommend supplements of these vitamins. Follow your doctor's instructions on the type and amount of vitamins you should take.

What Foods Should You Avoid Eating If You Have Primary Biliary Cholangitis?

You should avoid eating raw or undercooked shellfish, fish, meat, and unpasteurized milk. Bacteria or viruses from these foods may cause severe infections in people with liver disease.

If you have PBC, your doctor will recommend that you quit smoking and stop drinking alcohol or, at least, limit your intake. If you have PBC and cirrhosis, you should completely stop drinking alcohol.[2]

---

[2] "Primary Biliary Cholangitis (Primary Biliary Cirrhosis)," National Institute of Diabetes and Digestive and Kidney Diseases (NIDDK), March 2021. Available online. URL: www.niddk.nih.gov/health-information/liver-disease/primary-biliary-cholangitis. Accessed May 11, 2023.

Section 42.3 | Primary Sclerosing Cholangitis

WHAT IS PRIMARY SCLEROSING CHOLANGITIS?

Primary sclerosing cholangitis (PSC) is a chronic liver disease in which the bile ducts inside and outside the liver become inflamed and scarred and are eventually narrowed or blocked. When the bile ducts are narrowed or blocked, bile builds up in the liver and causes further liver damage. This damage can lead to cirrhosis and, eventually, liver failure. Medical experts believe PSC is an autoimmune disease, in which the immune system attacks normal, healthy bile duct cells.

HOW COMMON IS PRIMARY SCLEROSING CHOLANGITIS?

Researchers estimate about 5–16 people out of every 100,000 have PSC.

WHO IS MORE LIKELY TO DEVELOP PRIMARY SCLEROSING CHOLANGITIS?

Primary sclerosing cholangitis is more commonly diagnosed in people who:
- are between the ages of 30 and 40 although PSC may occur at any age
- are male (PSC affects twice as many males as females.)
- have inflammatory bowel disease (IBD), most commonly ulcerative colitis

WHAT OTHER HEALTH PROBLEMS DO PEOPLE WITH PRIMARY SCLEROSING CHOLANGITIS HAVE?

People with PSC may have other health problems, including the following:
- IBD (About 7 out of 10 people who have PSC also have IBD.)
- gallstones
- autoimmune hepatitis
- other autoimmune diseases, such as type 1 diabetes, celiac disease, and thyroid diseases

WHAT ARE THE COMPLICATIONS OF PRIMARY SCLEROSING CHOLANGITIS?

Primary sclerosing cholangitis can lead to liver complications such as cirrhosis, cancers, and bile duct infection.

Liver Complications

Primary sclerosing cholangitis can damage the liver, leading to cirrhosis and its complications.

Cirrhosis

In cirrhosis, scar tissue replaces healthy liver tissue and prevents your liver from working normally. As cirrhosis gets worse, the liver begins to fail.

Portal Hypertension

Portal hypertension most often occurs when scar tissue in the liver slows the normal flow of blood, which causes high blood pressure in the portal vein. The portal vein is the large blood vessel that carries blood from your stomach, intestines, spleen, gallbladder, and pancreas to the liver.

When portal hypertension reaches a certain level, it can cause additional complications, such as:

- swelling in the legs, ankles, or feet, called "edema"
- buildup of fluid in the abdomen, called "ascites"
- enlarged veins—called "varices"—in the esophagus, stomach, or intestines, which can lead to gastrointestinal (GI) bleeding if the veins burst
- confusion or difficulty thinking caused by a buildup of toxins in the brain, called "hepatic encephalopathy"

Liver Failure

Cirrhosis may eventually lead to liver failure, also called "end-stage liver disease." With liver failure, your liver is badly damaged and stops working. People with liver failure may require a liver transplant.

Cancer

PSC can increase the chance of developing certain cancers, including the following:

- Bile duct cancer is the most common type of cancer in people who have PSC. People with PSC have a 10–20 percent chance of developing bile duct cancer at some point in their lives.
- People with PSC have an increased chance of getting gallbladder cancer.
- People with cirrhosis due to PSC have an increased chance of getting liver cancer.
- People with PSC and IBD have an increased chance of getting colorectal cancer.

Bile Duct Infection

People with PSC may develop a bacterial infection in narrowed or blocked bile ducts. Medical procedures that affect the bile ducts, such as endoscopic retrograde cholangiopancreatography, increase the chance of bile duct infection.

Other Complications

Other complications of PSC may include:

- low levels of fat-soluble vitamins A, D, E, and K
- osteoporosis, or loss of calcium from the bones

WHAT ARE THE SYMPTOMS OF PRIMARY SCLEROSING CHOLANGITIS?

Symptoms of PSC may include the following:

- pain in the abdomen, or belly
- itchy skin
- diarrhea
- yellowish color of the whites of the eyes and skin, called "jaundice"
- feeling tired or weak
- fever

PSC may lead to a bile duct infection. Symptoms of a bile duct infection include the following:

- chills
- fever
- new or worsening jaundice
- pain in the upper right side of the abdomen

As the disease gets worse, you may develop cirrhosis. Symptoms of cirrhosis may include the following:

- swelling of the abdomen from a buildup of fluid, called "ascites"
- confusion or difficulty thinking caused by a buildup of toxins in the brain, called "hepatic encephalopathy"
- GI bleeding caused when enlarged veins—called "varices"—burst in the esophagus, stomach, or intestines
- other symptoms of cirrhosis, such as edema, jaundice, and weight loss

Because PSC gets worse slowly, you can have the disease for years before you have any symptoms. Many people have no symptoms when they are first diagnosed with PSC.

WHAT CAUSES PRIMARY SCLEROSING CHOLANGITIS?

Experts are not sure what causes PSC. Studies suggest that several factors may play a role, including the following:

- genes
- immune system problems
- changes in the bacteria in the digestive tract, also called "gut flora" or the "gut microbiome"
- bile duct injury caused by bile acids

HOW DO DOCTORS DIAGNOSE PRIMARY SCLEROSING CHOLANGITIS?

Doctors diagnose PSC based on medical and family history, a physical exam, and the results of medical tests.

Medical and Family History

The doctor will ask about your symptoms. He or she may also ask whether you have:

- a history of IBD, particularly ulcerative colitis
- a parent or sibling who has PSC or IBD
- a personal or family history of autoimmune diseases, such as autoimmune hepatitis, type 1 diabetes, celiac disease, and thyroid diseases

Physical Exam

Your doctor will examine your body, including your abdomen. He or she will check for:

- signs of cirrhosis and liver failure, such as jaundice, which can make the whites of the eyes and skin look yellow
- scratch marks from scratching itchy skin
- signs that the liver and spleen are larger than they should be
- tenderness or pain in the abdomen

WHAT TESTS DO DOCTORS USE TO DIAGNOSE PRIMARY SCLEROSING CHOLANGITIS?

Blood Tests

A health-care professional will take a blood sample from you and send the sample to a lab.

Liver tests can show abnormal levels of liver enzymes and other substances in your blood. Abnormal levels of certain liver enzymes may be a sign your liver or bile ducts are damaged.

Imaging Tests

To diagnose PSC, doctors typically order one of the following special imaging tests to examine the bile ducts:

- **Magnetic resonance cholangiopancreatography (MRCP).** MRCP uses a magnetic resonance imaging (MRI) machine to create pictures of the bile ducts. It is the most common test that doctors use to diagnose PSC.

- **Endoscopic retrograde cholangiopancreatography (ERCP).** ERCP combines upper GI endoscopy and x-rays to examine the bile and pancreatic ducts. Doctors may also use ERCP to treat narrowed bile ducts.
- **Percutaneous transhepatic cholangiography (PTC).** PTC is an x-ray of the bile ducts. A health-care professional inserts a needle through the skin and into the liver to inject a special dye into the bile ducts. The special dye lets a doctor see the bile ducts on the x-ray.

Doctors may also order other imaging tests to check for signs of PSC, other bile duct or liver problems, or complications. These tests include the following:

- **Ultrasound.** It uses a hand-held device, called a "transducer," that bounces safe, painless sound waves off organs to create an image of their structure.
- **Computed tomography (CT) scan.** This is a combination of x-rays and computer technology to create images of the liver.
- **Elastography.** This is a special test that measures the stiffness of the liver. Increased liver stiffness may be a sign of fibrosis or scarring.

Liver Biopsy

A liver biopsy is generally not needed to diagnose PSC. However, in some cases, doctors may order a liver biopsy to check for signs of other liver diseases, such as autoimmune hepatitis.

During a liver biopsy, a doctor will take small pieces of tissue from the liver. A pathologist will examine the tissue under a microscope.

Colonoscopy

For people who have PSC and have not already been diagnosed with IBD, doctors may recommend a colonoscopy to check for

IBD. Many people with PSC have mild IBD and do not have IBD symptoms.

HOW DO DOCTORS TREAT PRIMARY SCLEROSING CHOLANGITIS?

Currently, no cure or effective treatments for PSC exist. However, doctors can treat narrowed or blocked bile ducts and symptoms of PSC.

Narrowed or Blocked Bile Ducts

If bile ducts are narrowed or blocked, doctors may use ERCP to open them and help keep them open. To help keep ducts open, doctors sometimes place stents. Stents are tiny tubes that a doctor leaves in narrowed ducts for a short time to hold them open.

In some cases, doctors may use percutaneous transhepatic cholangiography to open narrowed or blocked bile ducts.

Itchy Skin

Doctors may recommend OTC medicines or prescribe medicines to treat itchy skin caused by PSC.

HOW DO DOCTORS TREAT THE COMPLICATIONS OF PRIMARY SCLEROSING CHOLANGITIS?

Liver Complications

Doctors may recommend treatments for liver complications of PSC.

Cirrhosis or Portal Hypertension

If PSC leads to cirrhosis or portal hypertension, doctors can treat the health problems related to these conditions with medicines, medical procedures, or surgery.

Liver Failure

If cirrhosis leads to liver failure, you may need a liver transplant.

Cancer

PSC increases the risk of developing several types of cancer. Your doctor may recommend tests to check for signs of cancer. Finding cancer at an early stage improves the chance of curing the cancer.

- For adults with PSC, doctors may suggest imaging tests and blood tests to check for bile duct cancer and gallbladder cancer.
- For people with cirrhosis caused by PSC, doctors may suggest blood tests and an ultrasound or another type of imaging test to check for liver cancer.
- For people with PSC and IBD, doctors may suggest a colonoscopy to check for colorectal cancer.

Bile Duct Infection

To treat a bile duct infection, doctors may prescribe antibiotics. To help prevent bile duct infections, doctors may prescribe antibiotics for people with PSC before and after they have procedures, such as ERCP, that increase the risk of getting an infection.

WHAT SHOULD YOU EAT IF YOU HAVE PRIMARY SCLEROSING CHOLANGITIS?

People with PSC should eat a healthy, well-balanced diet. Good nutrition is important in all stages of PSC—including cirrhosis—to help the liver work properly and manage complications.

Your doctor can recommend a healthy diet that provides enough calories and nutrients. Your doctor may recommend taking dietary supplements of calcium and vitamin D to help prevent osteoporosis. For low levels of fat-soluble vitamins A, D, E, or K, your doctor may recommend taking supplements of these vitamins. Follow your doctor's instructions on the type and amount of vitamins you should take.[3]

---

[3] "Primary Sclerosing Cholangitis," National Institute of Diabetes and Digestive and Kidney Diseases (NIDDK), February 2022. Available online. URL: www.niddk.nih.gov/health-information/liver-disease/primary-sclerosing-cholangitis. Accessed May 11, 2023.

Chapter 43 | **Paraneoplastic Syndromes**

WHAT ARE PARANEOPLASTIC SYNDROMES?

Paraneoplastic syndromes are a group of rare disorders that occur when the immune system has a reaction to a cancerous tumor known as a "neoplasm."

The immune system is very important in keeping you healthy. It consists of cells, tissues, and organs that work together to help your body fight infections and other diseases. Scientists think paraneoplastic syndromes happen when cancer-fighting antibodies or white blood cells (WBCs; known as "T cells") mistakenly attack normal cells in the nervous system.

Paraneoplastic syndromes are most common in middle-aged or older adults. They more commonly occur in people with lung, ovarian, lymphatic, or breast cancer. These symptoms normally start before a tumor, or cancer-filled growth, is found. They slowly develop over a few days or weeks. The symptoms include the following:

- difficulty walking or swallowing
- loss of muscle tone
- loss of fine motor coordination
- slurred speech
- memory loss
- vision problems
- sleep disturbances
- dementia
- seizures
- sensory loss in the limbs
- vertigo or dizziness

Paraneoplastic syndromes include the following:
- Lambert-Eaton myasthenic syndrome (LEMS)
- Stiff-Person syndrome
- encephalomyelitis
- myasthenia gravis (MG)
- cerebellar degeneration
- limbic or brain stem encephalitis
- neuromyotonia
- opsoclonus
- sensory neuropathy

Treatment for paraneoplastic syndromes focuses on taking care of any tumor or cancer that is found in the body, followed by efforts to decrease the autoimmune response.

Plasmapheresis, a process that cleanses antibodies from the blood, may ease symptoms in people with paraneoplastic disorders that affect the peripheral nervous system. Speech and physical therapy may help individuals regain some functions.

There is no cure for paraneoplastic syndromes, and treatment will not stop neurological damage.

HOW CAN YOU OR YOUR LOVED ONE HELP IMPROVE CARE FOR PEOPLE WITH PARANEOPLASTIC SYNDROME?

Consider participating in a clinical trial so that clinicians and scientists can learn more about paraneoplastic syndromes and related disorders. Clinical research uses human volunteers to help researchers learn more about a disorder and perhaps find better ways to safely detect, treat, or prevent disease.

All types of volunteers are needed—those who are healthy or may have an illness or disease—of all different ages, sexes, races, and ethnicities to ensure that study results apply to as many people as possible and that treatments will be safe and effective for everyone who will use them.[1]

---

[1] "Paraneoplastic Syndromes," National Institute of Neurological Disorders and Stroke (NINDS), January 23, 2023. Available online. URL: www.ninds.nih.gov/health-information/disorders/paraneoplastic-syndromes. Accessed May 12, 2023.

Chapter 44 | **Pediatric Autoimmune Neuropsychiatric Disorders Associated with Streptococcal Infections**

WHAT IS PANDAS?

A child may be diagnosed with pediatric autoimmune neuropsychiatric disorders associated with streptococcal infections (PANDAS) when:

- obsessive-compulsive disorder (OCD), tic disorder, or both suddenly appear following a streptococcal (strep) infection, such as strep throat or scarlet fever
- the symptoms of OCD or tic symptoms suddenly become worse following a strep infection

The symptoms are usually dramatic, happen "overnight and out of the blue," and can include motor and/or vocal tics, obsessions, and/or compulsions. In addition to these symptoms, children may also become moody or irritable, experience anxiety attacks, or show concerns about separating from parents or loved ones.

WHAT CAUSES PANDAS?

Strep bacteria are very ancient organisms that survive in the human host by hiding from the immune system for as long as possible. They hide themselves by putting molecules on their cell wall so that they look nearly identical to molecules found in the child's heart, joints, skin, and brain tissues. This hiding is called "molecular mimicry" and allows the strep bacteria to evade detection for a long time.

However, the molecules on the strep bacteria are eventually recognized as foreign to the body, and the child's immune system reacts to them by producing antibodies. Because of the molecular mimicry by the bacteria, the immune system reacts not only to the strep molecules but also to the human host molecules that were mimicked; the antibody system "attacks" the mimicked molecules in the child's own tissues. Studies at the National Institute of Mental Health (NIMH) and elsewhere have shown that some cross-reactive "anti-brain" antibodies target the brain—causing OCD, tics, and the other neuropsychiatric symptoms of PANDAS.

CAN ADULTS DEVELOP PANDAS?

PANDAS is considered a pediatric disorder and typically first appears in childhood from the age of three to puberty. Reactions to strep infections are rare after the age of 12, but researchers recognize that PANDAS could occur, though rarely, among adolescents. It is unlikely that someone would experience these post-strep neuropsychiatric symptoms for the first time as an adult, but it has not been fully studied.

It is possible that adolescents and adults may have immune-mediated OCD, but this is not known. The research studies on immune-mediated OCD at the NIMH are restricted to children.

WHAT ARE THE SIGNS AND SYMPTOMS OF PANDAS?

Children with PANDAS often experience one or more of the following symptoms in conjunction with their OCD or tic disorder:
- symptoms of attention deficit hyperactivity disorder (ADHD), such as hyperactivity, inattention, and fidgeting
- separation anxiety (e.g., the child is "clingy" and has difficulty separating from his/her caregivers; the child

  may not want to be in a different room in the house
  from his or her parents)
- mood changes, such as irritability, sadness, and
  emotional lability (i.e., tendency to laugh or cry
  unexpectedly at what might seem the wrong moment)
- trouble sleeping
- nighttime bedwetting, daytime frequent urination, or
  both
- changes in motor skills such as changes in handwriting
- joint pains

What Is an Episodic Course of Symptoms?

Children with PANDAS seem to have dramatic ups and downs in the severity of their OCD and/or tics. OCD or tics that are almost always present at a relatively consistent level do not represent an episodic course. Many children with OCD or tics have good days and bad days, or even good weeks and bad weeks. However, children with PANDAS have a very sudden onset or worsening of their symptoms, followed by a slow, gradual improvement. If children with PANDAS get another strep infection, their symptoms suddenly worsen again. The increased symptom severity usually persists for at least several weeks but may last for several months or longer.

Your Child Has Had Strep Throat Before, and He or She Has Tics, Obsessive-Compulsive Disorder, or Both. Does That Mean He or She Has PANDAS?

No. Many children have OCD, tics, or both, and almost all school-aged children get strep throat at some point. In fact, the average grade-school student will have two or three strep throat infections each year.

PANDAS is considered as a diagnosis when there is a very close relationship between the abrupt onset or worsening of OCD, tics, or both and a strep infection. If strep is found in conjunction with two or three episodes of OCD, tics, or both, then the child may have PANDAS.

What Does an Elevated Anti-Strep Antibody Titer Mean? Is This Bad for Your Child?

The anti-strep antibody titer (i.e., the number of molecules in blood that indicates a previous infection) is a test that determines whether the child has had a previous strep infection.

An elevated anti-strep titer means the child has had a strep infection sometime within the past few months, and his or her body created antibodies to fight the strep bacteria.

Some children create lots of antibodies and have very high titers (up to 2,000), while others have more modest elevations. The height of the titer elevation does not matter, and elevated titers are not necessarily bad for your child. The test measures a normal, healthy response—the production of antibodies to fight off an infection. The antibodies stay in the body for some time after the infection is gone, but the amount of time that the antibodies persist varies greatly between individuals. Some children have "positive" antibody titers for many months after a single infection.

When Is a Strep Titer Considered to Be Abnormal or Elevated?

The lab at the National Institutes of Health considers strep titers between 0 and 400 to be normal. Other labs set the upper limit at 150 or 200. Because each lab measures titers in different ways, it is important to know the range used by the lab where the test was done—just ask where the lab draws the line between negative and positive titers.

HOW IS PANDAS DIAGNOSED?

The diagnosis of PANDAS is a clinical diagnosis, which means that there are no lab tests that can diagnose PANDAS. Instead, healthcare providers use diagnostic criteria for the diagnosis of PANDAS. At the present time, the clinical features of the illness are the only means of determining whether a child might have PANDAS.

The diagnostic criteria are:
- the presence of OCD, a tic disorder, or both
- the pediatric onset of symptoms (i.e., age three to puberty)

- an episodic course of symptom severity
- an association with group A beta-hemolytic streptococcal infection, such as a positive throat culture for strep or a history of scarlet fever
- an association with neurological abnormalities, such as physical hyperactivity, or unusual, jerky movements that are not in the child's control
- very abrupt onset or worsening of symptoms

If the symptoms have been present for more than a week, blood tests may be done to document a preceding streptococcal infection.

WHAT ARE THE TREATMENT OPTIONS FOR CHILDREN WITH PANDAS?
Treatment with Antibiotics

The best treatment for acute episodes of PANDAS is to treat the strep infection causing the symptoms (if it is still present) with antibiotics:

- A throat culture should be done to document the presence of strep bacteria in the throat.
- If the throat culture is positive, a single course of antibiotics will usually get rid of the strep infection and allow the PANDAS symptoms to subside.

If a properly obtained throat culture is negative, the clinician should make sure that the child does not have an occult (hidden) strep infection, such as a sinus infection (often caused by strep bacteria) or strep bacteria infecting the anus, vagina, or urethral opening of the penis. Although the latter infections are rare, they have been reported to trigger PANDAS symptoms in some patients and can be particularly problematic because they will linger for longer periods of time and continue to provoke the production of cross-reactive antibodies.

The strep bacteria can be harder to eradicate in the sinuses and other sites, so the course of antibiotic treatment may need to be longer than that used for strep throat.

Tips for Parents or Caregivers

Sterilize or replace toothbrushes during and following the antibiotic treatment to make sure that the child is not reinfected with strep.

It might also be helpful to ask a health-care provider to perform throat cultures on the child's family members to make sure that none are "strep carriers," who could serve as a source of the strep bacteria.

HOW CAN YOU MANAGE NEUROPSYCHIATRIC SYMPTOMS OF PANDAS?

Children with PANDAS-related obsessive-compulsive symptoms will benefit from standard medications and/or behavioral therapies, such as cognitive-behavioral therapy (CBT). OCD symptoms are treated best with a combination of CBT and a selective serotonin reuptake inhibitor (SSRI) medication, and tics respond to a variety of medications.

Children with PANDAS appear to be unusually sensitive to the side effects of SSRIs and other medications, so it is important to "start slow and go slow!!" when using these medications. In other words, clinicians should prescribe a very small starting dose of the medication and increase it slowly enough that the child experiences as few side effects as possible. If PANDAS symptoms worsen, the SSRI dosage should be decreased promptly. However, SSRIs and other medications should not be stopped abruptly, as that could also cause difficulties.[1]

---

[1] "PANDAS—Questions and Answers," National Institute of Mental Health (NIMH), 2019. Available online. URL: www.nimh.nih.gov/health/publications/pandas. Accessed May 23, 2023.

Chapter 45 | **Autoimmune Renal and Kidney Disorders**

Chapter Contents

Section 45.1 | Glomerular Diseases

Many diseases affect kidney function by attacking the glomeruli, the tiny units within the kidney where blood is cleaned. Glomerular diseases include many conditions with a variety of genetic and environmental causes, but they fall into the following two major categories:

- **Glomerulonephritis.** It describes the inflammation of the membrane tissue in the kidney that serves as a filter, separating wastes and extra fluid from the blood.
- **Glomerulosclerosis.** It describes the scarring or hardening of the tiny blood vessels within the kidney.

Although glomerulonephritis and glomerulosclerosis have different causes, they both can lead to kidney failure.

WHAT ARE THE KIDNEYS, AND WHAT DO THEY DO?

The two kidneys are bean-shaped organs located just below the rib cage, one on each side of the spine. Every day, the two kidneys filter about 120–150 quarts of blood to produce about 1–2 quarts of urine, composed of wastes and extra fluid.

Blood enters the kidneys through arteries that branch inside the kidneys into tiny clusters of looping blood vessels. Each cluster is called a "glomerulus," which comes from a Greek word meaning filter. The plural form of the word is "glomeruli." There are approximately 1 million glomeruli, or filters, in each kidney. The glomerulus is attached to the opening of a small fluid-collecting tube called a "tubule." Blood is filtered in the glomerulus, and extra fluid and wastes pass into the tubule and become urine. Eventually, the urine drains from the kidneys into the bladder through larger tubes called "ureters" (refer to Figure 45.1).

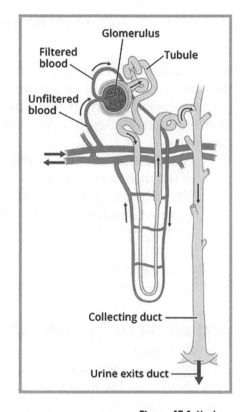

Figure 45.1. Nephron

National Institute of Diabetes and Digestive and Kidney Diseases (NIDDK)

Each glomerulus and tubule unit is called a "nephron." Each kidney is composed of about 1 million nephrons. In healthy nephrons, the glomerular membrane that separates the blood vessel from the tubule allows waste products and extra water to pass into the tubule while keeping blood cells and protein in the bloodstream.

HOW DO GLOMERULAR DISEASES INTERFERE WITH KIDNEY FUNCTION?

Glomerular diseases damage the glomeruli, letting protein and sometimes red blood cells (RBCs) leak into the urine. Sometimes, a glomerular disease also interferes with the clearance of waste products by the kidney, so they begin to build up in the blood. Furthermore, loss of blood proteins such as albumin in the urine can result in a fall in their level in the bloodstream. In normal blood, albumin acts like a sponge, drawing extra fluid from the body into the bloodstream, where it remains until the kidneys remove it. But, when albumin leaks into the urine, the blood loses its capacity to absorb extra fluid from the body. Fluid can accumulate outside the circulatory system in the face, hands, feet, or ankles and cause swelling.

WHAT ARE THE SYMPTOMS OF GLOMERULAR DISEASE?

The signs and symptoms of glomerular disease include:
- albuminuria, large amounts of protein in the urine
- hematuria, blood in the urine
- reduced glomerular filtration rate, inefficient filtering of wastes from the blood
- hypoproteinemia, low blood protein
- edema, swelling in parts of the body

One or more of these symptoms can be the first sign of kidney disease. But how would you know, for example, whether you have proteinuria? Before seeing a doctor, you may not. But some of these symptoms have signs, or visible manifestations:
- Proteinuria may cause foamy urine.
- Blood may cause the urine to be pink or cola-colored.
- Edema may be obvious in hands and ankles, especially at the end of the day, or around the eyes when awakening in the morning, for example.

WHAT CAUSES GLOMERULAR DISEASE?

A number of different diseases can result in glomerular disease. It may be the direct result of an infection or a drug toxic to the kidneys, or it may result from a disease that affects the entire body, such as diabetes or lupus. Many different kinds of diseases can cause swelling or scarring of the nephron or glomerulus. Sometimes, glomerular disease is idiopathic, meaning that it occurs without an apparent associated disease.

The categories presented below can overlap: that is, a disease might belong to two or more of the categories. For example, diabetic nephropathy is a form of glomerular disease that can be placed in two categories: systemic diseases, since diabetes itself is a systemic disease, and sclerotic diseases, because the specific damage done to the kidneys is associated with scarring.

Autoimmune Diseases

When the body's immune system functions properly, it creates protein-like substances called "antibodies" and "immunoglobulins" to protect the body against invading organisms. In an autoimmune disease, the immune system creates autoantibodies, which are antibodies or immunoglobulins that attack the body itself. Autoimmune diseases may be systemic and affect many parts of the body, or they may affect only specific organs or regions.

Systemic lupus erythematosus (SLE) affects many parts of the body: primarily the skin and joints but also the kidneys. Because women are more likely to develop SLE than men, some researchers believe that a sex-linked genetic factor may play a part in making a person susceptible although viral infection has also been implicated as a triggering factor. "Lupus nephritis" is the name given to kidney disease caused by SLE, and it occurs when autoantibodies form or are deposited in the glomeruli, causing inflammation. Ultimately, the inflammation may create scars that keep the kidneys from functioning properly. Conventional treatment for lupus nephritis includes a combination of two drugs: cyclophosphamide, a cytotoxic agent that suppresses the immune system, and prednisolone, a corticosteroid used to reduce inflammation. A newer immunosuppressant, mycophenolate mofetil (MMF), has been used instead of cyclophosphamide. Preliminary studies indicate that MMF may be as effective as cyclophosphamide and has milder side effects.

Goodpasture syndrome involves an autoantibody that specifically targets the kidneys and the lungs. Often, the first indication that patients have the autoantibody is when they cough up blood. But lung damage in Goodpasture syndrome is usually

446

superficial compared with progressive and permanent damage to the kidneys. Goodpasture syndrome is a rare condition that affects mostly young men but also occurs in women, children, and older adults. Treatments include immunosuppressive drugs and a blood-cleansing therapy called "plasmapheresis" that removes the autoantibodies.

Immunoglobulin A (IgA) nephropathy is a form of glomerular disease that results when IgA forms deposits in the glomeruli, where it creates inflammation. IgA nephropathy was not recognized as a cause of glomerular disease until the late 1960s when sophisticated biopsy techniques were developed that could identify IgA deposits in kidney tissue.

The most common symptom of IgA nephropathy is blood in the urine, but it is often a silent disease that may go undetected for many years. The silent nature of the disease makes it difficult to determine how many people are in the early stages of IgA nephropathy when specific medical tests are the only way to detect it. This disease is estimated to be the most common cause of primary glomerulonephritis—that is, glomerular disease not caused by a systemic disease such as lupus or diabetes mellitus. It appears to affect men more than women. Although IgA nephropathy is found in all age groups, young people rarely display signs of kidney failure because the disease usually takes several years to progress to the stage where it causes detectable complications.

No treatment is recommended for early or mild cases of IgA nephropathy when the patient has normal blood pressure and less than 1 g of protein in 24-hour urine output. When proteinuria exceeds 1 g/day, treatment is aimed at protecting kidney function by reducing proteinuria and controlling blood pressure. Blood pressure medicines—angiotensin-converting enzyme inhibitors (ACE inhibitors) or angiotensin receptor blockers (ARBs)—that block a hormone called "angiotensin" are most effective at achieving those two goals simultaneously.

Hereditary Nephritis (Alport Syndrome)

The primary indicator of Alport syndrome is a family history of chronic glomerular disease although it may also involve hearing or vision impairment. This syndrome affects both men and women, but men are more likely to experience chronic kidney disease and sensory loss. Men with Alport syndrome usually first show evidence of renal insufficiency while in their 20s and reach total kidney failure by age 40. Women rarely have significant renal impairment, and hearing loss may be so slight that it can be detected only through testing with special equipment. Usually, men can pass the disease only to their daughters. Women can transmit the disease to either their sons or their daughters. Treatment focuses on controlling blood pressure to maintain kidney function.

Infection-Related Glomerular Disease

Glomerular disease sometimes develops rapidly after an infection in other parts of the body.

- **Acute poststreptococcal glomerulonephritis (PSGN).** It can occur after an episode of strep throat or, in rare cases, impetigo (a skin infection). *Streptococcus* bacteria do not attack the kidney directly, but an infection may stimulate the immune system to overproduce antibodies, which are circulated in the blood and finally deposited in the glomeruli, causing damage. PSGN can bring on sudden symptoms of swelling (edema), reduced urine output (oliguria), and blood in the urine (hematuria). Tests will show large amounts of protein in the urine and elevated levels of creatinine and urea nitrogen in the blood, thus indicating reduced kidney function. High blood pressure frequently accompanies reduced kidney function in this disease.

Poststreptococcal glomerulonephritis is most common in children between the ages of three and seven although it can strike at any age, and it most often affects boys. It lasts only a brief time and usually allows the kidneys to recover. In a few cases, however, kidney damage may be permanent, requiring dialysis or transplantation to replace renal function.

- **Bacterial endocarditis.** The infection of the tissues inside the heart is also associated with subsequent glomerular disease. Researchers are not sure whether the renal lesions that form after a heart infection are caused entirely by the immune response or whether some other disease mechanism contributes to kidney damage. Treating the heart infection is the most effective way of minimizing kidney damage. Endocarditis sometimes produces chronic kidney disease (CKD).
- **Human immunodeficiency virus (HIV).** The virus that leads to acquired immunodeficiency syndrome (AIDS) can also cause glomerular disease. Between 5 and 10 percent of people with HIV experience kidney failure, even before developing full-blown AIDS. HIV-associated nephropathy usually begins with heavy proteinuria and progresses rapidly (within a year of detection) to total kidney failure. Researchers are looking for therapies that can slow down or reverse this rapid deterioration of renal function, but some possible solutions involving immunosuppression are risky because of the patients' already compromised immune system.

Sclerotic Diseases

Glomerulosclerosis is scarring (sclerosis) of the glomeruli. In several sclerotic conditions, a systemic disease such as lupus or diabetes is responsible. Glomerulosclerosis is caused by the activation of glomerular cells to produce scar material. This may be stimulated by molecules called growth factors, which may be made by glomerular cells themselves or may be brought to the glomerulus by the circulating blood that enters the glomerular filter.

Diabetic nephropathy is the leading cause of glomerular disease and total kidney failure in the United States. Kidney disease is one of several problems caused by elevated levels of blood glucose, the central feature of diabetes. In addition to scarring the kidney, elevated glucose levels appear to increase the speed of blood flow into the kidney, putting a strain on the filtering glomeruli and raising blood pressure.

Diabetic nephropathy usually takes many years to develop. People with diabetes can slow down damage to their kidneys by controlling their blood glucose through healthy eating with moderate protein intake, physical activity, and medications. People with diabetes should also be careful to keep their blood pressure at a level below 140/90 mm Hg, if possible. Blood pressure medications called ACE inhibitors and ARBs are particularly effective at minimizing kidney damage and are now frequently prescribed to control blood pressure in patients with diabetes and in patients with many forms of kidney disease.

Focal segmental glomerulosclerosis (FSGS) describes scarring in scattered regions of the kidney, typically limited to one part of the glomerulus and to a minority of glomeruli in the affected region. FSGS may result from a systemic disorder, or it may develop as an idiopathic kidney disease without a known cause. Proteinuria is the most common symptom of FSGS, but since proteinuria is associated with several other kidney conditions, the doctor cannot diagnose FSGS on the basis of proteinuria alone. A biopsy may confirm the presence of glomerular scarring if the tissue is taken from the affected section of the kidney. But finding the affected section is a matter of chance, especially early in the disease process, when lesions may be scattered.

Confirming a diagnosis of FSGS may require repeat kidney biopsies. Arriving at a diagnosis of idiopathic, FSGS requires the identification of focal scarring and the elimination of possible systemic causes such as diabetes or an immune response to infection. Since idiopathic FSGS is, by definition, of unknown cause, it is difficult to treat. No universal remedy has been found, and most patients with FSGS progress to kidney failure over 5–20 years. Some patients with an aggressive form of FSGS reach kidney failure in two to three years. Treatments involving steroids or other immunosuppressive drugs appear to help some patients by decreasing proteinuria and improving kidney function. But these treatments are beneficial to only a minority of those to whom they are tried, and some patients experience even poorer kidney function as a result. ACE inhibitors and ARBs may also be used in FSGS to decrease proteinuria. Treatment should focus on controlling blood pressure and blood cholesterol levels, factors that may contribute to kidney scarring.

Other Glomerular Diseases

Membranous nephropathy, also called "membranous glomerulopathy," is the second most common cause of nephrotic syndrome (proteinuria, edema, high cholesterol) in U.S. adults after diabetic nephropathy. Diagnosis of membranous nephropathy requires a kidney biopsy, which reveals unusual deposits of immunoglobulin G and complement component 3, substances created by the body's immune system. Totally, 75 percent of cases are idiopathic, which means that the cause of the disease is unknown. The remaining 25 percent of cases are the result of other diseases such as systemic lupus erythematosus, hepatitis B or hepatitis C infection, or some forms of cancer. Drug therapies involving penicillamine, gold, or captopril have also been associated with membranous nephropathy. About 20–40 percent of patients with membranous nephropathy progress usually over decades to kidney failure, but most patients experience either complete remission or continued symptoms without progressive kidney failure. Doctors disagree about how aggressively to treat this condition since about 20 percent of patients recover without treatment. ACE inhibitors and ARBs are generally used to reduce proteinuria. Additional medication to control high blood pressure and edema is frequently required. Some patients benefit from steroids, but this treatment does not work for everyone. Additional immunosuppressive medications are helpful for some patients with progressive disease.

Minimal change disease (MCD) is the diagnosis given when a patient has nephrotic syndrome and the kidney biopsy reveals little or no change to the structure of glomeruli or surrounding tissues when examined by a light microscope. Tiny drops of a fatty substance called a lipid may be present, but no scarring has taken place within the kidney. MCD may occur at any age, but it is most common in childhood. A small percentage of patients with idiopathic nephrotic syndrome do not respond to steroid therapy. For these patients, the doctor may recommend a low-sodium diet and prescribe a diuretic to control edema. The doctor may recommend the use of nonsteroidal anti-inflammatory drugs to reduce proteinuria. ACE inhibitors and ARBs have also been used to reduce proteinuria in patients with steroid-resistant MCD. These patients may respond to larger doses of steroids, more prolonged use of steroids, or steroids in combination with immunosuppressant drugs, such as chlorambucil, cyclophosphamide, or cyclosporine.

HOW IS GLOMERULAR DISEASE DIAGNOSED?

Patients with glomerular disease have significant amounts of protein in the urine, which may be referred to as a "nephrotic range" if levels are very high. RBCs in the urine are a frequent finding as well, particularly in some forms of glomerular disease. Urinalysis provides information about kidney damage by indicating levels of protein and RBCs in the urine. Blood tests measure the levels of waste products such as creatinine and urea nitrogen to determine whether the filtering capacity of the kidneys is impaired. If these lab tests indicate kidney damage, the doctor may recommend ultrasound or an x-ray to see whether the shape or size of the kidneys is abnormal. These tests are called "renal imaging." But since glomerular disease causes problems at the cellular level, the doctor will probably also recommend a kidney biopsy—a procedure in which a needle is used to extract small pieces of tissue for examination with different types of microscopes, each of which shows a different aspect of the tissue. A biopsy may be helpful in confirming glomerular disease and identifying the cause.[1]

[1] "Glomerular Diseases," National Institute of Diabetes and Digestive and Kidney Diseases (NIDDK), April 2014. Available online. URL: www.niddk.nih.gov/health-information/kidney-disease/glomerular-diseases. Accessed May 12, 2023.

Section 45.2 | Immunoglobulin A Nephropathy

WHAT IS IMMUNOGLOBULIN A NEPHROPATHY?

Immunoglobulin A (IgA) nephropathy, also known as "Berger disease," is a kidney disease that occurs when IgA deposits build up in the kidneys, causing inflammation that damages kidney tissues. IgA is an antibody—a protein made by the immune system to protect the body from foreign substances such as bacteria or viruses. Most people with IgA nephropathy receive care from a nephrologist, a doctor who specializes in treating people with kidney disease.

HOW DOES IMMUNOGLOBULIN A NEPHROPATHY AFFECT THE KIDNEYS?

Immunoglobulin A nephropathy affects the kidneys by attacking the glomeruli. The glomeruli are sets of looping blood vessels in nephrons—the tiny working units of the kidneys that filter wastes and remove extra fluid from the blood. The buildup of IgA deposits inflames and damages the glomeruli, causing the kidneys to leak blood and protein into the urine. The damage may lead to scarring of the nephrons that progresses slowly over many years. Eventually, IgA nephropathy can lead to end-stage kidney disease, sometimes called "end-stage renal disease" (ESRD), which means the kidneys no longer work well enough to keep a person healthy. When a person's kidneys fail, he or she needs a transplant or blood-filtering treatment called "dialysis."

WHAT CAUSES IMMUNOGLOBULIN A NEPHROPATHY?

Scientists think that IgA nephropathy is an autoimmune kidney disease, meaning that the disease is due to the body's immune system harming the kidneys.

People with IgA nephropathy have an increased blood level of IgA that contains less of a special sugar, galactose, than normal.

This galactose-deficient IgA is considered "foreign" by other antibodies circulating in the blood. As a result, these other antibodies attach to the galactose-deficient IgA and form a clump. This clump is also called an "immune complex." Some of the clumps become stuck in the glomerulus of the nephron and cause inflammation and damage.

For some people, IgA nephropathy runs in families. Scientists have recently found several genetic markers that may play a role in the development of the disease. IgA nephropathy may also be related to respiratory or intestinal infections and the immune system's response to these infections.

HOW COMMON IS IMMUNOGLOBULIN A NEPHROPATHY, AND WHO IS MORE LIKELY TO GET THE DISEASE?

Immunoglobulin A nephropathy is one of the most common kidney diseases, other than those caused by diabetes or high blood pressure.

IgA nephropathy can occur at any age although the first evidence of kidney disease most frequently appears when people are in their teens to late 30s. IgA nephropathy in the United States is twice as likely to appear in men than in women. While found in people all over the world, IgA nephropathy is more common among Asians and Caucasians.

A person may be more likely to develop IgA nephropathy if:
- he or she has a family history of IgA nephropathy or IgA vasculitis—a disease that causes small blood vessels in the body to become inflamed and leak
- he is a male in his teens to late 30s
- he or she is Asian or Caucasian

WHAT ARE THE SIGNS AND SYMPTOMS OF IMMUNOGLOBULIN A NEPHROPATHY?

In its early stages, IgA nephropathy may have no symptoms; it can be silent for years or even decades. Once symptoms appear, the most common one is hematuria, or blood in the urine. Hematuria can be a sign of damaged glomeruli. Blood in the urine may appear during or soon after a cold, sore throat, or other respiratory infection.

The amount of blood may be:

- visible with the naked eye (The urine may turn pink or the color of tea or cola. Sometimes, a person may have dark or bloody urine.)
- so small that it can only be detected using special medical tests

Another symptom of IgA nephropathy is albuminuria—when a person's urine contains an increased amount of albumin, a protein typically found in the blood, or large amounts of protein in the urine. Albumin is the main protein in the blood. Healthy kidneys keep most proteins in the blood from leaking into the urine. However, when the glomeruli are damaged, large amounts of protein leak out of the blood into the urine.

When albumin leaks into the urine, the blood loses its capacity to absorb extra fluid from the body. Too much fluid in the body may cause edema, or swelling, usually in the legs, feet, or ankles and less often in the hands or face. Foamy urine is another sign of albuminuria. Some people with IgA nephropathy have both hematuria and albuminuria.

After 10–20 years with IgA nephropathy, about 20–40 percent of adults develop end-stage kidney disease. Signs and symptoms of end-stage kidney disease may include:

- high blood pressure
- little or no urination
- edema
- feeling tired
- drowsiness
- generalized itching or numbness
- dry skin
- headaches
- weight loss
- appetite loss
- nausea
- vomiting
- sleep problems
- trouble concentrating
- darkened skin
- muscle cramps

WHAT ARE THE COMPLICATIONS OF IMMUNOGLOBULIN A NEPHROPATHY?

Complications of IgA nephropathy include the following:
- high blood pressure
- acute kidney failure—sudden and temporary loss of kidney function
- chronic kidney failure—reduced kidney function over a period of time
- nephrotic syndrome—a collection of symptoms that indicate kidney damage, which include albuminuria, lack of protein in the blood, and high blood cholesterol levels
- heart or cardiovascular problems
- Henoch-Schönlein purpura

HOW IS KIDNEY DISEASE DIAGNOSED?

A health-care provider diagnoses kidney disease with:
- a medical and family history
- a physical exam
- a urine test
- a blood test

Medical and Family History

Taking a medical and family history may help a health-care provider diagnose kidney disease.

Physical Exam

A physical exam may help diagnose kidney disease. During a physical exam, a health-care provider usually:
- measures the patient's blood pressure
- examines the patient's body for swelling

Urine Tests

- **Dipstick test for albumin and blood**. A dipstick test performed on a urine sample can detect the presence of albumin and blood. The patient provides a urine sample in a special container in a health-care provider's office or a commercial facility. A nurse or technician can test the sample in the same location, or he or she can send it to a lab for analysis. The test involves placing a strip of chemically treated paper, called a "dipstick," into the patient's urine sample. Patches on the dipstick change color when albumin or blood is present in urine.

- **Urine albumin-to-creatinine ratio (UACR).** A health-care provider uses this measurement, which compares the amount of albumin with the amount of creatinine in a urine sample, to estimate 24-hour albumin excretion. A patient may have chronic kidney disease if the UACR is greater than 30 mg of albumin for each gram of creatinine (30 mg/g).

Blood Test

A blood test involves having blood drawn at a health-care provider's office or a commercial facility and sending the sample to a lab for analysis. A health-care provider may order a blood test to estimate how much blood a patient's kidneys filter each minute—a measurement called the "estimated glomerular filtration rate" (eGFR). Depending on the results, the test can indicate the following:

- eGFR of 60 or above is in the normal range.
- eGFR below 60 may indicate kidney disease.
- eGFR of 15 or below may indicate kidney failure.

HOW IS IMMUNOGLOBULIN A NEPHROPATHY DIAGNOSED?

Currently, health-care providers do not use blood or urine tests as reliable ways to diagnose IgA nephropathy; therefore, the diagnosis of IgA nephropathy requires a kidney biopsy.

A kidney biopsy is a procedure that involves taking a small piece of kidney tissue for examination with a microscope. A health-care provider performs a kidney biopsy in a hospital or an outpatient center with light sedation and a local anesthetic. The health-care provider uses imaging techniques such as ultrasound or a computerized tomography scan to guide the biopsy needle into the kidney. A pathologist—a doctor who specializes in examining tissues to diagnose diseases—examines the kidney tissue with a microscope. Only a biopsy can show the IgA deposits in the glomeruli. The biopsy can also show how much kidney damage has already occurred. The biopsy results can help the health-care provider determine the best course of treatment.

HOW IS IMMUNOGLOBULIN A NEPHROPATHY TREATED?

Researchers have not yet found a specific cure for IgA nephropathy. Once the kidneys are scarred, they cannot be repaired. Therefore, the ultimate goal of IgA nephropathy treatment is to prevent or delay end-stage kidney disease. A health-care provider may prescribe medications to:

- control a person's blood pressure and slow the progression of kidney disease
- remove extra fluid from a person's blood
- control a person's immune system
- lower a person's blood cholesterol levels

HOW CAN A PERSON PREVENT IMMUNOGLOBULIN A NEPHROPATHY?

Researchers have not found a way to prevent IgA nephropathy. People with a family history of IgA nephropathy should talk with their health-care provider to find out what steps they can take to keep their kidneys healthy, such as controlling their blood pressure and keeping their blood cholesterol at healthy levels.

Eating, Diet, and Nutrition

Researchers have not found that eating, diet, and nutrition play a role in causing or preventing IgA nephropathy. Health-care providers may recommend that people with kidney disease, such as IgA nephropathy, make dietary changes such as:

- limiting dietary sodium, often from salt, to help reduce edema and lower blood pressure

- decreasing liquid intake to help reduce edema and lower blood pressure
- eating a diet low in saturated fat and cholesterol to help control high levels of lipids, or fats, in the blood

Health-care providers may also recommend that people with kidney disease eat moderate or reduced amounts of protein although the benefit of reducing protein in a person's diet is still being researched. Proteins break down into waste products the kidneys must filter from the blood. Eating more protein than the body needs may burden the kidneys and cause kidney function to decline faster. However, protein intake that is too low may lead to malnutrition, a condition that occurs when the body does not get enough nutrients. People with kidney disease on a restricted protein diet should receive blood tests that can show nutrient levels.

Some researchers have shown that fish oil supplements containing omega-3 fatty acids may slow kidney damage in some people with kidney disease by lowering blood pressure. Omega-3 fatty acids may help reduce inflammation and slow kidney damage due to IgA nephropathy. To help ensure coordinated and safe care, people should discuss their use of complementary and alternative medical practices, including their use of dietary supplements and probiotics, with their health-care provider.

People with IgA nephropathy should talk with a health-care provider about dietary changes to best manage their individual needs.[2]

---

[2] "IgA Nephropathy," National Institute of Diabetes and Digestive and Kidney Diseases (NIDDK), November 2015. Available online. URL: www.niddk.nih.gov/health-information/kidney-disease/iga-nephropathy. Accessed May 11, 2023.

Section 45.3 | Lupus Nephritis

WHAT IS LUPUS NEPHRITIS?

Lupus nephritis is a type of kidney disease caused by systemic lupus erythematosus (SLE or lupus). Lupus is an autoimmune disease—a disorder in which the body's immune system attacks the body's own cells and organs. Kidney disease caused by lupus may get worse over time and lead to kidney failure. If your kidneys fail, you will need dialysis or a kidney transplant to maintain your health.

What Do Your Kidneys Do?

The kidneys' main job is to filter extra water and wastes out of your blood to make urine. To keep your body working properly, the kidneys balance the salts and minerals—such as calcium, phosphorus, sodium, and potassium—that circulate in the blood. Your kidneys also make hormones that help control blood pressure, make red blood cells (RBCs), and keep your bones strong (refer to Figure 45.2).

WHO GETS LUPUS NEPHRITIS?

Lupus is much more common in women than in men and most often strikes during the childbearing years. Nine out of ten people who have lupus are women. Lupus is also more common in people of African or Asian backgrounds. African Americans and Asian Americans are about two to three times more likely to develop lupus than Caucasians. In the United States, 1 out of every 250 African American women will develop lupus.

HOW COMMON IS LUPUS NEPHRITIS?

Kidney damage is one of the more common health problems caused by lupus. In adults who have lupus, as many as 5 out of 10 will have kidney disease. In children who have lupus, 8 of 10 will have kidney disease.

Kidney

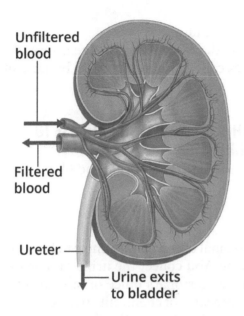

Unfiltered blood

Filtered blood

Ureter

Urine exits to bladder

Figure 45.2. Kidney

National Institute of Diabetes and Digestive and Kidney Diseases (NIDDK)

WHO IS MORE LIKELY TO DEVELOP LUPUS NEPHRITIS?

African Americans, Hispanics/Latinos, and Asian Americans are more likely to develop lupus nephritis than Caucasians. Lupus nephritis is more common in men than in women.

WHAT ARE THE SYMPTOMS OF LUPUS NEPHRITIS?

The symptoms of lupus nephritis may include foamy urine and edema—swelling that occurs when your body has too much fluid, usually in the legs, feet, or ankles, and less often in the hands or face. You may also develop high blood pressure.

Kidney problems often start at the same time or shortly after lupus symptoms appear and can include the following:
- joint pain or swelling
- muscle pain
- fever with no known cause
- a red rash, often on the face and across the nose and cheeks, sometimes called a "butterfly rash" because of its shape

WHAT TESTS DO HEALTH-CARE PROFESSIONALS USE TO DIAGNOSE LUPUS NEPHRITIS?

Lupus nephritis is diagnosed through urine and blood tests and a kidney biopsy.

Urine Test

Your health-care professional uses a urine sample to look for blood and protein in your urine. You collect the urine sample in a container in a health-care professional's office or lab. For the test, a nurse or technician places a strip of chemically treated paper, called a "dipstick," into the urine. Patches on the dipstick change color when blood or protein is present. A high level of protein or a high number of RBCs in the urine means kidney damage. The urine will also be examined under a microscope to look for kidney cells.

Blood Test

Your health-care professional uses a blood test to check your kidney function. The blood test measures creatinine, a waste product from the normal breakdown of muscles in your body. Your kidneys remove creatinine from your blood. Health-care professionals use the amount of creatinine in your blood to estimate your glomerular filtration rate (GFR). As kidney disease gets worse, the level of creatinine goes up.

Kidney Biopsy

A kidney biopsy is a procedure that involves taking a small piece of kidney tissue for examination under a microscope. A doctor performs the biopsy in a hospital using imaging techniques such as ultrasound or a computed tomography (CT) scan to guide the biopsy needle into the kidney. Health-care professionals numb the area to limit pain and use light sedation to help you relax during the procedure.

The kidney tissue is examined in a lab by a pathologist—a doctor who specializes in diagnosing diseases. A kidney biopsy can:
- confirm a diagnosis of lupus nephritis
- find out how far the disease has progressed
- guide treatment

The American College of Rheumatology recommends biopsies for people with signs of active lupus nephritis who have not yet been treated. Early diagnosis and prompt treatment may help protect your kidneys.

HOW DO DOCTORS TREAT LUPUS NEPHRITIS?
Health-care professionals treat lupus nephritis with medicines that suppress your immune system, so it stops attacking and damaging your kidneys. The goals of treatment are to:
- reduce inflammation in your kidneys
- decrease immune system activity
- block your body's immune cells from attacking the kidneys directly or making antibodies that attack the kidneys

Medicines
Your health-care professional may prescribe a corticosteroid, usually prednisone; a medicine to suppress your immune system, such as cyclophosphamide or mycophenolate mofetil (MMF); and hydroxychloroquine, a medicine for people who have SLE.

Lupus nephritis can cause high blood pressure in some people. You may need more than one kind of medicine to control your blood pressure. Blood pressure medicines include:
- angiotensin-converting enzyme (ACE) inhibitors and angiotensin receptor blockers (ARBs), with drug names that end in "pril" or "sartan"
- diuretics

- beta-blockers
- calcium channel blockers

ACE inhibitors and ARBs may help protect your kidneys, and diuretics help your kidneys remove fluid from your body.

WHAT ARE THE COMPLICATIONS OF LUPUS NEPHRITIS?

Treatment works well to control lupus nephritis, so you may not have complications. Between 10 and 30 percent of people who have lupus nephritis develop kidney failure.

The most severe form of lupus nephritis, called "diffuse proliferative nephritis," can cause scars to form in the kidneys. Scars are permanent, and kidney function often declines as more scars form. Early diagnosis and treatment may help prevent long-lasting damage.

People who have lupus nephritis are at high risk of cancer, primarily B-cell lymphoma—a type of cancer that begins in the cells of the immune system. They are also at high risk of heart and blood vessel problems.[3]

---

[3] "Lupus and Kidney Disease (Lupus Nephritis)," National Institute of Diabetes and Digestive and Kidney Diseases (NIDDK), January 2017. Available online. URL: www.niddk.nih.gov/health-information/kidney-disease/lupus-nephritis. Accessed May 12, 2023.

Chapter 46 | **Sarcoidosis**

WHAT IS SARCOIDOSIS?

Sarcoidosis is a condition that develops when groups of cells in your immune system form red and swollen (inflamed) lumps called "granulomas" in various organs in the body. The inflammation that leads to these granulomas can be caused either by infections or by certain things you come into contact with in your environment.

Sarcoidosis can affect any organ. Most often, it affects the lungs and lymph nodes in the chest. You may feel extremely tired or have a fever. You may also have other symptoms depending on what organ is affected. Your doctor will diagnose sarcoidosis in part by ruling out other diseases that have similar symptoms.

Not everyone needs treatment. Treatment will depend on your symptoms and which organs are affected. Medicines can help treat the inflammation or lower your body's immune response. Many people recover with few or no long-term problems. Sometimes, the disease causes permanent scarring (fibrosis) in the lungs or other organs and can lead to life-threatening heart or lung problems.

SYMPTOMS OF SARCOIDOSIS

Many people who have sarcoidosis have no symptoms, or they may feel unwell but without any obvious symptoms. Others may be depressed, feel very tired, or have a general feeling of discomfort. You may also faint or have unexplained weight loss (refer to Figure 46.1).

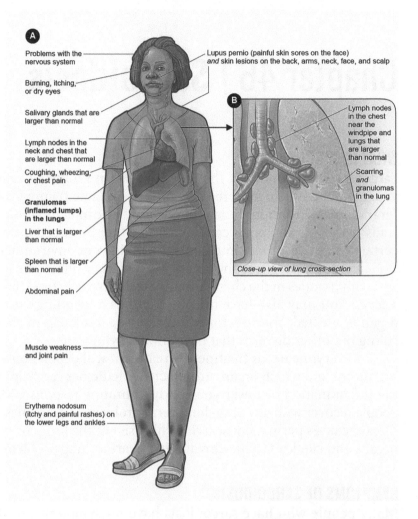

Figure 46.1. Symptoms of Sarcoidosis

National Heart, Lung, and Blood Institute (NHLBI)

Lofgren Syndrome

Lofgren syndrome is a classic set of symptoms of sarcoidosis that includes the following:

- swollen lymph nodes in your chest, neck, chin, armpits, or groin

- a rash of small, itchy, or painful bumps called "erythema nodosum" that most commonly appear on your head, neck, or legs
- blurred vision, eye pain or redness, light sensitivity, or watery eyes
- joint pain, stiffness, or swelling
- fever

Some people have Lofgren syndrome when they first develop sarcoidosis. This is most common in women between the ages of 30 and 40. It usually goes away completely within two years.

Sarcoidosis in the Lungs

If you have sarcoidosis in the lungs, you may experience the following symptoms:

- wheezing
- coughing
- shortness of breath
- chest pain

However, you can have sarcoidosis in the lungs without these symptoms. For example, skin rashes or sores can include erythema nodosum (explained above) or lupus pernio. Lupus pernio causes skin sores that usually affect the face, especially the nose, cheeks, lips, and ears. These sores usually last a long time. Lupus pernio affects African American people more often than other groups.

Other Symptoms

You may have other symptoms based on which organs are affected:

- larger than normal liver or spleen or jaundice, which can make your eyes or skin yellow
- nervous system problems, such as
  - headache
  - dizziness
  - vision problems
  - seizures

- mood swings
- hallucinations
- delusions
- nerve pain
- heart palpitations or an irregular heartbeat
- abdominal pain, nausea, or vomiting
- muscle pain or soreness
- swollen salivary glands

CAUSES OF SARCOIDOSIS

Your immune system creates inflammation to help defend you against germs and sickness. But, in sarcoidosis, inflammation goes off track, and the cells in your immune system form lumps, called "granulomas," in your body. Over time, inflammation may lead to permanent scarring of organs.

Studies suggest that some immune system triggers can lead to sarcoidosis in certain people. Triggers can include infections without symptoms or coming into contact with substances in the environment. Your genes can affect how your immune system reacts to a trigger.

RISK FACTORS FOR SARCOIDOSIS

There are many risk factors for sarcoidosis. Some risk factors, such as where you work, can be changed. But your age, family history, and many other risk factors cannot be changed.

- **Age**. You can get sarcoidosis at any age, but the risk goes up as you get older, especially after the age of 55.
- **Environment**. Living or working near insecticides, mold, or other substances that may cause inflammation raises your risk. You may be around these substances if you are in health care or the automotive industry or are a farmer or firefighter.
- **Family history and genetics**. Having a close relative with sarcoidosis raises your risk.
- **Medicines**. Certain types of human immunodeficiency virus (HIV) medicines and monoclonal antibodies

used to treat cancer or an overactive immune system can raise your risk.

- **Race or ethnicity**. Your risk is higher if you are of African or Scandinavian descent.
- **Sex**. Women are more likely to have sarcoidosis, although men can also have it.

Other medical conditions, such as lymphoma, a type of blood cancer, can also lead to sarcoidosis.

DIAGNOSIS OF SARCOIDOSIS

Sarcoidosis is diagnosed based on your symptoms, a physical exam, and imaging tests or a biopsy. Before diagnosing you with sarcoidosis, your health-care provider will rule out other possible conditions.

Stages of Sarcoidosis

Doctors use stages to describe sarcoidosis of the lung or lymph nodes of the chest. The stages are based on where the lumps, or granulomas, are found and whether there is scarring on imaging tests. Stage IV is the most serious and means you have permanent scarring in the lungs.

Medical History and Physical Exam

Bring a list of symptoms with you to your appointment. Tell your provider if you live or work near insecticides or mold or have other risk factors for sarcoidosis. During the physical exam, your provider may do the following:

- Check your temperature.
- Check to see if your lymph nodes, spleen, or liver are swollen.
- Listen to your chest with a stethoscope as you breathe in and out.
- Look for rashes or sores on your body, such as the scalp and lower legs.

Diagnostic Tests and Procedures

There are no screening tests to determine who will develop sarcoidosis. If you are at risk for sarcoidosis, your provider may talk to you about trying to avoid certain substances in your environment that can trigger granulomas.

Your health-care provider may have you undergo certain tests and procedures to diagnose sarcoidosis:

- Chest x-rays look for granulomas or scarring in the lungs and heart. This will also help figure out the stage of the disease. Often, sarcoidosis is found because a chest x-ray is done for another reason.
- Biopsy of the skin, lymph nodes, lungs, or other affected organs may help confirm your sarcoidosis diagnosis. Your doctor will do a bronchoscopy to get the biopsy sample from your lungs or lymph nodes in your chest.
- Blood tests check your blood counts, hormone levels, and how well your kidneys are working.
- Other imaging tests look for granulomas or inflammation in the heart, eyes, lymph nodes, or other areas. These may include magnetic resonance imaging (MRI) or an ultrasound.

The tests below look at how sarcoidosis is affecting the body:

- Neurological tests, such as electromyography, evoked potentials, spinal taps, or nerve conduction tests, look for problems with the nervous system caused by sarcoidosis.
- Eye exams look for eye damage, which can occur without symptoms in a person with sarcoidosis.
- Lung function tests check whether you have breathing problems.
- Heart tests monitor how well your heart is working. Sarcoidosis only rarely affects the heart, but cardiac sarcoidosis may be life-threatening. Tests may include electrocardiography (ECG or EKG), echocardiography, or cardiac MRI.

TREATMENT FOR SARCOIDOSIS

The goal of treatment for sarcoidosis is remission, which means the condition still exists but does not cause problems. Not everyone who is diagnosed with sarcoidosis needs treatment. Sometimes, the condition goes away on its own. Your treatment will depend on your symptoms, which organs are affected, and whether those organs are working well.

Medicine

Your doctor may prescribe medicines to lower inflammation or treat an overactive immune response. Immune-lowering medicines can raise the risk of infections. Talk with your provider about the benefits and risks of these medicines.

Corticosteroids to Treat Inflammation

The corticosteroid (steroid hormone medicine) prednisone is the most common treatment for sarcoidosis. Corticosteroids can be taken as pills or be injected, inhaled, or taken as eye drops or other topical medicines.

Corticosteroids can have serious side effects with long-term use, especially if taken in high doses. Side effects of the corticosteroid pill may include high blood sugar or blood pressure, mood changes, weight gain, and increased appetite. The pill also raises the risk of cataracts (clouding of the eye), glaucoma (damage to a nerve in the eye from high pressure), or osteoporosis (bone thinning). The common side effects from inhaled corticosteroids include a hoarse voice or a mouth infection called "thrush."

Medicines to Lower Your Immune System Response

- Medicines used to treat severe rheumatoid arthritis (RA) include methotrexate, azathioprine, and leflunomide. You usually take this as a pill or an injection (shot). Side effects may include liver damage or blood problems.
- Monoclonal antibodies, also called "immunotherapy," are used to treat cancer or an overactive immune system. These

include rituximab, infliximab, golimumab, and adalimumab. Your doctor will give you the medicine as a shot or through an intravenous (IV) line. Side effects are rare but can include a life-threatening immune reaction, heart problems, low blood counts, or a higher risk of certain cancers.

- Medicines used to treat malaria include hydroxychloroquine or chloroquine. Side effects may include eye damage, heart problems, and low blood sugar.
- Corticotropin (a hormone medicine) is given as a shot. It may be used when prednisone does not work or has serious side effects. Side effects of this medicine may include high blood pressure, problems controlling blood sugar, increased appetite, or mood changes.
- Pentoxifylline is taken as a pill. It is normally prescribed to improve blood flow. Side effects may include nausea.

Medicines to Treat Other Symptoms
- Antibiotics treat sarcoidosis of the skin. Examples include minocycline, tetracycline, and doxycycline. Side effects may include dizziness and gastrointestinal tract problems.
- Colchicine treats joint pain from sarcoidosis. You take this medicine as a pill. It is usually prescribed for gout. Side effects include nausea, vomiting, diarrhea, and stomach cramps or pain.

Treating Complications
If untreated, or if the treatment does not work, sarcoidosis can cause serious health problems. Your doctor may recommend the following medicines or procedures. Ask your doctor about the benefits and risks of any treatment.

LIVING WITH SARCOIDOSIS
Manage Your Condition
Even if you do not have symptoms of sarcoidosis, you should see your health-care provider for ongoing care. For example, your provider will monitor you for side effects from long-term use of corticosteroids or other medicines.

If the disease is not worsening, you may be watched closely to see whether the disease goes away on its own. If the disease does start to get worse, your doctor can prescribe treatment.

Remission and Flares

If your sarcoidosis goes into remission, your doctor may carefully stop your medicines. However, you will still need to watch for a flare. If you do have a flare, you may need another round of treatment.

Flares can be hard to predict. Most often, they happen within six months of stopping treatment. The longer you go without symptoms, the less likely you are to have a flare.

Tests for Complications

Some people have sarcoidosis that persists or comes back for many years after diagnosis. This may be called "chronic," "severe," "advanced," "refractory," or "progressive sarcoidosis." Your provider may order tests to keep track of your condition and check for complications.

Know When to Seek Medical Care

Watch for the warning signs of complications that may require emergency medical treatment. These include signs of changes in vision that may be a sign of brain tumors. Other complications that require immediate medical attention include kidney failure, cardiac arrest, and sudden shortness of breath or muscle weakness.

Make Healthy Lifestyle Changes

A healthy lifestyle may help you feel better and prevent sarcoidosis from getting worse.

- **Get regular physical activity**. Extreme tiredness can make it hard to exercise if you have sarcoidosis. However, physical activity can improve energy and help with other symptoms, such as shortness of breath and muscle weakness. Try to stay active but talk with your doctor about what level of physical activity is right for you.

- **Quit smoking**. If you smoke, quit. Also, try to avoid other lung irritants, such as dust, chemicals, and secondhand smoke. Visit Smoking and Your Heart at www.nhlbi.nih.gov/health/heart/smoking. For free help quitting smoking, you may call the National Cancer Institute's Smoking Quitline at 877-44U-QUIT (877-448-7848).
- **Try to get enough good-quality sleep**. Experts recommend that adults get seven to nine hours of sleep per day.

Take Care of Your Mental Health

Sarcoidosis may make you feel lonely, anxious, or depressed. You may continue to feel very tired even after your treatment has ended. But certain activities or treatments may help improve your mental health:

- Counseling, particularly cognitive therapy, can be helpful.
- Joining a patient support group may help you adjust to living with sarcoidosis. You can see how other people manage similar symptoms and their condition. Talk with your provider about local support groups or check with an area medical center.
- Talk to your doctor about medicines or other treatments. Antidepressants or other treatments may improve your quality of life (QOL).
- Support from family and friends can help relieve stress and anxiety. Let your loved ones know how you feel and what they can do to help you.[1]

---

[1] "What Is Sarcoidosis?" National Heart, Lung, and Blood Institute (NHLBI), March 24, 2022. Available online. URL: www.nhlbi.nih.gov/health/sarcoidosis. Accessed May 12, 2023.

Chapter 47 | Autoimmune Skin Disorders

Chapter Contents

WHAT IS ALOPECIA AREATA?

Alopecia areata is a disease that happens when the immune system attacks hair follicles and causes hair loss. Hair follicles are the structures in skin that form hair. While hair can be lost from any part of the body, alopecia areata usually affects the head and face. Hair typically falls out in small, round patches about the size of a quarter, but in some cases, hair loss is more extensive. Most people with the disease are healthy and have no other symptoms.

The course of alopecia areata varies from person to person. Some have bouts of hair loss throughout their lives, while others only have one episode. Recovery is unpredictable too, with hair regrowing fully in some people but not others.

There is no cure for alopecia areata, but there are treatments that help hair grow back more quickly. There are also resources to help people cope with hair loss.

Who Gets Alopecia Areata?

Anyone can have alopecia areata. Men and women get it equally, and it affects all racial and ethnic groups. The onset can be at any age, but most people get it in their teens, twenties, or thirties. When it occurs in children younger than 10, it tends to be more extensive and progressive.

If you have a close family member with the disease, you may have a higher risk of getting it, but for many people, there is no family history. Scientists have linked a number of genes to the disease, which suggests that genetics plays a role in alopecia areata. Many of the genes they have found are important for the functioning of the immune system.

People with certain autoimmune diseases, such as psoriasis, thyroid disease, or vitiligo, are more likely to get alopecia areata, as are those with allergic conditions such as hay fever. It is possible that emotional stress or an illness can bring on alopecia areata in people who are at risk, but in most cases, there is no obvious trigger.

TYPES OF ALOPECIA AREATA

There are three main types of alopecia areata:

- **Patchy alopecia areata**. In this type, which is the most common, hair loss happens in one or more coin-sized patches on the scalp or other parts of the body.
- **Alopecia totalis**. People with this type lose all or nearly all of the hair on their scalp.
- **Alopecia universalis**. In this type, which is rare, there is a complete or nearly complete loss of hair on the scalp, face, and rest of the body.

SYMPTOMS OF ALOPECIA AREATA

Alopecia areata primarily affects hair, but in some cases, there are nail changes as well. People with the disease are usually healthy and have no other symptoms.

Hair Changes

Alopecia areata typically begins with a sudden loss of round or oval patches of hair on the scalp, but any part of the body may be affected, such as the beard area in men or the eyebrows or eyelashes. Around the edges of the patch, there are often short broken hairs or "exclamation point" hairs that are narrower at their base than their tip. There is usually no sign of a rash, redness, or scarring on the bare patches. Some people say they feel tingling, burning, or itching on patches of skin right before the hair falls out.

When a bare patch develops, it is hard to predict what will happen next. The possibilities include the following:

- The hair regrows within a few months. It may look white or gray at first but may regain its natural color over time.
- Additional bare patches develop. Sometimes, hair regrows in the first patch while new bare patches are forming.
- Small patches join to form larger ones. In rare cases, hair is eventually lost from the entire scalp.

- There is a progression to complete loss of body hair. This is rare.

In most cases, the hair regrows, but there may be subsequent episodes of hair loss. The hair tends to regrow on its own more fully in people with:
- less extensive hair loss
- later age of onset
- no nail changes
- no family history of the disease

Nail Changes
Nail changes such as ridges and pits occur in some people, especially those who have more extensive hair loss.

CAUSES OF ALOPECIA AREATA
In alopecia areata, the immune system mistakenly attacks hair follicles, causing inflammation. Researchers do not fully understand what causes the immune attack on hair follicles, but they believe that both genetic and environmental (nongenetic) factors play a role.

DIAGNOSIS OF ALOPECIA AREATA
Doctors usually diagnose alopecia areata by the following:
- examining the areas where the hair has been lost and looking at your nails
- examining your hair and hair follicle openings using a handheld magnifying device
- asking about your medical and family history

Other health conditions can cause hair to fall out in the same pattern as alopecia areata. To determine if another condition is causing the hair loss, your doctor may order blood tests or a skin biopsy.

TREATMENT FOR ALOPECIA AREATA

For many people, hair grows back without any type of treatment. For people with milder cases, no treatment may be needed. Some people with severe cases opt to forego treatment as well and may instead consider products that conceal hair loss, such as hairpieces or wigs.

If you choose to seek treatment, your doctor will take into account your age and the extent of hair loss when making a treatment plan. A Janus kinase (JAK) inhibitor was recently approved to treat adult patients with severe alopecia areata. In addition, medications that have been approved for other conditions may be used to treat the disease. These include corticosteroids, immunosuppressants, and other medications that stimulate hair regrowth. The main goal of therapy is to stop the immune system's attack on hair follicles and to stimulate the regrowth of hair.

Who Treats Alopecia Areata?

Alopecia areata is treated by the following:
- dermatologists, who specialize in conditions of the skin, hair, and nails

Other specialists who may be involved in your care include the following:
- mental health professionals, who can help with the psychosocial challenges caused by having a medical condition
- primary care doctors, such as family physicians or internal medicine specialists, who coordinate care between the different health providers and treat other problems as they arise

LIVING WITH ALOPECIA AREATA

Alopecia areata does not cause physical disability, but it may affect your sense of well-being. There are many things you can do to cope with the effects of this disease, including the following.

Get Support

- Learn as much as you can about the disease and talk with others who are dealing with it. Having a support network can help you deal with difficult times.
- Visit a mental health professional if emotional problems arise. People with alopecia areata may have higher levels of stress, and depression and anxiety are more common in people with the disease.

Protect Bare Skin and Stay Comfortable

- Use sunscreens for any bare areas.
- Wear wigs, hairpieces, hats, or scarves to protect your scalp from the sun and to keep the head warm.
- Wear eyeglasses or sunglasses to protect your eyes from the sun and dust if you have lost hair from your eyebrows or eyelashes.

Consider Cosmetic Solutions

- Wear a wig, hairpiece, or bandana to cover up hair loss. Alternatively, some people choose to shave their heads to mask patchy hair loss.
- Use fake eyelashes or apply stick-on eyebrows if you lose hair from your eyelashes or eyebrows. Makeup or tattoos can also disguise the loss of eyebrow hair.

People with alopecia areata have a higher risk of certain diseases such as thyroid disease, atopic dermatitis, or other autoimmune diseases, so it is important to visit your primary care doctor regularly. The sooner these diseases are diagnosed, the easier they are to control.[1]

---

[1] "Alopecia Areata," National Institute of Arthritis and Musculoskeletal and Skin Diseases (NIAMS), April 2021. Available online. URL: www.niams.nih.gov/health-topics/alopecia-areata. Accessed May 12, 2023.

Section 47.2 | Lichen Planus

Lichen planus is a chronic inflammatory skin condition affecting different body parts, including the skin, mucous membranes, nails, and scalp. It is characterized by flat, itchy, purple bumps on the skin and white, lacy patches on the oral and genital mucosa. This condition is noncontagious and cannot be transmitted from one person to another.

CAUSES OF LICHEN PLANUS

The exact cause of this skin condition is unknown, but it is thought to be an immune disorder where the immune system accidentally attacks the skin and mucous membrane cells. Several other factors contribute to its development. Some of the possible causes and factors are as follows:

- **Autoimmune reactions**. Lichen planus occurs when the immune system mistakenly attacks the cells of the moist linings of the mouth, throat, or other areas including the skin.
- **Genetic factors**. Familial bullous lichen planus can be inherited although lichen planus, in general, is not a hereditary disease.
- **Viral infections**. Certain types of herpes and hepatitis C viruses increase the likelihood of developing lichen planus.
- **Allergic reactions**. Various reactions arising from allergic responses to different substances trigger and worsen the condition of lichen planus.
- **Stress and emotional factors**. Increased severity of oral lichen planus has been directly linked to feelings of excessive mental pressure and worry.
- **Medications**. Certain drugs such as diuretics and malaria prevention medication can lead to a rash resembling lichen planus.
- **Oral health factors**. Although an uncommon condition, oral lichen planus can be caused by dental fillings.

SYMPTOMS OF LICHEN PLANUS

The symptoms of lichen planus can vary from mild to severe and affect different body parts such as the legs, arms, trunk, scalp, nails, mouth, and genitals. The common symptoms of lichen planus vary depending on the affected area:

- Nail problems occur in various forms, such as shiny flat bumps, dark lines from the tip to the base, nail splitting or thinning, formation of grooves, and so on.
- Mouth symptoms include painful ulcers, bluish-white spots, and a lacy line network that gradually grows. There may also be a lacy line network/patches on the tongue, lips, gums, and inside of the cheeks.
- Skin problems present themselves as bumpy and itchy, with red or purple spots that feel firm to the touch. The affected area could look scaly with blisters or sores with white lines on the skin.
- The female genital symptoms include a burning sensation and soreness around the vulva. The male genital symptoms include nonitchy rash, shiny flat-topped bumps, or white or purple ring-shaped patches on the glans.

Other potential symptoms include dryness or a strange metallic taste in the mouth. Sometimes, although not very common, lichen planus can cause small bumps, bald spots, itchiness, redness, and hair thinning on the scalp.

RISK FACTORS FOR LICHEN PLANUS

Lichen planus can affect anyone, and it is estimated that about 1–2 percent of the worldwide population is affected by this condition. Some specific risk factors associated with lichen planus are as follows:

- **Age**. Lichen planus is more common in adults over 40, and the risk of developing it increases with age.
- **Gender**. Both men and women can be afflicted by skin lichen planus, but women are more likely than men to acquire it in their mouth.

- **Oral involvement**. The mouth is affected in approximately 50 percent of all cases of lichen planus.

DIAGNOSIS OF LICHEN PLANUS

The health-care provider is most likely to take an exhaustive medical history and perform a physical exam of skin or mouth lesions and may order some tests to confirm the diagnosis. These tests may include the following:

- **Blood tests**. Blood may be tested for health problems related to lichen planus, such as hepatitis C.
- **Biopsy**. A tiny sample of the questionable tissue is taken out and tested in the lab to see if it has the same cell patterns as lichen planus.
- **Patch tests**. The person's skin is covered with a sticky layer that contains small amounts of various substances. After a couple of days, a health-care provider examines the skin under these patches to see if there is any reaction. This helps the health-care provider figure out if the person is allergic to a particular substance.

A dermatologist or a dentist may sometimes identify lichen planus during a routine checkup. Additional blood tests may also be necessary to rule out other diseases.

TREATMENT FOR LICHEN PLANUS

Although lichen planus cannot be totally healed, therapy focuses on minimizing symptoms and assisting damaged areas to recover. Typically, skin lichen planus tends to go away within 24–36 weeks. However, oral and genital lichen planus may last longer. Treatment options include:

- antihistamines to alleviate itching
- corticosteroids, either topical or oral, to reduce swelling or immunological reactions
- psoralen with ultraviolet A (PUVA) light therapy to treat the skin

- retinoic acid, which can be either applied to the skin or given orally
- immune-modulating medicines, used when other treatments are not effective enough and the disease condition is quite serious, impacting the patient's daily life

If lichen planus develops in the mouth and causes burning, pain, ulcers, or sores, it can be treated first with numbing agents such as ointment, mouthwash, or gel. Other treatment options for severe cases may include medicines that calm the immune system or corticosteroid pills or injections. Side effects of these treatments vary, so it is important to discuss them with a health-care provider. If the disease affects mucous membranes and nails, it tends to be harder to treat and may require follow-up care. If the health-care provider thinks that lichen planus is related to a trigger, additional testing or treatment may be necessary.

MANAGEMENT AND PROGNOSIS OF LICHEN PLANUS

Lichen planus is a nonharmful skin and mouth condition that usually gets better with treatment. If lichen planus is caused by a medication you are taking, stopping the medication should make the rash go away.

Self-care approaches such as taking a lukewarm bath; applying a cool, damp cloth; and avoiding scratching the affected skin or injuring your nails can help reduce itching and pain. You can also use hydrocortisone cream or ointment to relieve symptoms under medical supervision.

Brushing and flossing your teeth on a regular basis is critical, if you have oral lichen planus, to keep your mouth clean and healthy. However, you should contact your health-care provider if your skin or mouth lesions change in appearance or the condition worsens despite treatment.

References

ADAM, "Lichen Planus," MedlinePlus, November 18, 2022. Available online. URL: https://medlineplus.gov/ency/article/000867.htm. Accessed May 4, 2023.

Amanda Oakley. "Monitoring Immune-Modulating Drugs Used in Dermatology," DermNet, February 13, 2016. Available online. URL: https://dermnetnz.org/topics/monitoring-immune-modulating-drugs-used-in-dermatology. Accessed May 29, 2023.

"Lichen Planus," Mayo Foundation for Medical Education and Research (MFMER), April 4, 2023. Available online. URL: www.mayoclinic.org/diseases-conditions/lichen-planus/symptoms-causes/syc-20351378. Accessed May 4, 2023.

"Lichen Planus," NHS Inform, January 31, 2023. Available online. URL: www.nhsinform.scot/illnesses-and-conditions/skin-hair-and-nails/lichen-planus. Accessed May 4, 2023.

"Lichen Planus: Overview," American Academy of Dermatology Association (AAD), March 23, 2011. Available online. URL: www.aad.org/public/diseases/a-z/lichen-planus-overview. Accessed May 4, 2023.

"Patch Testing," Mayo Foundation for Medical Education and Research (MFMER), October 1, 2015. Available online. URL: www.mayoclinic.org/diseases-conditions/contact-dermatitis/multimedia/patch-testing/img-20008265. Accessed May 29, 2023.

Simarpreet V. Sandhu, et al. "Oral Lichen Planus and Stress: An Appraisal," National Center for Biotechnology Information (NCBI), 2014. Available online. URL: www.ncbi.nlm.nih.gov/pmc/articles/PMC4147812. Accessed May 29, 2023.

Section 47.3 | Pemphigus

WHAT IS PEMPHIGUS?

Pemphigus is a disease that causes blistering of the skin and the inside of the mouth, nose, throat, eyes, and genitals.

Pemphigus is an autoimmune disease in which the immune system mistakenly attacks cells in the top layer of the skin (epidermis) and the mucous membranes. People with the disease produce antibodies against desmogleins, proteins that bind skin cells to one another. When these bonds are disrupted, the skin becomes fragile, and fluid can collect between its layers, forming blisters. There is no cure for pemphigus, but in many cases, it is controllable with medications.

Who Gets Pemphigus?

You are more likely to get pemphigus if you have certain risk factors. These include the following:

- **Ethnic background**. While pemphigus occurs across ethnic and racial groups, some populations are at a greater risk for certain types of the disease. People of Jewish (especially Ashkenazi), Indian, Southeast European, or Middle Eastern descent are more susceptible to pemphigus vulgaris.
- **Geographic location**. Pemphigus vulgaris is the most common type worldwide, but pemphigus foliaceus is more common in some places, such as certain rural regions of Brazil and Tunisia.
- **Sex and age**. Women get pemphigus vulgaris more frequently than men, and the age of onset is usually between 50 and 60 years old. Pemphigus foliaceus generally affects men and women equally, but in some populations, women get the disease more frequently than men. While the age of onset of pemphigus foliaceus is usually between 40 and 60 years old, in some areas, symptoms may begin in childhood.

- **Genes**. Scientists believe that the higher frequency of the disease in certain populations is partly due to genetics. For example, evidence shows that certain variants in a family of immune system genes, called "human leukocyte antigens (HLAs)," are linked to a higher risk of pemphigus vulgaris and pemphigus foliaceus.
- **Medications**. In rare cases, pemphigus has resulted from taking certain medicines, such as certain antibiotics and blood pressure medications. Medicines that contain a chemical group called a "thiol" have also been linked to pemphigus.
- **Cancer**. Rarely, the development of a tumor—in particular a growth in a lymph node, tonsil, or thymus gland—can trigger the disease.

TYPES OF PEMPHIGUS

There are two major forms of pemphigus, and they are categorized based on the layer of skin where the blisters form and where the blisters are found on the body. The type of antibody that attacks the skin cells also helps define the type of pemphigus. The following are the two main forms of pemphigus:

- **Pemphigus vulgaris**. It is the most common type in the United States. Blisters form in the mouth and other mucosal surfaces, as well as on the skin. They develop within a deep layer of the epidermis and are often painful. There is a subtype of the disease called "pemphigus vegetans," in which blisters form mainly in the groin and under the arms.
- **Pemphigus foliaceus**. It is less common and only affects the skin. The blisters form in the upper layers of the epidermis and may be itchy or painful.

Other rare forms of pemphigus include the following:
- **Paraneoplastic pemphigus**. This type is characterized by sores in the mouth and on the lips, but blisters or inflamed lesions usually also develop on the skin and other mucosal surfaces. Severe lung problems may

occur with this type. People with this type of disease usually have a tumor, and the disease may improve if the tumor is surgically removed.

- **Immunoglobulin A (IgA) pemphigus**. A type of antibody called IgA causes this form. Blisters or pimple-like bumps often appear in groups or rings on the skin.
- **Drug-induced pemphigus**. Certain medicines, such as some antibiotics and blood pressure medications, as well as drugs that contain a chemical group called a "thiol," may bring on pemphigus-like blisters or sores. The blisters and sores usually go away when you stop taking the medication.

Pemphigoid is a disease that is different from pemphigus but shares some of its features. Pemphigoid produces a split where the epidermis and the underlying dermis meet, causing deep, rigid blisters that do not break easily.

SYMPTOMS OF PEMPHIGUS

The main symptom of pemphigus is blistering of the skin and, in some cases, the mucosal surfaces, such as the inside of the mouth, nose, throat, eyes, and genitals. The blisters are fragile and tend to burst, causing crusty sores. Blisters on the skin may join together, forming raw-looking areas that are prone to infection and that ooze large amounts of fluid. The symptoms vary somewhat depending on the type of pemphigus:

- Pemphigus vulgaris blisters often start in the mouth, but later on, they can develop on the skin. The skin may become so fragile that it peels off by rubbing a finger on it. Mucosal surfaces such as those of the nose, throat, eyes, and genitals may also be affected. Blisters form within the deep layer of the epidermis, and they are often painful.
- Pemphigus foliaceus only affects the skin. Blisters often appear first on the face, scalp, chest, or upper back, but they may eventually spread to other areas of the skin on the body. The affected areas of the skin may become

inflamed and peel off in layers or scales. The blisters form in the upper layers of the epidermis, and they may be itchy or painful.

CAUSES OF PEMPHIGUS

Pemphigus is an autoimmune disorder that happens when the immune system attacks healthy skin. Immune molecules called "antibodies" target proteins called "desmogleins," which help link neighboring skin cells to one another. When these connections are broken, skin becomes fragile, and fluid can collect between layers of cells, forming blisters.

Normally, the immune system protects the body from infection and disease. Researchers do not know what causes the immune system to turn on the body's own proteins, but they believe that both genetic and environmental factors are involved. Something in the environment may trigger pemphigus in people who are at risk because of their genetic makeup. In rare cases, pemphigus may be caused by a tumor or by certain medications.

DIAGNOSIS OF PEMPHIGUS

Early diagnosis is important, so if you have blisters on the skin or in the mouth that do not go away, it is important to see a doctor as soon as you can. Your doctor may try to rule out other conditions first since pemphigus is a rare disease. Your doctor may do the following:

- **Take your medical history and give you a physical exam**. A dermatologist (a doctor who specializes in conditions of the skin, hair, and nails) may ask you about your medical history and look at the appearance and location of blisters. He or she may run a finger or cotton swab over the surface of your skin to see if it shears off easily.
- **Take a tissue sample**. Your doctor may take a sample from one of your blisters to:
  - examine it under the microscope to look for cell separation and to determine the layer of the skin in which the cells are separated
  - determine which antibodies attacked the skin

- **Take a blood sample**. Antibody levels in your blood can help determine the severity of the disease. This blood test may also be used later on to see if treatment is working.

TREATMENT FOR PEMPHIGUS

There is no cure for pemphigus, but treatment can control the disease in most people. The initial goal of treatment is to clear existing blisters and help prevent relapses. Treatment typically depends on the severity and stage of the disease.

Symptoms of pemphigus may go away after many years of treatment, but most people need to continue taking medications to keep the disease under control. Treatment for pemphigus may involve the following medications:

- **Corticosteroids**. These anti-inflammatory medicines are a mainstay of treatment for pemphigus. They may be applied topically as a cream or ointment or can be administered either by mouth or by injection (systemically). Most people will be prescribed systemic corticosteroids, at least initially, to bring the disease under control. Because they are potent drugs, your doctor will prescribe the lowest dose possible to achieve the desired benefit.
- **Immunosuppressants**. These medicines help suppress or curb the overactive immune system.
- **Biologic response modifiers**. These immunomodulators target specific immune messages and interrupt the signal, helping to stop the immune system from attacking the skin.
- **Antibiotics, antivirals, and antifungal medications**. These medications are used to control or prevent infections.

If the above treatments do not work or pemphigus is severe, other treatments may be considered. These treatments include:

- **Plasmapheresis or immunoadsorption**. It removes damaging antibodies from the blood

491

- **Intravenous immunoglobulin therapy**. During this therapy, you are given pooled antibodies from 1,000 or more healthy blood donors

Be sure to report any problems or side effects from medications to your doctor. In some cases, a person with pemphigus may need to be hospitalized to treat health problems that the disease or its treatment can cause. Widespread sores on the skin can result in dehydration or infection, and painful blisters in the mouth can make it difficult to eat. In the hospital, you may be given intravenous (IV) therapy to replace lost fluids, get much-needed nutrition, and treat infection.

Who Treats Pemphigus?
The following health-care providers may diagnose and treat pemphigus:
- dermatologists, who specialize in conditions of the skin, hair, and nails
- dentists, who can tell you how to take care of your gums and teeth if you have blisters in your mouth
- mental health professionals, who help people cope with difficulties in the home and workplace that may result from their medical conditions
- ophthalmologists, in cases where the eyes are affected, who specialize in treating disorders and diseases of the eye
- primary care doctors, such as a family physician or internal medicine specialist, who coordinate care between different health-care providers and treat other problems as they arise

LIVING WITH PEMPHIGUS
Blisters in the mouth may make brushing and flossing your teeth painful, so talk to your dentist about ways to keep your teeth and gums healthy. Avoid foods that irritate your mouth blisters. Your dermatologist may recommend baths and wound dressings to help heal the sores and blisters.

Pemphigus and its treatments can be debilitating and cause lost time at work, weight loss, sleep problems, and emotional distress. A mental health professional or a support group may help you cope with the disease. Remember to follow the recommendations of your health-care providers.[2]

Section 47.4 | Psoriasis

WHAT IS PSORIASIS?

Psoriasis is a chronic (long-lasting) disease in which the immune system becomes overactive, causing skin cells to multiply too quickly. Patches of skin become scaly and inflamed, most often on the scalp, elbows, or knees, but other parts of the body can be affected as well. Scientists do not fully understand what causes psoriasis, but they know that it involves a mix of genetic and environmental factors.

The symptoms of psoriasis can sometimes go through cycles, flaring for a few weeks or months followed by periods when they subside or go into remission. There are many ways to treat psoriasis, and your treatment plan will depend on the type and severity of the disease. Most forms of psoriasis are mild or moderate and can be successfully treated with creams or ointments. Managing common triggers, such as stress and skin injuries, can also help keep the symptoms under control. Having psoriasis carries the risk of getting other serious conditions, including the following:

- psoriatic arthritis, a chronic form of arthritis that causes pain, swelling, and stiffness of the joints and places where tendons and ligaments attach to bones (entheses)
- cardiovascular events, such as heart attacks and strokes
- mental health problems, such as low self-esteem, anxiety, and depression

---

[2] "Pemphigus," National Institute of Arthritis and Musculoskeletal and Skin Diseases (NIAMS), January 2021. Available online. URL: www.niams.nih.gov/health-topics/pemphigus. Accessed May 12, 2023.

- certain cancers, Crohn's disease, diabetes, metabolic syndrome, obesity, osteoporosis, uveitis (inflammation of the middle of the eye), liver disease, and kidney disease

Who Gets Psoriasis?

Anyone can get psoriasis, but it is more common in adults than in children. It affects men and women equally.

TYPES OF PSORIASIS

There are different types of psoriasis, including the following:

- **Plaque psoriasis**. This is the most common kind, and it appears as raised, red patches of skin that are covered by silvery-white scales. The patches usually develop in a symmetrical pattern on the body and tend to appear on the scalp, trunk, and limbs, especially the elbows and knees.
- **Guttate psoriasis**. This type usually appears in children or young adults and looks like small, red dots, typically on the torso or limbs. Outbreaks are often triggered by an upper respiratory tract infection, such as strep throat.
- **Pustular psoriasis**. In this type, pus-filled bumps called "pustules" surrounded by red skin appear. It usually affects the hands and feet, but there is a form that covers most of the body. Symptoms can be triggered by medications, infections, stress, or certain chemicals.
- **Inverse psoriasis**. This form appears as smooth, red patches in folds of skin, such as beneath the breasts or in the groin or armpits. Rubbing and sweating can make it worse.
- **Erythrodermic psoriasis**. This is a rare but severe form of psoriasis characterized by red, scaly skin over most of the body. It can be triggered by a bad sunburn or taking certain medications, such as corticosteroids. Erythrodermic psoriasis often develops in people

who have a different type of psoriasis that is not well controlled, and it can be very serious.

SYMPTOMS OF PSORIASIS

Symptoms of psoriasis vary from person to person, but some common ones are:

- patches of thick, red skin with silvery-white scales that itch or burn, typically on the elbows, knees, scalp, trunk, palms, and soles of the feet
- dry, cracked skin that itches or bleeds
- thick, ridged, pitted nails

Some patients have a related condition called "psoriatic arthritis," which is characterized by stiff, swollen, painful joints. If you have symptoms of psoriatic arthritis, it is important to see your doctor soon because this is one of the most destructive forms of arthritis.

The symptoms of psoriasis tend to come and go. You may find that there are times when your symptoms get worse, called "flares," followed by times when you feel better.

CAUSES OF PSORIASIS

Psoriasis is an immune-mediated disease, which means that your body's immune system starts overacting and causing problems. If you have psoriasis, immune cells become active and produce molecules that set off the rapid production of skin cells. This is why skin in people with the disease is inflamed and scaly. Scientists do not fully understand what triggers the faulty immune cell activation, but they know that it involves a combination of genetic and environmental factors. Many people with psoriasis have a family history of the disease, and researchers have pinpointed some of the genes that may contribute to its development. Nearly all of them play a role in the function of the immune system. Some external factors that may increase the chances of developing psoriasis include:

- infections, especially streptococcal and human immunodeficiency virus (HIV) infections

- certain medicines, such as drugs for treating heart disease, malaria, or mental health problems
- smoking
- obesity

DIAGNOSIS OF PSORIASIS

To diagnose psoriasis, your doctor usually examines your skin, scalp, and nails for signs of the condition. They may also ask questions about your health and history, such as whether you:
- experience symptoms such as itchy or burning skin
- had a recent illness or experienced severe stress
- take certain medicines
- have relatives with the disease
- experience joint tenderness

This information will help the doctor figure out if you have psoriasis and, if so, identify which type. To rule out other skin conditions that look like psoriasis, your doctor may take a small skin sample to examine under a microscope.

TREATMENT FOR PSORIASIS

While there is currently no cure for psoriasis, there are treatments that keep symptoms under control so that you can resume daily activities and sleep better. There are different types of treatment, and your doctor will work with you to decide which is best for you, taking into consideration the type of psoriasis you have, how severe it is, where it is on your body, and the possible side effects of medications. Your treatment may include the following.

Medications

- **Topical therapies**. Creams, ointments, lotions, foams, or solutions, especially those containing corticosteroids, are commonly used to treat people with mild-to-moderate disease. Other topical therapies include vitamin D–based medicines, retinoids (related to vitamin A), coal tar, and anthralin (another tar product).

- **Injected or oral therapies**:
  - **Methotrexate**. This medicine is in a class called "antimetabolites," and it is available in an oral or injected form. It suppresses the immune system and slows down cell growth and division.
  - **Retinoids**. These compounds, which are related to vitamin A, may help some people with moderate-to-severe psoriasis. They can be used in combination with phototherapy.
  - **Biologic response modifiers**. These medications are injected and block specific immune molecules, helping to decrease or stop inflammation.
  - **Immunosuppressants**. These medicines are normally used for severe cases, and they work by suppressing the immune system.
  - **Phosphodiesterase 4 (PDE4) inhibitors**. These target enzymes inside immune cells and suppress the rapid turnover of skin cells and inflammation.

Phototherapy

This treatment involves having a doctor shine an ultraviolet light on your skin in their office. A doctor may also prescribe a home ultraviolet light unit. Phototherapy is usually used when large areas of the skin are affected by the disease.

LIVING WITH PSORIASIS

Psoriasis can affect a person's day-to-day life, including work and sleep. However, health-care providers understand the impact of the disease and can work with you to help reduce the symptoms. In addition to going to your doctor regularly, here are some things you can do to help manage your symptoms:

- **Keep your skin well moisturized**. Bathe in lukewarm water and use mild soap that has added oils. After bathing, apply heavy moisturizing lotions while your skin is still damp.

- **Maintain a healthy weight**. Obesity makes the symptoms of psoriasis worse.
- **Quit smoking**. If work with your doctor to make a plan to quit. Studies have shown that the more a person smokes, the worse the symptoms tend to be.
- **Moderate your use of alcohol**. Some studies suggest that excessive alcohol consumption aggravates symptoms.
- **Expose your skin to small amounts of sunlight**. Limited sunlight can alleviate symptoms, but too much can make them worse, so consult your doctor for advice.
- **Avoid known triggers**. Try to identify things that trigger psoriasis flares and work to avoid them. Some people have found that stress, cold weather, skin injuries, certain medicines, and infections spark flares.
- **Join a support group or visit a mental health provider**. The scaly patches of the skin can make many people feel self-conscious about their appearance. Psoriasis can affect a person's mental health, increasing the risk of anxiety and depression. Seeking out support can help you learn more about coping and living with the disease.[3]

Section 47.5 | **Scleroderma**

WHAT IS SCLERODERMA?

Scleroderma is an autoimmune connective tissue and rheumatic disease that causes inflammation in the skin and other areas of the body. When an immune response tricks tissues into thinking they are injured, it causes inflammation, and the body makes too much collagen, leading to scleroderma. Too much collagen in your skin and other tissues causes patches of tight, hard skin. Scleroderma involves many systems in your body. The following definitions can

---

[3] "Psoriasis," National Institute of Arthritis and Musculoskeletal and Skin Diseases (NIAMS), September 2020. Available online. URL: www.niams.nih.gov/health-topics/psoriasis. Accessed May 12, 2023.

help you better understand how the disease affects each of those systems.

- A connective tissue disease is one that affects tissues such as skin, tendons, and cartilage. Connective tissue supports, protects, and provides structure to other tissues and organs.
- Autoimmune diseases happen when the immune system, which normally helps protect the body from infection and disease, attacks its own tissues.
- Rheumatic disease refers to a group of conditions characterized by inflammation or pain in the muscles, joints, or fibrous tissue.

The following are the two major types of scleroderma:

- **Localized scleroderma**. This type only affects the skin and the structures directly under the skin.
- **Systemic scleroderma**. Also called "systemic sclerosis," this type affects many systems in the body. This is the more serious type of scleroderma and can damage your blood vessels and internal organs, such as the heart, lungs, and kidneys.

There is no cure for scleroderma. The goal of treatment is to relieve symptoms and stop the progression of the disease. Early diagnosis and ongoing monitoring are important.

What Happens in Scleroderma?

The cause of scleroderma is unknown. However, researchers think that the immune system overreacts and causes inflammation and injury to the cells that line blood vessels. This triggers connective tissue cells, especially a cell type called "fibroblasts," to make too much collagen and other proteins. The fibroblasts live longer than normal, causing a buildup of collagen in the skin and other organs, leading to the signs and symptoms of scleroderma.

Who Gets Scleroderma?

Anyone can get scleroderma; however, some groups have a higher risk of developing the disease. The following factors may affect your risk:

- **Sex.** Scleroderma is more common in women than in men.
- **Age.** The disease usually appears between the ages of 30 and 50 and is more common in adults than in children.
- **Race.** Scleroderma can affect people of all races and ethnic groups, but the disease can affect African Americans more severely. The following are a few examples:
  - The disease is more common in African Americans than in European Americans.
  - African Americans with scleroderma develop the disease earlier than other groups.
  - African Americans are more likely to have more skin involvement and lung disease than other groups.

TYPES OF SCLERODERMA

The types of scleroderma are as follows (see also Figure 47.1):

- **Localized scleroderma.** This type affects the skin and underlying tissues and generally appears in one or both of the following patterns:
  - **Morphea or patches of scleroderma.** This may be a half-inch or larger in diameter.

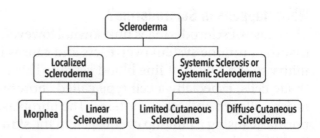

Figure 47.1. Types of Scleroderma

National Institute of Arthritis and Musculoskeletal and Skin Diseases (NIAMS)

- **Linear scleroderma.** The scleroderma thickening occurs in a line. This usually extends down an arm or leg but sometimes runs down the forehead and face.
- **Systemic scleroderma.** Sometimes called "systemic sclerosis," this type affects your skin, tissues, blood vessels, and major organs. Doctors usually divide systemic scleroderma into the following two types:
  - **Limited cutaneous scleroderma.** This comes on gradually and affects the skin on your fingers, hands, face, lower arms, and legs below the knees.
  - **Diffuse cutaneous scleroderma.** This comes on more rapidly and starts as being limited to the fingers and toes but then extends beyond the elbows and knees to the upper arms, trunk, and thighs. This type usually has more internal organ damage.

SYMPTOMS OF SCLERODERMA

The symptoms of scleroderma vary from person to person depending on the type of scleroderma you have. Localized scleroderma typically causes patches of thick, hard skin in one of the following two patterns:

- **Morphea.** It causes patches of skin to thicken into firm, oval-shaped areas. These areas may have a yellow, waxy appearance surrounded by a reddish or bruise-like edge. The patches may stay in one area or spread to other areas of the skin. The disease usually becomes inactive over time, but you may still have darkened patches of the skin. Some people also develop fatigue (feeling tired).
- **Linear scleroderma.** It causes lines of thickened or different-colored skin to run down your arm and leg and, rarely, on the forehead.

Systemic scleroderma, also known as "systemic sclerosis," may come on quickly or gradually and may also cause problems with your internal organs in addition to the skin. Many people with this type of scleroderma have fatigue.

- Limited cutaneous scleroderma comes on gradually and usually affects the skin on your fingers, hands, face, lower arms, and legs below the knees. It can also cause problems with your blood vessels and esophagus. The limited form has internal organ involvement, but it is generally milder than the diffuse form. People with limited cutaneous scleroderma often have all or some of the symptoms that some doctors call CREST, which stands for the following symptoms:
  - **Calcinosis**. This is the formation of calcium deposits in the connective tissues, which can be detected by x-ray.
  - **Raynaud phenomenon**. This is a condition in which the small blood vessels of the hands or feet contract in response to cold or anxiety, causing color changes in fingers and toes (white, blue, and/ or red).
  - **Esophageal dysfunction**. This refers to the impaired function of the esophagus (the tube connecting the throat and the stomach) that occurs when smooth muscles in the esophagus lose normal movement.
  - **Sclerodactyly**. This refers to the thick and tight skin on the fingers, resulting from deposits of excess collagen within skin layers.
  - **Telangiectasia**. This is a condition caused by the swelling of tiny blood vessels, in which small red spots appear on the hands and face.
- Diffuse cutaneous scleroderma comes on suddenly, usually with skin thickening on your fingers or toes. The skin thickening then spreads to the rest of your body above the elbows and/or knees. This type can damage your internal organs, such as:
  - anywhere along your digestive system
  - your lungs
  - your kidneys
  - your heart

Although CREST historically refers to limited scleroderma, people with the diffuse form of scleroderma can also have CREST features.

CAUSES OF SCLERODERMA

Researchers do not know the exact cause of scleroderma, but they suspect that several factors may contribute to the disease:

- **Genetic makeup**. Genes can increase the chance for certain people to develop scleroderma and play a role in determining the type of scleroderma they have. You cannot inherit the disease, and it is not passed from the parent to the child like some genetic diseases. However, first-degree relatives of people with scleroderma are at a higher risk of developing scleroderma than the general population.
- **Environment**. Researchers suspect that exposure to some environmental factors, such as viruses or chemicals, may trigger scleroderma.
- **Immune system changes**. Abnormal immune or inflammatory activity in your body triggers cell changes that cause the production of too much collagen.
- **Hormones**. Women develop most types of scleroderma more often than men. Researchers suspect that hormonal differences between women and men might play a part in the disease.

DIAGNOSIS OF SCLERODERMA

It can be difficult for doctors to diagnose scleroderma because the symptoms vary from person to person and are similar to other diseases. There is no single test to diagnose the disease; instead, doctors use a combination of the following to help diagnose scleroderma. Your doctor may:

- ask about your medical history
- ask about your current and past symptoms
- perform a physical exam

Your doctor may recommend additional testing such as:
- ordering laboratory tests to check for certain antibodies that mistakenly target and react to your own tissues (Some of the antibodies may be common in people with scleroderma. However, antibodies may develop due to other factors, so a blood test alone does not diagnose scleroderma.)
- performing a skin biopsy

If you have symptoms that suggest problems with organs, such as the heart, lungs, or kidneys, your doctor may order additional testing. Early diagnosis of organ involvement helps doctors treat and manage the disease. Testing may include:
- computerized tomography (CT), which uses a scanner to take images of the lungs and other organs
- echocardiogram, which uses sound waves to create moving pictures of your heart

TREATMENT FOR SCLERODERMA

Your treatment depends on the type of scleroderma you have, your symptoms, and which tissues and organs are affected. Treatment can help control the symptoms and limit the damage. Your doctor may recommend medications, including:
- anti-inflammatory medications to manage pain and reduce swelling
- corticosteroid topical creams to treat skin changes, including tightness and itching
- corticosteroids given by mouth, injection, or intravenous (IV) infusion to help manage joint pain or inflammation (Because they are potent medications, your doctor will prescribe the lowest dose possible to achieve the desired benefit and to avoid side effects.)
- immunosuppressants, which may suppress the overactive immune system and can help control symptoms of the disease (Your doctor may prescribe oral, IV, or topical immunosuppressants.)

- vasodilators to help blood vessels dilate (widen), which may prevent lung and kidney damage and treat Raynaud phenomenon

WHO TREATS SCLERODERMA?

Most people will see a rheumatologist for scleroderma treatment. A rheumatologist is a doctor who specializes in rheumatic diseases such as arthritis and other inflammatory or autoimmune disorders. Dermatologists, who specialize in conditions of the skin, hair, and nails, play an important role in treating the disease, particularly for people with localized scleroderma.

Because scleroderma can affect many different organs and organ systems, you may have several different doctors providing your care. These health-care providers may include:

- cardiologists, who specialize in treating diseases of the heart and blood vessels
- dental providers, who can treat complications from the thickening of tissues of the mouth and face
- gastroenterologists, who treat digestive problems
- mental health professionals, who provide counseling and treat mental health disorders such as depression and anxiety
- nephrologists, who treat kidney disease
- occupational therapists, who teach how to safely perform activities of daily living
- orthopedists, who treat and perform surgery for bone and joint diseases or injuries
- primary care providers, including physicians, nurse practitioners, and physician assistants
- physical therapists, who teach ways to build muscle strength
- pulmonologists, who treat lung disease and problems
- speech-language pathologists, who specialize in the treatment of speech and communication disorders

LIVING WITH SCLERODERMA

Depending on the type of scleroderma you have and your symptoms, living with the disease may be hard. To help, try to take an active part in treating your scleroderma. The following tips and suggestions may help:

- **Keep warm**. Your body regulates its temperature through the skin. So dress in layers, wear gloves and socks, and avoid cold rooms and weather when possible.
- **Try to avoid cold or wet environments**. It may trigger Raynaud phenomenon symptoms.
- **Quit smoking**. If you smoke, quit. Nicotine and smoking cause blood vessels to contract, which can make some symptoms worse and cause lung problems.
- **Apply sunscreen**. Before you go outdoors, it is important to apply sunscreen to protect against further damage from the sun's rays.
- **Use moisturizers**. Applying moisturizer on your skin helps lessen stiffness.
- **Use humidifiers**. It helps moisten the air in your home in colder winter climates. Clean humidifiers often to stop bacteria from growing in the water.
- **Avoid hot baths and showers**. Hot water dries the skin.
- **Avoid harsh soaps, household cleaners, and caustic chemicals**. Wear rubber gloves if you use such products.
- **Exercise regularly**. Exercise, especially swimming, stimulates blood circulation to affected areas.
- **Visit the dentist**. It is important to visit dentist regularly for checkups.
- **Reach out for support**. There are online and community support groups that you can reach out for help and support.
- **Keep the lines of communication open**. Talk to your family and friends to help them understand the disease.
- **Talk to a mental health professional**. Get help from a professional to coping with a chronic illness.

Some types of scleroderma can affect parts of the digestive system. Doctors may prescribe heartburn, constipation, and motility medications to help manage these symptoms. Here are some tips to help if you have digestive symptoms:

- Eat small, frequent meals.
- After meals, stay upright for three hours. Try to avoid reclining or slouching.
- Eat moist, soft foods and chew them well. If you have difficulty swallowing or if your body does not absorb nutrients properly, your doctor may prescribe a special diet.
- Drink less alcohol and caffeine.
- Stay hydrated.
- When it is time to sleep, raise the head of your bed with blocks. Using several pillows is not as helpful as raising the head of the bed by using blocks or special wedges.[4]

Section 47.6 | Vitiligo

WHAT IS VITILIGO?

Vitiligo is a chronic (long-lasting) autoimmune disorder that causes patches of skin to lose pigment or color. This happens when melanocytes—skin cells that make pigment—are attacked and destroyed, causing the skin to turn a milky-white color. In vitiligo, the white patches usually appear symmetrically on both sides of your body, such as on both hands or both knees.

Sometimes, there can be a rapid loss of color or pigment and even cover a large area. The segmental subtype of vitiligo is much less common and happens when the white patches are only on one segment or side of your body, such as a leg, one side of the face, or

---

[4] "Scleroderma," National Institute of Arthritis and Musculoskeletal and Skin Diseases (NIAMS), February 2020. Available online. URL: www.niams.nih.gov/health-topics/scleroderma. Accessed May 12, 2023.

arm. This type of vitiligo often begins at an early age and progresses for 6–12 months and then usually stops.

Vitiligo is an autoimmune disease. Normally, the immune system works throughout your body to fight off and defend your body from viruses, bacteria, and infections. In people with autoimmune diseases, the immune cells attack the body's own healthy tissues by mistake. People with vitiligo may be more likely to develop other autoimmune disorders as well. A person with vitiligo occasionally may have family members who also have the disease. Although there is no cure for vitiligo, treatments can be very effective at stopping the progression and reversing its effects, which may help skin tone appear more even.

Who Gets Vitiligo?

Anyone can get vitiligo, and it can develop at any age. However, for many people with vitiligo, the white patches begin to appear before the age of 20 and can start in early childhood.

Vitiligo seems to be more common in people who have a family history of the disorder or who have certain autoimmune diseases, including the following:
- Addison disease
- pernicious anemia
- psoriasis
- rheumatoid arthritis
- systemic lupus erythematosus (SLE)
- thyroid disease
- type 1 diabetes

SYMPTOMS OF VITILIGO

The main symptom of vitiligo is loss of natural color or pigment, called "depigmentation." The depigmented patches can appear anywhere on your body and can affect:
- skin, which develops milky-white patches, often on the hands, feet, arms, and face (However, the patches can appear anywhere.)

- hair, which can turn white in areas where the skin is losing pigment (This can happen on the scalp, eyebrows, eyelashes, beard, and body hair.)
- mucous membranes, such as the inside of your mouth or nose

People with vitiligo can also develop:
- low self-esteem or a poor self-image from concerns about appearance, which can affect the quality of life (QOL)
- uveitis, a general term that describes inflammation or swelling in the eye
- inflammation in the ear

CAUSES OF VITILIGO

Scientists believe that vitiligo is an autoimmune disease in which the body's immune system attacks and destroys the melanocytes. In addition, researchers continue to study how family history and genes may play a role in causing vitiligo. Sometimes, an event—such as a sunburn, emotional distress, or exposure to a chemical—can trigger vitiligo or make it worse.

DIAGNOSIS OF VITILIGO

To diagnose vitiligo, your doctor will ask about your family history and perform a thorough physical exam. The exam may include a close evaluation of your skin. Sometimes, doctors use Wood lamp, also known as a "black light," which is an ultraviolet light that the doctor shines on your skin. If you have vitiligo, the light makes affected areas of your skin appear chalky and bright.

Other tests can include:
- blood tests to check for other autoimmune diseases
- an eye exam to check for uveitis, an inflammation of part of the eye that sometimes occurs with vitiligo
- a skin biopsy, which means taking a small sample of your skin to be examined under a microscope

(Doctors can examine the tissue for the missing melanocytes seen in the depigmented skin of a person with vitiligo.)

TREATMENT FOR VITILIGO

Your doctor may prescribe a medication that focuses on stopping the immune system from destroying the melanocytes and improving the skin's appearance. In most cases, the goals of your treatment are to:

- slow or stop the disease from progressing
- encourage the regrowth of melanocytes
- restore color to the white patches of skin, which can help the skin color look more even

It is important to remember that treatments may take time, and not everyone responds. In addition, the results from treatments can vary from one part of the body to another, and new patches may appear in the meantime. Sometimes, doctors will recommend more than one treatment to get the best results.

Treatments can include the following:

- Medicines or medicated skin creams, such as corticosteroids or a calcineurin inhibitor, may be able to return color to the white patches of the skin.
- Use of light (phototherapy) may help return color to the skin. There are several different forms of light therapy. Doctors may use light boxes to treat large areas of vitiligo and use laser treatments on more localized areas.
- Depigmentation or removing color from dark areas of the skin is done so that they match the white patches. Doctors usually recommend this treatment for people who have vitiligo on more than half of their bodies. Depigmentation tends to be permanent and can take more than a year to complete. As with other treatments, it is very important to limit exposure to sunlight during and after treatment.

- Dermatologists may consider surgical techniques for long-standing segmental vitiligo or vitiligo of any type for which other treatments do not work. Surgery is typically not recommended when vitiligo is spreading or for people who scar easily or develop keloids, which are raised scars that grow larger than the wound that caused the scar.

LIVING WITH VITILIGO

Living with vitiligo can be hard. Some people with the disorder feel embarrassed, sad, ashamed, or upset about the changes in their appearance. Sometimes, this can lead to low self-esteem and depression. Seeking advice and help from a mental health professional can help you cope with the disorder and treat depression.

In addition to the treatments your doctor recommends, you can help manage the disease by:

- protecting your skin from the sun (Use sunscreen and wear clothes to help protect your skin from sunburn and long-term damage.)
- wearing cosmetics, such as self-tanning lotions or dyes, to cover depigmented patches of skin (Talk to your doctor about which lotion or dye you should use.)
- finding a doctor who has experience treating people with vitiligo
- learning about the disorder and treatments to help you make decisions about care
- talking with other people who have vitiligo (Consider finding a vitiligo support group in your area or through an online community.)
- reaching out to family and friends for support[5]

---

[5] "Vitiligo," National Institute of Arthritis and Musculoskeletal and Skin Diseases (NIAMS), October 2022. Available online. URL: www.niams.nih.gov/health-topics/vitiligo. Accessed May 12, 2023.

Part 5 | Hypersensitive Immune Responses

Chapter 48 |
Hypersensitivity

Hypersensitivity refers to an excessive response of the body's immune system to typically harmless substances such as pollen, food, or certain environmental substances or even to parts of the body as if they are dangerous. Hypersensitivity can cause different reactions, such as allergies or autoimmune diseases. The responses range from mild reactions, such as a rash, to severe reactions, such as organ damage or anaphylactic shock.

Hypersensitivity reactions occur only in people who have already been exposed to a particular substance. Though there may not have been any symptoms during the first contact, the body would have started preparing to fight the substance by producing special cells or proteins. The next time the substance comes in contact with the body, these cells and proteins fight the foreign particles, and symptoms appear.

The following are the four types of hypersensitivity reactions:

- **Type 1 hypersensitivity (also called "immediate hypersensitivity").** This is the most common and rapid allergic reaction. It occurs within a few seconds or minutes after someone comes into contact with an allergen from sources such as food, environment, animals, or drugs.
  - Type I hypersensitivity happens in the following two stages:
    - The first stage, also known as the "sensitization stage," is when our body recognizes the antigen for the first time, but we do not feel any symptoms at this stage.

- The second stage, also called the "late-phase reaction," happens when we come into contact with the same antigen again after our body has already recognized it. This time, our body reacts strongly, and we may experience symptoms such as sneezing, itching, runny nose, or swelling. In type I hypersensitivity, the body produces an antibody called "immunoglobulin E" (IgE) in response to previous exposure to the allergen. These IgE antibodies attach to cells called "mast cells." When a person has a repeat exposure to the same allergen, it binds to the IgE on these cells, causing them to release chemicals such as histamine. These chemicals cause allergic symptoms, which may include skin rashes, itchy and red eyes, difficulty breathing, vomiting, diarrhea, and cramps. The reaction happens quickly, within minutes of exposure, and can be mild or severe. Most allergies are this type of hypersensitivity.

- **Type II hypersensitivity**. Certain proteins in our blood called "antibodies" stick to the outside of specific cells in our body, making them vulnerable to being destroyed by our immune system. Certain medicines, such as penicillin, cephalosporins, and methyldopa, can cause type II hypersensitivity in some people. This happens because the drug changes the body's proteins into foreign substances that the immune system does not recognize as "self" and reacts negatively and attacks its cells instead of protecting them. This typically happens in a condition called "hemolytic disease of the newborn," where a mother's antibodies attack the baby's red blood cells (RBCs). Other common reactions include anemia, nephritis, and, sometimes, paralysis.

- **Type III hypersensitivity**. This response occurs when the antibodies bind to antigens that are floating freely in the blood, forming clusters called "complexes" that trigger inflammation in the body. These complexes accumulate at the base of some tissues, such as the joints and kidneys, and create a large reaction that causes swelling. This response can harm neighboring cells and tissues, making them unable to function normally. The most common reaction in this type is serum sickness, where immune complexes are deposited in blood vessel walls and cause inflammation. Conditions such as systemic lupus erythematosus (SLE) and rheumatoid arthritis (RA) can arise as a result of type III hypersensitivity.

- **Type IV hypersensitivity**. In type IV hypersensitivity, our immune system reacts after being exposed to an antigen for the second time. T cells release inflammatory chemicals that cause an allergic reaction, such as a rash or itchiness on our skin, and assist in fighting illness when our immune system identifies an invading pathogen. They accomplish this by recognizing and directly destroying bacteria or viruses or signaling other cells to assist. In certain situations, this process can cause inflammation or damage to our own cells. It occurs in diseases such as tuberculosis (TB), where the immune response is delayed, leading to increased sensitivity. The TB skin test also relies on this type of heightened sensitivity. Similarly, contact dermatitis occurs when the skin comes in contact with an allergen to which the skin is allergic.

Some individuals may experience intense allergic reactions to substances such as mold, pollen, food, animal bites, or drugs. The development of new tools such as microarrays, a tool used to detect thousands of genes at the same time, and human leukocyte antigen tetramers, a tool used to isolate allergen-specific T cells, assists health-care professionals in pinpointing the exact trigger behind the hypersensitivity reactions. Providing a targeted treatment plan helps health-care providers treat the patient more effectively.

References

Agrawal, Amogh. "Hypersensitivity: Summary," The Calgary Guide to Understanding Disease, April 23, 2019. Available online. URL: https://calgaryguide.ucalgary.ca/ hypersensitivity-summary. Accessed May 9, 2023.

Basu, Shibani and Banik, Bimal Krishna. "Hypersensitivity: An Overview," OMICS Publishing Group, October 23, 2018. Available online. URL: www.omicsonline.org/ open-access/hypersensitivity-an-overview-105371.html. Accessed May 9, 2023.

"Hypersensitivity," Biology Online, July 24, 2022. Available online. URL: www.biologyonline.com/dictionary/ hypersensitivity. Accessed May 9, 2023.

Justiz Vaillant, Angel A; Vashisht, Rishik; and Zito, Patrick M. "Immediate Hypersensitivity Reactions," National Center for Biotechnology Information (NCBI), March 7, 2023. Available online. URL: www.ncbi.nlm.nih. gov/books/NBK513315. Accessed May 9, 2023.

Speller, Jess. "Hypersensitivity Reactions," TeachMePhysiology, January 17, 2022. Available online. URL: https://teachmephysiology.com/immune-system/ immune-responses/hypersensitivity-reactions. Accessed May 9, 2023.

Chapter 49 | **Anaphylaxis (Type 1)**

WHAT IS ANAPHYLAXIS?

Anaphylaxis is a serious allergic reaction that involves more than one organ system (e.g., skin, respiratory tract, and/or gastrointestinal (GI) tract). It can begin very rapidly, and symptoms may be severe or life-threatening. Figure 49.1 explains allergic reactions mediated by immunoglobulin E (IgE).

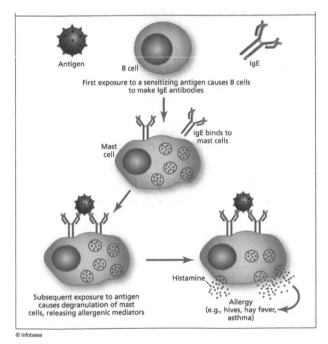

© Infobase

Figure 49.1. Immunoglobulin E–Mediated Allergic Reactions

Infobase

CAUSES OF ANAPHYLAXIS

The most common causes of anaphylaxis are reactions to foods (especially peanuts), medications, and stinging insects. Sometimes, anaphylaxis occurs without an identifiable trigger. This is called "idiopathic anaphylaxis."

SYMPTOMS OF ANAPHYLAXIS

Anaphylaxis includes a wide range of symptoms that can occur in many combinations and may be difficult to recognize. Some symptoms are not life-threatening, but the most severe ones restrict breathing and blood circulation. Many of the body's organs can be affected:

- skin: itching, hives, redness, swelling
- nose: sneezing, stuffy nose, runny nose
- mouth: itching, swelling of the lips or tongue
- throat: itching, tightness, difficulty swallowing, swelling of the back of the throat
- chest: shortness of breath, cough, wheezing, chest pain, tightness
- heart: weak pulse, passing out, shock
- GI tract: vomiting, diarrhea, cramps
- nervous system: dizziness or fainting

How Soon after Exposure Will Symptoms Occur?

Symptoms can begin within minutes to hours after exposure to the allergen. Sometimes, the symptoms go away, only to return anywhere from 8 to 72 hours later. When you begin to experience symptoms, seek immediate medical attention because anaphylaxis can be life-threatening.

How Do You Know If a Person Is Having an Anaphylactic Reaction?

Anaphylaxis is likely if a person experiences two or more of the following symptoms within minutes to several hours after exposure to an allergen:

- hives, itchiness, or redness all over the body and swelling of the lips, tongue, or back of the throat

- trouble breathing
- severe GI symptoms such as abdominal cramps, diarrhea, or vomiting
- dizziness or fainting (signs of a drop in blood pressure)

If you are experiencing symptoms of anaphylaxis, seek immediate treatment and tell your health-care professional if you have a history of allergic reactions.

Can Anaphylaxis Be Predicted?

Anaphylaxis caused by an allergic reaction is highly unpredictable. The severity of one attack does not predict the severity of subsequent attacks. Any anaphylactic reaction can become dangerous quickly and must be evaluated immediately by a health-care professional.

TREATMENT FOR ANAPHYLAXIS

If you or someone you know is having an anaphylactic episode, health experts advise using an auto-injector, if available, to inject epinephrine (a hormone that increases the heart rate, constricts the blood vessels, and opens the airways) into the thigh muscle and calling 911 if you are not in a hospital. If you are in a hospital, summon a resuscitation team.

If epinephrine is not given promptly, rapid decline and death could occur within 30–60 minutes. Epinephrine acts immediately but does not last long in the body, so it may be necessary to give repeat doses.

After epinephrine has been given, the patient can be placed in a reclining position with feet elevated to help restore normal blood flow.

A health-care professional may also give the patient any of the following secondary treatments:

- medications to open the airways
- antihistamines to relieve itching and hives
- corticosteroids (a class of drugs used to treat inflammatory diseases) to prevent prolonged inflammation and long-lasting reactions

- additional medications to constrict blood vessels and increase heart rate
- supplemental oxygen therapy
- intravenous (IV) fluids

Conditions such as asthma, chronic lung disease, and cardio-vascular disease (CVD) may increase the risk of death from ana-phylaxis. Medications such as those that treat high blood pressure may also worsen symptom severity and limit response to treatment.

Antihistamines should be used only as a secondary treatment. Giving antihistamines instead of epinephrine may increase the risk of a life-threatening allergic reaction.

EMERGENCY MANAGEMENT

Before leaving emergency medical care, your health-care profes-sional should provide the following:

- an epinephrine auto-injector or a prescription for two doses and training in how to use the auto-injector
- a follow-up appointment or an appointment with a clinical specialist such as an allergist or immunologist
- information on where to get medical identification jewelry or an anaphylaxis wallet card that alerts others of the allergy
- education about allergen avoidance, recognizing the symptoms of anaphylaxis, and giving epinephrine
- an anaphylaxis emergency action plan

If you or someone you know has a history of severe allergic reactions or anaphylaxis, your health-care professional should remember to keep you S.A.F.E.:

- **Seek support**. Your health-care professional should tell you the following:
  - Anaphylaxis is a life-threatening condition.
  - The symptoms of the current episode may occur again (sometimes up to three days later).
  - You are at risk of anaphylaxis in the future.

- At the first sign of symptoms, give yourself epinephrine and then immediately call an ambulance or have someone else take you to the nearest emergency facility.
- **Allergen identification and avoidance.** Before you leave the hospital, your health-care professional should have:
  - made efforts to identify the allergen by taking your medical history
  - explained the importance of getting additional testing to confirm what triggered the reaction, so you can successfully avoid it in the future
- **Follow-up with specialty care.** Your health-care professional should encourage you to consult a specialist for an allergy evaluation.
- **Epinephrine for emergencies.** Your health-care professional should give you the following:
  - an epinephrine auto-injector or a prescription and training on how to use an auto-injector
  - advice to routinely check the expiration date of the auto-injector[1]

---

[1] "Anaphylaxis," National Institute of Allergy and Infectious Diseases (NIAID), April 23, 2015. Available online. URL: www.niaid.nih.gov/topics/anaphylaxis/Pages/default.aspx. Accessed May 29, 2023.

Chapter 50 | **Blood Transfusion Reaction (Type 2)**

KEY FACTS

- Each day, lifesaving blood transfusions are needed in hospitals and emergency treatment facilities across the United States.
- Annually, in the United States, there are nearly 11 million blood donors and more than 14 million units of blood transfused.
- Most patients do not experience any side effects from blood transfusions. On rare occasions, blood transfusions can cause adverse reactions in patients receiving blood.
- Although the U.S. blood supply is safer than ever before, some bacteria, viruses, prions, and parasites can be transmitted by blood transfusions.
- Each donor is screened for risk of transmissible disease by a questionnaire prior to donating blood, and each unit of blood donated in the United States is routinely screened for various infectious disease pathogens using assays approved by the U.S. Food and Drug Administration (FDA).

SCREENING DONATED BLOOD

Blood donors are asked a set of standard questions prior to donating blood to assist in determining if they are in good health and free of any diseases that could be transmitted by blood transfusion. If the donor's answers indicate they are not well or are at risk of having a disease transmissible by blood transfusion, they are not allowed to donate blood.

If the donor is eligible to donate, the donated blood is tested for blood type (ABO group) and rhesus (Rh; positive or negative). This is to make sure that patients receive blood that matches their blood type. Before transfusion, the donor and blood unit are also tested for certain additional proteins (antibodies) that may cause adverse reactions in a person receiving a blood transfusion.

All blood for transfusion is tested for evidence of certain infectious disease pathogens, such as hepatitis B and C viruses and human immunodeficiency virus (HIV). The tests used to screen donated blood are listed in Table 50.1.

Table 50.1. Infectious Disease Pathogen and the Laboratory Tests Used to Screen Donated Blood

Infectious Disease Pathogen	Laboratory Tests Used	Frequency of Tests
Hepatitis B virus (HBV)	• Hepatitis B surface antigen (HBsAg) assay • Total antibody to hepatitis B core antigen (anti-HBc) assay • Nucleic acid testing for HBV	Every donation
Hepatitis C virus (HCV)	• Antibody to hepatitis C virus (anti-HCV) assay • Nucleic acid testing for HCV • Enzyme-linked immunosorbent assay (ELISA) for HCV	Every donation
Human immunodeficiency virus (HIV) types 1 and 2	• Antibodies to HIV-1 and HIV-2 (anti-HIV-1 and anti-HIV-2) assay • Nucleic acid testing for HIV-1	Every donation
Human T-lymphotropic virus (HTLV) types I and II	• Antibodies to human T-lymphotropic virus types I and II (anti-HTLV-I/II) assay	Every donation
Treponema pallidum (syphilis)	• Anti-treponemal antibody detection	Every donation

526

Table 50.1. Continued

Infectious Disease Pathogen	Laboratory Tests Used	Frequency of Tests
West Nile virus (WNV)	• Nucleic acid testing for WNV	Every donation
Trypanosoma cruzi (Chagas disease)	• Anti–*T. cruzi* assay	All first-time donors tested
Cytomegalovirus (CMV)	• Anti–CMV assay	Performed on some donations for special-needs recipients
Babesia	• Nucleic acid test for *Babesia* species and antibody test for *B. microti*	Performed on donations in *Babesia*-endemic regions
Bacterial contamination	• Risk control strategies	As specified by FDA guidance (www.fda.gov/regulatory-information/search-fda-guidance-documents/bacterial-risk-control-strategiesblood-collection-establishments-andtransfusion-services-enhance)

ADVERSE REACTIONS ASSOCIATED WITH BLOOD TRANSFUSIONS

The chance of having a reaction to a blood transfusion is very small. The most common adverse reactions from blood transfusions are allergic and febrile reactions, which make up over half of all adverse reactions reported. Rare but serious adverse reactions include infection caused by bacterial contamination of the blood products and immune reactions due to problems in blood type matching between the donor and the recipient.

The following is a list of blood-transfusion-associated adverse reactions that are tracked through the National Healthcare Safety Network (NHSN) Hemovigilance Module (www.cdc.gov/nhsn/biovigilance/blood-safety/index.html?CDC_AA_refVal=https%3A%2F%2Fwww.cdc.

527

gov%2Fnhsn%2Facute-care-hospital%2Fbio-hemo%2Findex. html):

- **Allergic reaction**. An allergic reaction results from an interaction of an allergen in the transfused blood with preformed antibodies in the person receiving the blood transfusion. In some instances, the infusion of antibodies from the donor may be involved. The reaction may present only with irritation of the skin and/or mucous membranes but can also involve serious symptoms such as difficulty breathing.
- **Acute hemolytic transfusion reaction (AHTR)**. An AHTR is the rapid destruction of red blood cells (RBCs) that occurs during, immediately after, or within 24 hours of a transfusion when a patient is given an incompatible blood type. The recipient's body immediately begins to destroy the donated RBCs, resulting in fever, pain, and sometimes severe complications such as kidney failure.
- **Delayed hemolytic transfusion reaction (DHTR)**. A DHTR occurs when the recipient develops antibodies to RBC antigen(s) between 24 hours and 28 days after a transfusion. Symptoms are usually milder than in AHTRs and may even be absent. A DHTR is diagnosed with laboratory testing to detect specific antibodies.
- **Delayed serologic transfusion reaction (DSTR)**. A DSTR occurs when a recipient develops new antibodies against RBCs between 24 hours and 28 days after a transfusion without clinical symptoms or laboratory evidence of hemolysis. Since this is by definition a reaction with no clinical symptoms, the severity of the reaction cannot be graded.
- **Febrile nonhemolytic transfusion reaction (FNHTR)**. FNHTRs are the most common reaction reported after a transfusion. An FNHTR is characterized by fever and/or chills in the absence of hemolysis (breakdown of RBCs) occurring in the patient during or up to four hours after a transfusion. These reactions are

generally mild and respond quickly to treatment. Fever can be a symptom of a more severe reaction with more serious causes and should be fully investigated.

- **Hypotensive transfusion reaction.** A hypotensive transfusion reaction is a drop in systolic blood pressure occurring soon after a transfusion begins that responds quickly to the cessation of the transfusion and supportive treatment. Hypotension can also be a symptom of a more severe reaction and should be fully investigated.

- **Post-transfusion purpura (PTP).** PTP is a rare but potentially fatal condition that occurs when a transfusion recipient develops antibodies against platelets, resulting in the rapid destruction of both transfused platelets and the patient's own platelets and a severe decline in the platelet count. PTP usually occurs 5–12 days after a transfusion and is more common in women than in men.

- **Transfusion-associated circulatory overload (TACO).** TACO occurs when the volume of blood or blood components transfused cannot be effectively processed by the recipient. TACO can occur due to an excessively high infusion rate and/or volume or due to an underlying heart or kidney condition. Symptoms may include difficulty breathing, cough, and fluid in the lungs.

- **Transfusion-related acute lung injury (TRALI).** TRALI is a serious but rare reaction that occurs when fluid builds up in the lungs but is not related to excessive volume of blood or blood products transfused. The symptoms include acute respiratory distress with no other explanation for lung injury, such as pneumonia or trauma, occurring within six hours of transfusion. The mechanism of TRALI is not well-understood, but it is thought to be associated with the presence of antibodies in donor blood.

- **Transfusion-associated dyspnea (TAD).** TAD is the onset of respiratory distress within 24 hours of transfusion that cannot be defined as TACO, TRALI, or an allergic reaction.
- **Transfusion-associated graft versus host disease (TAGVHD).** TAGVHD is a rare complication of transfusion that occurs when donor T lymphocytes (the "graft") introduced by the blood transfusion rapidly increase in number in the recipient (the "host") and then attack the recipient's own cells. The symptoms include fever, a characteristic rash, enlargement of the liver, and diarrhea that occur between two days and six weeks after transfusion. Though very rare, this inflammatory response is difficult to treat and often results in death.
- **Transfusion-transmitted infection (TTI).** A TTI occurs when a bacterium, parasite, virus, or other potential pathogen is transmitted in donated blood to the transfusion recipient.[1]

---

[1] "Blood Safety Basics," Centers for Disease Control and Prevention (CDC), August 30, 2022. Available online. URL: www.cdc.gov/bloodsafety/basics.html. Accessed May 12, 2023.

Chapter 51 | **Serum Sickness (Type 3)**

Serum sickness is a delayed response to certain medications or to foreign proteins, particularly the substances found in antiserums. Serum is the clear portion of blood that does not contain red or white blood cells but does contain proteins, electrolytes, antibodies, antigens, hormones, and other substances. An antiserum is produced in certain animals and humans with an already-developed immunity to a particular disease; this is then used to treat the specific condition in other animals or individuals. The same method is used to treat stings or bites of venomous animals.

While vaccines may also be prepared from serum in a similar fashion, they are intended to prevent illness by "teaching" the body to develop immunity to a particular disease; antiserums (the liquid component of blood that contains antibodies) are primarily used to stimulate the immune system to combat an existing infection or disease.

In serum sickness, as with an allergy, the body erroneously identifies the medicine or foreign protein as a threat, and the immune system responds by attacking it with its antibodies. These combine with the antigens (foreign substances) to form immune complexes that can collect on the blood vessels, heart, and other body parts to cause the illness.

Serum sickness resulting from animal-based antiserums is becoming less common because of the decrease in the use of foreign serum proteins in the treatment of human diseases. However, the condition still occurs with some regularity and is most prevalent as a reaction to various medications.

CAUSES OF SERUM SICKNESS

Penicillin reaction is one of the most common causes of serum sickness, affecting an estimated 10 percent of patients treated. Other medications that can trigger the response include various other antibiotics, thiazides (used to treat hypertension and edema), aspirin, fluoxetine (used to treat depression), and, occasionally, vaccines. Serum sickness can also be caused by bee or wasp stings; by antivenoms made to treat bites from venomous snakes, spiders, insects, or fish; and by antiserums used in the treatment of conditions such as tetanus and rabies.

SYMPTOMS OF SERUM SICKNESS

Serum sickness usually happens a few days to three weeks after an individual takes a medicine or antiserum for the first time. However, some people may experience symptoms in as little as one to three days if they have already been exposed to the medicine. In some individuals, it can also develop as quickly as one hour after exposure.

The symptoms of serum sickness include:
- fever
- skin rash
- joint pain
- itching
- swollen lymph nodes
- soft tissue swelling
- flushed skin
- diarrhea
- blurred vision
- shortness of breath
- arthritis
- nausea
- low blood pressure
- general malaise

DIAGNOSIS OF SERUM SICKNESS

To diagnose serum sickness, a doctor generally begins by collecting the patient's history, particularly asking about medications taken and any recent insect bites or stings. A physical exam may reveal lymph nodes that are enlarged and sore, skin rashes, or reactions at an injection site. Laboratory tests may include blood work to detect antibodies that have developed to counter foreign proteins, a urine test to see if it contains blood or proteins, and biopsies of rashes or skin eruptions.

TREATMENT FOR SERUM SICKNESS

The initial step to treat serum sickness is to discontinue using the medication or antiserum responsible for the reaction. Serum sickness commonly resolves without long-term complications once the triggering therapy is discontinued.

To manage symptoms, medication can be used in different forms:

- To alleviate itching and rash, corticosteroids can be applied to the skin.
- Antihistamines can help reduce the duration of illness and alleviate rash and itching.
- Joint pain can be relieved with nonsteroidal anti-inflammatory drugs (NSAIDs) such as ibuprofen or naproxen.
- Severe cases may require corticosteroids taken orally.

Sometimes, a medical treatment called "plasma exchange" may be needed to get rid of harmful substances such as autoantibodies and proteins from the body.

High doses of intravenous (IV) corticosteroids are often administered for three days, followed by reduced doses of oral steroids based on clinical response. Avoiding the use of the triggering medication or antiserum in the future is important to prevent future reactions.

COMPLICATIONS OF SERUM SICKNESS

With proper treatment, the symptoms of serum sickness generally improve in 7–10 days, and a full recovery can be expected within

30 days. Although the condition is usually not life-threatening, it is important to consult a physician when symptoms appear since serum sickness can, on occasion, lead to severe disorders.

Some possible complications include the following:
- recurrence from future exposure to the causative substance
- inflammation of the blood vessels
- angioedema (swelling of the face, arms, and legs)
- nervous system disorders, such as Guillain-Barré syndrome and peripheral neuritis
- anaphylaxis (a potentially fatal allergic reaction)
- kidney disorders
- heart inflammation

PREVENTION OF SERUM SICKNESS

Although there is no definite way to prevent serum sickness altogether, the most effective approach to avoid it is to refrain from using the medication or antiserum injection that initially triggered it. However, for those who do not have a known sensitivity to a specific substance, it can be challenging to anticipate a reaction until it actually occurs. Nevertheless, there are a few strategies that a physician can employ to prevent the development or recurrence of the condition potentially.

For example, prior to injecting the antiserum, the health-care provider could try a skin prick sensitivity test using diluted antiserum to check if any reaction occurs.

Serum sickness usually goes away by itself in a few weeks, but it can be very uncomfortable. If an individual has symptoms of serum sickness, they should go to the health-care provider and seek medical attention right away to get diagnosed and treated promptly. It is extremely important to act quickly to prevent worsening of the condition.

References

ADAM, "Serum Sickness," MedlinePlus, January 25, 2022. Available online. URL: https://medlineplus.gov/ency/article/000820.htm. Accessed April 18, 2023.

Alissa, Hassan M. "Serum Sickness," MedScape, July 19, 2022. Available online. URL: http://emedicine.medscape.com/article/332032-overview#a3. Accessed April 18, 2023.

Dewlyn, Dyall-Smith. "Serum Sickness," DermNet, October 4, 2010. Available online. URL: www.dermnetnz.org/topics/serum-sickness. Accessed April 18, 2023.

Lucchetti, Lorenzo. "What to Know about Serum Sickness," Medical News Today, October 26, 2022. Available online. URL: www.medicalnewstoday.com/articles/serum-sickness. Accessed April 18, 2023.

Ronis, Tova. "Pediatric Serum Sickness," MedScape, July 17, 2018. Available online. URL: http://emedicine.medscape.com/article/887954-overview. Accessed April 18, 2023.

Santos-Longhurst, Adrienne. "Understanding Serum Sickness," Healthline, November 13, 2018. Available online. URL: www.healthline.com/health/serum-sickness. Accessed April 18, 2023.

Chapter 52 | Transplant Rejection (Type 4)

The immune system is the body's tool that fights infection and disease. It works by seeing harmful cells as "foreign" and attacking them. When you receive a donor's stem cells (the "graft"), the stem cells recreate the donor's immune system in your body (the "host").

"Graft versus host disease" (GVHD) is the term used when this new immune system from the donor attacks your body. Your donor's cells see your body as "foreign" and attack it, which causes damage. GVHD can range from mild to moderate to severe.

Acute GVHD usually occurs within the first 100 days after your transplant or infusion of T cells (in a donor lymphocyte infusion (DLI)). Acute GVHD commonly affects your skin, liver, and gastrointestinal (GI) tract. Chronic GVHD can happen 60–100 days after transplant and can reoccur for several years after transplant.

WHAT ARE THE SIGNS AND SYMPTOMS OF GRAFT VERSUS HOST DISEASE?

First, make sure to report all new or worsening symptoms to your National Institutes of Health (NIH) clinical center doctor:

- skin GVHD:
  - red rash
  - itching
  - darkening of the skin
- liver GVHD:
  - elevated liver enzymes determined through blood tests

- yellowing of the skin and whites of the eyes
- abdominal pain
- GI GVHD:
  - watery diarrhea
  - stomach cramps (especially before and during bowel movements and after eating)
  - persistent nausea

HOW CAN YOU MANAGE THE SYMPTOMS OF GRAFT VERSUS HOST DISEASE?

Along with your treatment plan, there are also things that you can do to help manage GVHD:

- skin care:
  - Avoid scratching.
  - Use moisturizing lotion.
  - Avoid perfumed lotions.
  - Avoid hot showers.
  - Use sunscreen with a sun protection factor (SPF) 30 or greater.
  - Avoid prolonged sun exposure.
  - Wear long sleeves and pants.
- diarrhea:
  - Follow the diet prescribed by your doctor and dietitian to prevent worsening diarrhea.
  - Avoid spicy foods.
  - To avoid skin problems (such as irritation) around your rectal area, it is very important to keep this area clean. Clean this area well after each bout of diarrhea. Tell your nurse if this area gets red, cracked, painful, or infected.
- preventing infection:
  - Wash your hands often.
  - Stay away from sick family members and friends.
  - Your doctor may ask you to wear a mask.
  - Notify your doctor if you have fevers, chills, or redness/pain at your catheter site.

CAN YOU PREVENT GRAFT VERSUS HOST DISEASE?

There is nothing you can do to prevent GVHD. However, skin GVHD can be triggered and worsened by sun exposure. Wearing a hat, long sleeves, long pants, and sunscreen will help control skin GVHD caused by sun damage. Avoiding sun exposure is the best prevention.

GVHD cannot be predicted, but depending on the type of stem cell transplant you received, your doctor may place you on immunosuppressive medications (medications that decrease the immune system's ability to fight infections) to lessen GVHD.

Medications such as cyclosporine, tacrolimus, and sirolimus suppress the immune system to lessen harmful GVHD. You may be required to take these medications for several months after your transplant. It is important to take these medications as prescribed and to report any side effects.

HOW IS GRAFT VERSUS HOST DISEASE DIAGNOSED?

Diagnosis is based on symptoms, laboratory results, and tissue biopsies. Diagnosis of GVHD is difficult because early symptoms are often the same as other side effects and complications after the transplant. It is important that you report any changes in your skin or bowel patterns to your health-care provider.

WHAT IS THE TREATMENT FOR GRAFT VERSUS HOST DISEASE?

Treatment aims at decreasing the donor's immune reaction against your body. You will be given immunosuppressive medication to decrease this reaction. Steroids, such as prednisone and methylprednisolone, are first-line treatments for GVHD. But steroids weaken your immune system and the ability to fight infection. Therefore, depending on how severe your GVHD is, your doctor may want you to be admitted to the hospital for treatment.[1]

---

[1] Clinical Center, "Graft Versus Host Disease (GVHD): A Guide for Patients and Families after Stem Cell Transplant," National Institutes of Health (NIH), January 24, 2005. Available online. URL: www.cc.nih.gov/ccc/patient_education/pepubs/gvh.pdf. Accessed May 29, 2023.

Part 6 | Diagnostic Tests for Immune Disorders

Chapter 53 | **Getting a Proper Diagnosis of Autoimmune Disease**

Diagnosing autoimmune diseases is usually challenging because the symptoms are very general and can be attributed to other illnesses. Symptoms such as fatigue, fever, depression, and difficulty concentrating are common to many autoimmune diseases. Sometimes, health-care providers may think these symptoms are caused by stress, worry, or other conditions.

Detecting the presence of an autoimmune disease can be difficult since these diseases show up suddenly and very unexpectedly. Also, there are over 80 autoimmune diseases that make it complicated to test for each one as the diagnosis differs for all of them.

WHAT ARE AUTOIMMUNE DISEASES?

Autoimmune diseases result from the body being attacked by the immune system instead of protecting it. There is no clarity on why this happens. Many autoimmune diseases are thought to be triggered when the body is exposed to foreign agents. These can range from infections to food, such as iodine and gluten, to toxins, such as smoke, drugs, hair dyes, and chemicals at home or at the workplace.

SYMPTOMS OF AUTOIMMUNE DISEASES

Autoimmune diseases affect any type of tissue or organ in the body. The symptoms depend on which part of the body is being attacked and the type of disorder. The symptoms of autoimmune disorders are often nonspecific and may linger for a considerable length of time. They can include the following:

- difficulty concentrating
- fatigue
- heart palpitations
- low-grade fever
- miscarriage
- muscle and joint pain
- rashes
- shortness of breath
- weakness
- weight loss

Autoimmune diseases are generally chronic and not fatal. The objective of treatment is to control the disease and not necessarily to cure it.

HINDRANCES IN DIAGNOSING AN AUTOIMMUNE DISEASE
Some of the hurdles faced in diagnosing an autoimmune disease are as follows:

- Symptoms may be delayed or completely absent. For example, symptoms of celiac disease may be present in children as young as nine months of age or remain latent until well into adulthood.
- Many symptoms are common to a number of autoimmune diseases, as well as other disorders. Joint pain is one such common symptom, but some diseases are systemic and can cause pain anywhere in the body.
- One autoimmune condition can mask another, which increases the difficulty of making a diagnosis.
- Some people tend to disregard pain and avoid consulting a doctor, thinking that their symptoms are too mild or that they are too young to be afflicted with conditions such as rheumatoid arthritis.
- Autoimmune diseases mimic one another. For instance, multiple sclerosis (MS) looks similar to lupus and other neurological conditions. This makes it difficult to rule out one or the other.

- Autoimmune disease symptoms are present differently in different individuals, so doctors cannot depend on symptoms alone to diagnose correctly.

METHODS OF DIAGNOSIS

The diagnosis of autoimmune disorders involves an array of blood tests, urinalysis, assessment of symptoms, medical history review, and physical examinations. Diagnostic tests can help in making a diagnosis but are often not definitive on their own.

Blood tests, such as inflammation tests and the antinuclear antibody (ANA) test, can help detect autoantibodies. These autoantibodies are harmful substances that attack the body's own tissues.

HOW TO HELP ENSURE AN ACCURATE DIAGNOSIS

The following are a few things a patient can do to help the doctor make an accurate diagnosis. These include the following:

- **Knowing your family's medical history**. Autoimmune diseases are known to be inherited, but the diseases can overlap, and there is a chance that you may have a different disease than another person in your family. Talk to your relatives and gather information to see if someone in the family has a history of autoimmune disease. Let your doctor know about it, so he or she can take genetic factors into consideration when making a diagnosis.
- **Maintaining a journal of symptoms**. Autoimmune diseases come with numerous symptoms, and you may not remember them in detail when you see your doctor. Although symptoms may seem unrelated, the combination could be important in making a diagnosis. So keep a diary and note all the symptoms you experienced, the time they occurred, the food and drink you had, and the medications you were taking. Do not forget to take the journal with you when you visit the doctor.
- **Finding a knowledgeable physician**. Ask your friends and relatives for recommendations to good physicians

who will be able to make an accurate diagnosis. Discuss your symptoms with health-care professionals at a health agency and community health meetings. Agencies specializing in autoimmune diseases maintain referral lists, which can help you find the right doctor. "Autoimmunology" as a medical specialty does not exist, so it may take some work to identify a physician who will be able to treat your major symptoms under their area of specialization.

- **Getting a comprehensive clinical examination**. To diagnose an autoimmune disease, the health-care provider may conduct an exhaustive medical history, perform a thorough physical examination, and run different medical tests to gather information and analyze the symptoms. During the examination, the patient can ask questions and relate concerns regarding tests, such as cost, alternatives, preparation, discomfort, and insurance options. It is important to understand that test results can be uncertain at times, so additional testing and long-term observation may be required.

- **Seeking a second opinion**. When your physician does not accurately figure out the cause of the symptoms, it might be a good idea to schedule a visit with a different health-care provider. Be sure to take your test results when seeing a second physician. And, if you are referred to a psychologist by a doctor who dismisses your symptoms as stress-related and you feel you are not under undue stress, it would be wise to consult another physician.

- **Consulting a specialist**. If your doctor thinks you may have an autoimmune disease, ask him or her to refer you to a physician specializing in treating your primary symptoms. Although diagnosis may still not be easy or fast, a specialist is the best person to diagnose the disease based on the specific symptoms you are experiencing.

- **Considering other disorders**. There is a chance that you may have more than one autoimmune condition.

>Talk to your doctor about making a fresh diagnosis if the treatment is ineffective. Consult another doctor and, after providing your complete history and test results, request the doctor to investigate other illnesses.

Finally, since the symptoms associated with autoimmune diseases can be varied, unrelated, and inconclusive, it is vital to be aware that diagnosis can be a long and sometimes arduous process. According to a survey by the American Autoimmune Related Disease Association (AARDA), people with autoimmune disorders typically have to wait about four years to find out what is causing their health problems. So patience may be required, but effective diagnosis and treatment can be achieved with proper attention from knowledgeable medical professionals.

References

"Autoimmune Diseases," Boston Children's, March 11, 2015. Available online. URL: www.childrenshospital.org/conditions/autoimmune-diseases. Accessed April 18, 2023.

"Autoimmune Diseases," Cleveland Clinic, July 21, 2021. Available online. URL: https://my.clevelandclinic.org/health/diseases/21624-autoimmune-diseases. Accessed April 18, 2023.

"Do You Know Your Family AQ?" American Autoimmune Related Diseases Association (AARDA), December 31, 2016. Available online. URL: https://autoimmune.org/wp-content/uploads/2016/12/AARDA-Do_you_know_your_family_AQ-DoubleSided.pdf. Accessed April 18, 2023.

Gordon, Sherri. "Top 5 Reasons to Get a Second Opinion," VeryWell Health, March 28, 2020. Available online. URL: www.verywellhealth.com/top-reasons-to-get-a-second-opinion-4144734. Accessed April 18, 2023.

Lawrence, Jean. "Life with an Autoimmune Disease," WebMD, November 10, 2003. Available online.

URL: www.webmd.com/women/features/life-with-autoimmune-disease. Accessed April 18, 2023.

Marshall, Amy Sarah. "The Detective Work of Autoimmune Disease," UVA Health, October 31, 2014. Available online. URL: https://blog.uvahealth.com/2014/10/31/detective-work-autoimmune-disease. Accessed April 18, 2023.

MedlinePlus, "Autoimmune Diseases," National Institutes of Health (NIH), October 15, 2021. Available online. URL: https://medlineplus.gov/autoimmunediseases.html. Accessed April 18, 2023.

Watson, Stephanie. "Autoimmune Diseases: Types, Symptoms, Causes, and More," Healthline, July 15, 2022. Available online. URL: www.healthline.com/health/autoimmune-disorders. Accessed April 18, 2023.

Chapter 54 | **Allergy Tests**

Allergies occur when your immune system overreacts to something in the environment, such as pollen or dust. Allergic reactions may result in the following:

- atopic dermatitis
- blocked sinuses
- cough, more in the nighttime
- expiratory wheeze
- itchy and watery eyes
- runny nose
- sneezing
- urticarial rash

These allergic reactions are caused by allergens, which are substances that tend to cause an allergic reaction. The following are the three primary types of allergens:

- **Contact allergens**. Also known as "contact dermatitis," these allergens cause skin reactions such as itching, redness, swelling, and blistering when a person's skin touches certain substances, such as soaps, jewelry, waxes, detergents, hair dye, or poison ivy.
- **Inhaled allergens**. These allergens cause allergies when they come into contact with the membranes of the nostrils, throat, or lungs. Sneezing is the initial reaction caused when inhaling dust or pollen, sometimes followed by a wheeze.
- **Ingested allergens**. These allergens cause allergies when you consume an allergen such as peanuts or seafood. Vomiting is an example of a reaction caused when you consume any ingested allergen. This will

be associated with itching, urticarial rash, and even wheezing.

Various tests can determine what kind of substance is causing an allergic reaction. The health-care provider will decide on the testing procedure based on your symptoms. The previous medical history is reviewed to see if any previous medical conditions and medications are involved in causing allergic reactions.

SKIN TESTS

Skin tests are used to identify potential allergens that cause the allergy. Skin tests are performed by applying possible allergy triggers on your skin and then observing the body's reactions to these possible triggers. Skin tests are also used to determine allergies caused by food since food allergy testing is complex. The types of skin tests are as follows.

Skin Prick Test

A skin prick test is used to detect immediate allergy reactions by pricking your skin with a lancet and inserting small droplets of allergens in specified locations. This test is frequently used to discover allergies to substances such as pollen or certain foods. If you are allergic to the substance, there will be swelling, redness, or other reactions in the area. It might take 15–20 minutes for any allergic reactions to manifest. The reaction caused in the spot disappears in a few hours.

Intradermal Test

The intradermal test is similar to the skin prick test, except that the allergen solution is injected into the skin rather than pricking it. This test is more sensitive, detecting milder allergic reactions. It can, however, be uncomfortable and may cause more severe allergic reactions. It is usually performed only when a skin prick test is insufficient and does not produce any satisfactory results (allergic reactions).

Skin Scratch Test

The health-care provider performs a skin scratch test if the skin prick test results are unclear. This test involves removing a small layer of your skin and then rubbing the allergen over the exposed flesh. The health-care provider will observe the reactions of your skin. However, the skin scratch test is considered less reliable because it can lead to nonallergic skin irritation.

Patch Test

The patch test does not include needles but does consist of patches filled with allergens. This test is used to identify allergies where symptoms appear half a day to three days after exposure to the allergen. The triggers are usually single substances found in medications, jewelry, cosmetics, gloves, or other latex materials. During the test, a patch with the suspected allergens is applied to the back for a day. If there is no reaction, the skin is checked again after 24 hours and sometimes again after three days. A contact allergy is determined and confirmed if your skin is inflamed or has itching, redness, swelling, or blistering.

Blood Test

The health-care provider may recommend a blood test if the skin test causes a severe allergic reaction. Blood tests are also done if the skin tests are inconclusive.

The health-care provider draws your blood and tests it for the presence of a specific antibody, such as immunoglobulin E (IgE). If you have any allergy, the number of IgE antibodies will be found to be more than the normal value. However, the number of IgE antibodies can also be increased due to smoking or a parasite infestation.

CHALLENGE TESTS

The challenge test, typically performed for potential medication or food allergies, takes place in a medical facility where you will be exposed to small and gradually increasing amounts of a suspected allergen through inhalation or ingestion over several hours. The presence of an allergy can be tested in a similar way on the eyes or lungs. The challenge test is usually done under close medical supervision since this test can cause severe allergic reactions.

Once allergy testing has been done, the health-care provider will determine the type of allergen responsible for the allergy and prescribe medications to ease your symptoms.

References

"Allergy Diagnosis," Asthma and Allergy Foundation of America (AAFA), October 15, 2015. Available online. URL: https://aafa.org/allergies/allergy-diagnosis. Accessed April 19, 2023.

Kerr, Michael. "Ingested vs. Contact vs. Inhaled Allergies," Healthline, February 28, 2018. Available online. URL: www.healthline.com/health/allergies/ingested-contact-inhaled. Accessed April 19, 2023.

Krans, Brian. "Allergy Testing: Types, Risks, and Next Steps," Healthline, December 21, 2021. Available online. URL: www.healthline.com/health/allergy-testing. Accessed April 19, 2023.

More, Daniel. "How Allergies Are Diagnosed," Asthma and Allergy Foundation of America (AAFA), October 14, 2022. Available online. URL: www.verywellhealth.com/diagnosis-of-allergies-82640. Accessed April 19, 2023.

National Center for Biotechnology Information (NCBI), "What Kinds of Allergy Tests Are There?" U.S. National Library of Medicine (NLM), April 23, 2020. Available online. URL: www.ncbi.nlm.nih.gov/books/NBK367583. Accessed April 19, 2023.

"Package Insert—TRUE TEST," U.S. Food and Drug Administration (FDA), August 28, 2017. Available online. URL: www.fda.gov/media/83084/download. Accessed April 19, 2023.

Chapter 55 | **Genetic Testing**

WHAT IS GENETIC TESTING?

Genetic testing is a type of medical test that identifies changes in genes, chromosomes, or proteins. The results of a genetic test can confirm or rule out a suspected genetic condition or help determine a person's chance of developing or passing on a genetic disorder. More than 77,000 genetic tests are currently in use, and others are being developed.

Genetic testing is voluntary. Because testing has benefits as well as limitations and risks, the decision about whether to be tested is a personal and complex one. A geneticist or genetic counselor can help by providing information about the pros and cons of the test and discussing the social and emotional aspects of testing.

WHAT ARE THE DIFFERENT TYPES OF GENETIC TESTS?

A health-care provider will consider several factors when selecting the appropriate test, including what condition or conditions are suspected and the genetic variations typically associated with those conditions. If a diagnosis is unclear, a test that looks at many genes or chromosomes may be used. However, if a specific condition is suspected, a more focused test may be done. The following are a few types of genetic tests:

- **Molecular tests**. They look for changes in one or more genes. These types of tests determine the order of deoxyribonucleic acid (DNA) building blocks (nucleotides) in an individual's genetic code, a process called "DNA sequencing." These tests can vary in scope:

- **Targeted single variant**. Single variant tests look for a specific variant in one gene. The selected variant is known to cause a disorder (e.g., the specific variant in the hemoglobin subunit beta (*HBB*) gene that causes sickle cell disease (SCD)). This type of test is often used to test family members of someone who is known to have a particular variant to determine whether they have a familial condition. Also, direct-to-consumer genetic testing companies typically analyze a number of specific variants in particular genes (rather than finding all the variants in those genes) when providing health or disease risk information.
- **Single gene**. Single gene tests look for any genetic changes in one gene. These tests are typically used to confirm (or rule out) a specific diagnosis, particularly when there are many variants in the gene that can cause the suspected condition.
- **Gene panel**. Panel tests look for variants in more than one gene. This type of test is often used to pinpoint a diagnosis when a person has symptoms that may fit a wide array of conditions or when the suspected condition can be caused by variants in many genes (e.g., there are hundreds of genetic causes of epilepsy).
- **Whole exome sequencing/whole genome sequencing**. These tests analyze the bulk of an individual's DNA to find genetic variations. Whole exome or whole genome sequencing is typically used when single gene or panel testing has not provided a diagnosis or when the suspected condition or genetic cause is unclear. Whole exome or whole genome sequencing is often more cost- and time-effective than performing multiple single gene or panel tests.
- **Chromosomal tests**. It analyzes whole chromosomes or long lengths of DNA to identify large-scale changes. Changes that can be found include an

extra or missing copy of a chromosome (trisomy or monosomy, respectively), a large piece of a chromosome that is added (duplicated) or missing (deleted), or rearrangements (translocations) of segments of chromosomes. Certain genetic conditions are associated with specific chromosomal changes, and a chromosomal test can be used when one of these conditions is suspected (e.g., Williams syndrome is caused by a deletion of a section of chromosome 7).

- **Gene expression tests**. It looks at which genes are turned on or off (expressed) in different types of cells. When a gene is turned on (active), the cell produces a molecule called "messenger ribonucleic acid" (mRNA) from the instructions in the genes, and the mRNA molecule is used as a blueprint to make proteins. Gene expression tests study the mRNA in cells to determine which genes are active. Too much activity (overexpression) or too little activity (underexpression) of certain genes can be suggestive of particular genetic disorders, such as many types of cancer.
- **Biochemical tests**. They do not directly analyze DNA, but they study the amount or activity level of proteins or enzymes that are produced from genes. Abnormalities in these substances can indicate that there are changes in the DNA that underlie a genetic disorder (e.g., low levels of biotinidase enzyme activity are suggestive of biotinidase deficiency, which is caused by biotinidase (*BTD*) gene variants).

WHAT ARE THE USES OF GENETIC TESTING?

Genetic testing can provide information about a person's genetic background. The uses of genetic testing are as follows.

Newborn Screening

Newborn screening is used just after birth to identify genetic disorders that can be treated early in life. Millions of babies are tested each year in the United States. The U.S. Health Services and

Resource Administration recommends that states screen for a set of 35 conditions, which many states exceed.

Diagnostic Testing

Diagnostic testing is used to identify or rule out a specific genetic or chromosomal condition. In many cases, genetic testing is used to confirm a diagnosis when a particular condition is suspected based on physical signs and symptoms. Diagnostic testing can be performed before birth or at any time during a person's life, but it is not available for all genes or all genetic conditions. The results of a diagnostic test can influence a person's choices about health care and the management of the disorder.

Carrier Testing

Carrier testing is used to identify people who carry one copy of a gene mutation that, when present in two copies, causes a genetic disorder. This type of testing is offered to individuals who have a family history of a genetic disorder and to people in certain ethnic groups with an increased risk of specific genetic conditions. If both parents are tested, the test can provide information about a couple's risk of having a child with a genetic condition.

Prenatal Testing

Prenatal testing is used to detect changes in a fetus's genes or chromosomes before birth. This type of testing is offered during pregnancy if there is an increased risk that the baby will have a genetic or chromosomal disorder. In some cases, prenatal testing can lessen a couple's uncertainty or help them make decisions about a pregnancy. It cannot identify all possible inherited disorders and birth defects, however.

Preimplantation Testing

Preimplantation testing, also called "preimplantation genetic diagnosis" (PGD), is a specialized technique that can reduce the risk of having a child with a particular genetic or chromosomal disorder.

It is used to detect genetic changes in embryos that were created using assisted reproductive techniques (ARTs) such as in vitro fertilization (IVF). IVF involves removing egg cells from a woman's ovaries and fertilizing them with sperm cells outside the body. To perform preimplantation testing, a small number of cells are taken from these embryos and tested for certain genetic changes. Only embryos without these changes are implanted in the uterus to initiate a pregnancy.

Predictive and Presymptomatic Testing

Predictive and presymptomatic types of testing are used to detect gene mutations associated with disorders that appear after birth, often later in life. These tests can be helpful to people who have a family member with a genetic disorder but who have no features of the disorder themselves at the time of testing. Predictive testing can identify mutations that increase a person's risk of developing disorders with a genetic basis, such as certain types of cancer. Presymptomatic testing can determine whether a person will develop a genetic disorder, such as hereditary hemochromatosis (an iron overload disorder), before any signs or symptoms appear. The results of predictive and presymptomatic testing can provide information about a person's risk of developing a specific disorder and help with making decisions about medical care.

Forensic Testing

Forensic testing uses DNA sequences to identify an individual for legal purposes. Unlike the tests described above, forensic testing is not used to detect gene mutations associated with the disease. This type of testing can identify crime or catastrophe victims, rule out or implicate a crime suspect, or establish biological relationships between people (e.g., paternity).

HOW IS GENETIC TESTING DONE?

Once a person decides to proceed with genetic testing, a health-care provider can arrange testing. Genetic testing is often done as part of a genetic consultation. Genetic tests are performed on a sample of blood, hair, skin, amniotic fluid (the fluid that surrounds a fetus during pregnancy), or other tissue. For example, a procedure called a "buccal smear" uses a small brush or cotton swab to collect a sample of cells from the inside surface of the cheek. The sample is sent to a laboratory where technicians look for specific changes in chromosomes, DNA, or proteins, depending on the suspected disorder. The laboratory reports the test results in writing to a person's doctor or genetic counselor or directly to the patient if requested.

Newborn screening tests are done on a small blood sample, which is taken by pricking the baby's heel. Unlike other types of genetic testing, a parent will usually only receive the result if it is positive. If the test result is positive, additional testing is needed to determine whether the baby has a genetic disorder.

Before a person has a genetic test, it is important to understand the testing procedure, the benefits and limitations of the test, and the possible consequences of the test results. The process of educating a person about the test and obtaining permission is called "informed consent."

Individuals interested in direct-to-consumer genetic testing do not need to go through a health-care provider to obtain a test, but they can get it directly from the testing company. After undergoing direct-to-consumer genetic testing, people who test positive for a condition or are found to be at higher risk of developing a disorder are encouraged to follow up with a genetic counselor or other health-care provider.

WHAT IS INFORMED CONSENT?

"Informed" means that the person has enough information to make an educated decision about testing; "consent" refers to a person's voluntary agreement to have the test done.

In general, informed consent can only be given by adults who are competent to make medical decisions for themselves. For children and others who are unable to make their own medical decisions (such as people with impaired mental status), informed consent can be given by a parent, guardian, or other person legally responsible for making decisions on that person's behalf.

Genetic Testing

Informed consent for genetic testing is generally obtained by a doctor or genetic counselor during an office visit. The health-care provider will discuss the test and answer any questions. If the person wishes to have the test, he or she will then usually read and sign a consent form.

The following are a few items commonly included in an informed consent form:

- a general description of the test, including the purpose of the test and the condition for which the testing is being performed
- how the test will be carried out (e.g., a blood sample)
- what the test results mean, including positive and negative results, and the potential for uninformative results or incorrect results such as false positives or false negatives
- any physical or emotional risks associated with the test
- whether the results can be used for research purposes
- whether the results might provide information about other family members' health, including the risk of developing a particular condition or the possibility of having affected children
- how and to whom test results will be reported and under what circumstances results can be disclosed (e.g., to health insurance providers)
- status of the test specimen after the test is complete
- acknowledgment that the person undergoing testing has had the opportunity to discuss the test with a health-care provider
- the individual's signature and possibly that of a witness

The elements of informed consent may vary because some states have laws that specify factors that must be included (e.g., some states require disclosure that the test specimen will be destroyed within a certain period of time after the test is complete).

Informed consent is not a contract, so a person can change their mind at any time after giving initial consent. A person may choose not to go through with genetic testing even after the test sample has been collected. A person simply needs to notify the health-care provider if the decision has been made not to continue with the testing process.

HOW CAN YOU BE SURE A GENETIC TEST IS VALID AND USEFUL?

Before undergoing genetic testing, it is important to be sure that the test is valid and useful. A genetic test is valid if it provides an accurate result. Two main measures of accuracy apply to genetic tests: analytical validity and clinical validity. Another measure of the quality of a genetic test is its usefulness or clinical utility.

- **Analytical validity**. It refers to how well the test predicts the presence or absence of a particular gene or genetic change. In other words, can the test accurately detect whether a specific genetic variant is present or absent?
- **Clinical validity**. It refers to how well the genetic variant being analyzed is related to the presence, absence, or risk of a specific disease.
- **Clinical utility**. It refers to whether the test can provide helpful information about the diagnosis, treatment, management, or prevention of a disease.

All laboratories that perform health-related testing for disease prevention, diagnosis, or treatment, including genetic testing, are subject to federal regulatory standards called the "Clinical Laboratory Improvement Amendments" (CLIA) or even stricter state requirements. CLIA standards cover how tests are performed, the qualifications of laboratory personnel, and quality control and testing procedures for each laboratory. By controlling the quality of laboratory practices, CLIA standards are designed to ensure the analytical validity of genetic tests.

CLIA standards do not address the clinical validity or clinical utility of genetic tests. The Food and Drug Administration (FDA) requires information about the clinical validity of some genetic tests, particularly those tests that can influence a person's medical care. Additionally, states may require additional information on clinical validity for laboratory tests performed on people living in that state. Test takers, health-care providers, and health insurance companies are often the ones who determine the clinical utility of a genetic test.

It can be difficult to determine the quality of genetic tests sold directly to the public. Some providers of direct-to-consumer genetic tests are not CLIA-certified, and many direct-to-consumer genetic tests are not regulated by the FDA, so it can be difficult to tell whether the tests are valid. If providers of direct-to-consumer genetic tests offer easy-to-understand information about the scientific basis of their tests, it can help people make more informed decisions. It may also be helpful to discuss any concerns with a health-care provider before ordering a direct-to-consumer genetic test and after receiving the test results.

WHAT DO THE RESULTS OF GENETIC TESTS MEAN?

The results of genetic tests are not always straightforward, which often makes them challenging to interpret and explain. Therefore, it is important for patients and their families to ask questions about the potential meaning of genetic test results both before and after the test is performed. When interpreting test results, health-care providers consider a person's medical history, family history, and the type of genetic test that was done.

A positive test result means that the laboratory found a change in a particular gene, chromosome, or protein of interest. Depending on the purpose of the test, this result may confirm a diagnosis, indicate that a person is a carrier of a particular genetic variant, identify an increased risk of developing a disease (such as cancer), or suggest a need for further testing. Because family members have some genetic material in common, a positive test result may also have implications for certain blood relatives of the person undergoing testing. It is important to note that a positive result of a predictive or presymptomatic genetic test usually cannot establish the exact risk of developing a disorder. Also, health-care providers typically cannot use a positive test result to predict the course or severity of a condition. Rarely tests results can be false positive, which occurs when results indicate an increased risk for a genetic condition when the person is unaffected.

A negative test result means that the laboratory did not find a change that is known to affect health or development in the gene, chromosome, or protein under consideration. This result can indicate that a person is not affected by a particular disorder, is not a carrier of a specific genetic variant, or does not have an increased risk of developing a certain disease. It is possible, however, that the test missed a disease-causing genetic alteration because many tests cannot detect all genetic changes that can cause a particular disorder. Further testing, or retesting at a later date, may be required to confirm a negative result. Rarely tests results can be false negative, which occurs when the results indicate a decreased risk of a genetic condition when the person is actually affected.

In some cases, a test result might not give any useful information. This type of result is called "uninformative," "indeterminate," "inconclusive," or "ambiguous." Uninformative test results sometimes occur because everyone has common, natural variations in their DNA, called "polymorphisms," that do not affect health. If a genetic test finds a change in DNA that has not been confirmed to play a role in the development of a disease, known as a "variant of uncertain significance" (VUS or VOUS), it can be difficult to tell whether it is a natural polymorphism or a disease-causing variant. For these variants, there may not be enough scientific research to confirm or refute a disease association, or the research may be conflicting. An uninformative result cannot confirm or rule out a specific diagnosis, and it cannot indicate whether a person has an increased risk of developing a disorder. In some cases, testing other affected and unaffected family members can help clarify this type of result.

WHAT IS THE COST OF GENETIC TESTING, AND HOW LONG DOES IT TAKE TO GET THE RESULTS?

The cost of genetic testing can range from under $100 to more than $2,000, depending on the nature and complexity of the test. The cost increases if more than one test is necessary or if multiple family members must be tested to obtain a meaningful result. For newborn screening, costs vary by state. Some states cover part of the total cost, but most charge a fee of $30–$150 per infant.

From the date that a sample is taken, it may take a few days to weeks to receive the test results. Results from prenatal testing are usually available more quickly because time is an important consideration in making decisions about a pregnancy. The doctor or genetic counselor who orders a particular test can provide specific information about the cost and time frame associated with that test.

WILL HEALTH INSURANCE COVER THE COSTS OF GENETIC TESTING?

In many cases, health insurance plans will cover the costs of genetic testing when it is recommended by a person's doctor. Health insurance providers have different policies about which tests are covered, however. A person may wish to contact their insurance company before testing to ask about coverage.

Some people may choose not to use their insurance to pay for testing. Instead, they may opt to pay out-of-pocket for the test or pursue direct-to-consumer genetic testing if available. People considering genetic testing may want to find out more about their state's privacy protection laws before they ask their insurance company to cover the costs.

WHAT ARE THE BENEFITS OF GENETIC TESTING?

Genetic testing has potential benefits, whether the results are positive or negative for a gene mutation. Test results can provide a sense of relief from uncertainty and help people make informed decisions about managing their health care. For example, a negative result can eliminate the need for unnecessary checkups and screening tests in some cases. A positive result can direct a person toward available prevention, monitoring, and treatment options. Some test results can also help people make decisions about having children. Newborn screening can identify genetic disorders early in life so treatment can be started as early as possible.

WHAT ARE THE RISKS AND LIMITATIONS OF GENETIC TESTING?

The physical risks associated with most genetic tests are very small, particularly for those tests that require only a blood sample or buccal smear (a method that samples cells from the inside surface of the cheek). The procedures used for prenatal diagnostic testing (called "amniocentesis" and "chorionic villus sampling") carry a small but real risk of losing the pregnancy (miscarriage) because they require a sample of amniotic fluid or tissue from around the fetus.

Many of the risks associated with genetic testing involve the emotional, social, or financial consequences of the test results. People may feel angry, depressed, anxious, or guilty about their results. In some cases, genetic testing creates tension within a family because the results can reveal information about other family members in addition to the person who is tested. The possibility of genetic discrimination in employment or insurance is also a concern.

Genetic testing can provide only limited information about an inherited condition. The test often cannot determine if a person will show symptoms of a disorder, how severe the symptoms will be, or whether the disorder will progress over time. Another major limitation is the lack of treatment strategies for many genetic disorders once they are diagnosed.

A genetics professional can explain in detail the benefits, risks, and limitations of a particular test. It is important that any person who is considering genetic testing understand and weigh these factors before making a decision.

WHAT IS GENETIC DISCRIMINATION?

Genetic discrimination occurs when people are treated differently by their employer or insurance company because they have a gene mutation that causes or increases the risk of an inherited disorder. Fear of discrimination is a common concern among people considering genetic testing.

Several laws at the federal and state levels help protect people against genetic discrimination. In particular, a federal law called the "Genetic Information Nondiscrimination Act" (GINA) is designed to protect people from this form of discrimination.

GINA has two parts: Title I, which prohibits genetic discrimination in health insurance, and Title II, which prohibits genetic discrimination in employment. Title I makes it illegal for health insurance providers to use or require genetic information to make decisions about a person's insurance eligibility or coverage. This part of the law went into effect on May 21, 2009. Title II makes it illegal for employers to use a person's genetic information when making decisions about hiring, promotion, and several other terms of employment. This part of the law went into effect on November 21, 2009.

GINA and other laws do not protect people from genetic discrimination in every circumstance. For example, GINA does not apply when an employer has fewer than 15 employees. GINA also does not protect against genetic discrimination in forms of insurance other than health insurance, such as life, disability, or long-term care insurance.

HOW ARE GENETIC SCREENING TESTS DIFFERENT FROM GENETIC DIAGNOSTIC TESTS?

Screening tests evaluate an individual's risk of developing a genetic condition, while diagnostic tests identify genetic conditions. All genetic tests have both benefits and limitations.

Genetic screening tests are generally used in people who do not have signs or symptoms of a disorder. These tests estimate whether an individual's risk of having a certain condition is increased or decreased compared with the risk in other people in a similar population. A positive result means that a person's risk of developing the condition is higher than average. A negative screening test means that a person's risk is lower than average. However, having a positive screening result does not mean the individual has the condition. Because screening tests are only estimates, in some cases, the results indicate an increased risk for a genetic abnormality when the person is actually unaffected (false positive), or the results indicate a decreased risk for a genetic abnormality when the person is really affected (false negative). While genetic screening tests do not provide a conclusive answer, they can help guide the next steps, such as whether additional diagnostic testing is needed.

Genetic diagnostic tests are often used in people who have signs and symptoms. These tests are used to confirm or rule out suspected genetic conditions.

Diagnostic tests can also help inform a person's chance of developing a genetic condition or of passing on a genetic condition to their children. Diagnostic testing can be performed before birth or at any time during a person's life, but it is not available for all genes or all genetic conditions. The results of a diagnostic test can be used to guide a person's choices about health care and the management of the disorder. Examples of genetic screening tests are as follows:

- **Noninvasive prenatal testing/screening (NIPT/ NIPS)**. This screening test is performed before birth to help determine the risk that a fetus will be born with certain genetic abnormalities, such as Down syndrome and other chromosomal disorders.

- **Newborn screening**. In the United States, a screening test is performed on all newborns shortly after birth. This test can assess the risk of developing more than 35 genetic conditions. For many of these conditions, the test analyzes various protein and enzyme levels, which would be abnormal in affected individuals.

Examples of genetic diagnostic tests are as follows:

- **Molecular gene tests**. These tests determine the order of DNA building blocks (nucleotides) in an individual's genetic code, a process called "DNA sequencing." The purpose of these tests is to identify genetic changes that can cause disease.

- **Chromosomal tests**. These tests analyze whole chromosomes or long lengths of DNA to identify large-scale changes, such as an extra or missing copy of a chromosome (trisomy or monosomy, respectively) or abnormalities of large segments of chromosomes that underlie certain genetic conditions.[1]

---

[1] MedlinePlus, "What Is Genetic Testing?" National Institutes of Health (NIH), July 28, 2021. Available online. URL: https://medlineplus.gov/genetics/understanding/testing/genetictesting. Accessed May 12, 2023.

Chapter 56 | Immune Assessment Tests

Chapter Contents

Section 56.1 | Basic Tests to Evaluate Immune Status

The immune system recognizes and destroys antigens, which can be present on the surface of cells, bacteria, fungi, viruses, toxins, and foreign substances to defend the body. The health-care provider analyzes various symptoms of these illnesses and the patient's medical and family history to determine which lab tests are most appropriate for assessing immune system function. The following are some of the blood tests commonly used to diagnose underlying health conditions and initiate or monitor treatment.

COMPLETE BLOOD COUNT

A physician orders a complete blood count (CBC) to assess a patient's immune system function and overall health. This test checks the quantity and quality of three major components of blood: the red blood cells (RBCs), the white blood cells (WBCs), and the plasma. If the numbers of any of these components fall outside the healthy range, the person may require further medical assessment.

A doctor generally orders a CBC test when the patient exhibits symptoms such as inflammation, bleeding, bruising, fatigue, or weakness. The test can help detect a number of conditions, such as vitamin or mineral deficiencies, infections, bone marrow disorders, anemia, and leukemia, and can also monitor a medical condition after its diagnosis. It may also be used to ensure the effectiveness of treatment for a blood-related disorder or monitor treatment that can affect blood cell counts, such as chemotherapy or radiation therapy.

CBC test results include the following:

- **Red blood cell, hemoglobin, and hematocrit count**. These can indicate anemia, nutritional deficiency, or chronic kidney disease if the RBC level is below normal or conditions such as polycythemia vera (PCV), lung disease, or dehydration if the level is above normal.
- **White blood cell count**. If low, this can reveal issues such as autoimmune disorders, sepsis, dietary

deficiencies, or cancer, and if high, it can indicate conditions such as infection, inflammation, allergies, or asthma. If the WBC count is either high or low, it can be a sign of bone marrow disease or a reaction to certain medications.

- **Platelet count.** A low platelet count (thrombocytopenia) may indicate that you have certain health problems, such as a viral infection, liver disease, or a reaction to chemotherapy or radiation therapy. In contrast, a high platelet count (thrombocytosis) may indicate that you have other health issues, such as a shortage of RBCs, rheumatoid arthritis (RA), inflammatory bowel disease (IBD), or cancer.

A CBC is not considered a definitive test by itself but is typically ordered along with other diagnostic tests. Sometimes, depending on the CBC report, the doctor may order additional tests as a follow-up. A number of conditions can affect the CBC count, including factors such as the age of the patient or a recent blood transfusion.

IMMUNOGLOBULIN TEST

This test provides a measurement of immunoglobulins (antibodies) in the blood serum. Immunoglobulins are produced in plasma cells in response to foreign particles, such as bacteria, fungi, viruses, cancer cells, or animal dander. There are five major types: immunoglobulin A (IgA) antibodies, which protect body surfaces exposed to foreign particles; immunoglobulin G (IgG) antibodies, found in all body fluids to fight bacterial and viral infections; immunoglobulin M (IgM) antibodies, which are produced first in response to an infection and are found in lymph fluid and blood; immunoglobulin E (IgE) antibodies, are found in the lungs, skin, and mucous membranes, and are responsible for allergic reactions; and immunoglobulin D (IgD) antibodies, found in small amounts in the tissues that line the stomach or chest.

The test helps identify the presence of immunoglobulins in the blood, which, if detected, implies that the body is reacting to some foreign invader. Each of its types is produced to fight a specific condition, so identifying these immunoglobulins helps detect underlying disorders, such as infection, autoimmune diseases, allergies, and certain types of cancer. Test results can also be used to monitor treatment for *Helicobacter pylori* (*H. pylori*) bacteria or certain cancers that affect the bone marrow or to check the body's response to immunizations.

Some of the conditions that are detected through an immunoglobulin test are as follows:

- **Immunoglobulin A.** If low, it may indicate kidney injury (nephrotic syndrome), enteropathy, leukemia, or ataxia-telangiectasia. High levels may be a sign of monoclonal gammopathy of unknown significance (MGUS), multiple myeloma, autoimmune diseases, or liver diseases.

- **Immunoglobulin G.** Low IgG could be an indication of conditions such as macroglobulinemia, certain types of leukemia, or kidney damage (nephrotic syndrome), while a high reading might be a warning of chronic infections, such as human immunodeficiency virus (HIV) and hepatitis, as well as multiple myeloma or multiple sclerosis (MS).

- **Immunoglobulin M.** Some types of leukemia, multiple myeloma, or certain inherited types of immune diseases may cause low levels of IgM, and high results could indicate macroglobulinemia, parasite infection, mononucleosis, early viral hepatitis, RA, or nephrotic syndrome.

- **Immunoglobulin D.** High IgD levels may indicate multiple myeloma although this is much less common than IgA or IgG multiple myeloma.

- **Immunoglobulin E.** A low IgE reading could be a warning sign of ataxia-telangiectasia (a rare inherited disease that affects muscle coordination), while high levels might indicate allergic reactions, asthma, parasitic infection, atopic dermatitis (AD), certain autoimmune diseases, some types of cancer, or, in rare cases, multiple myeloma.

There are various factors that can change the outcome of an immunoglobulin test, so it is crucial for the health-care provider who orders the test to know about these factors:

- blood transfusions, if any, in the past six months
- vaccinations in the past six months, particularly those with booster doses
- drugs such as those used for heart failure, RA, seizures, or birth control
- radiation and chemotherapy for cancer
- radioactive scan, if any, in the past three days
- the use of alcohol or illegal drugs

COMPLEMENT TEST

A complement test is done to analyze the activity of a group of blood serum proteins in the immune system. This group of nine major proteins (labeled C1–C9) forms the complement system and helps antibodies fight against foreign microorganisms. Autoimmune disorders, too, will sometimes activate the antibodies, and in such cases, they will fight against the body's own tissues, which it considers to be foreign invaders.

When a patient shows symptoms of conditions such as cryoglobulinemia, RA, lupus, kidney disease, myasthenia gravis (MG), or an infectious disease such as meningitis, the doctor may order a total complement measurement or one or all of the more targeted tests (C1, C3, and C4). The doctor can then assess the underlying condition's progression by examining the test results for the activity of specific complement proteins and, additionally, monitor the effectiveness of its treatment. A total complement test may also be used to detect some infectious diseases and cancers or may be ordered when a patient has a family history of complement deficiency.

A complement test shows low activity for health conditions that include autoimmune disorders, such as lupus, or a flare-up of an autoimmune disease, cirrhosis, hepatitis, glomerulonephritis (kidney disease), or hereditary angioedema (rapid swelling that affects the face, limbs, or some internal organs). Low complement activity can also be a sign of malnutrition, an underlying infection, or rejection of a transplanted kidney. Disorders identified through a higher-than-normal measure of complement activity include thyroiditis, sarcoidosis, myocardial infarction, juvenile rheumatoid arthritis (JRA), cancer, or ulcerative colitis.

Typically, a lack of early complement proteins (C1–C4) makes the individual more susceptible to infections, particularly those caused by fungi, and some parasitic infections, such as malaria, identified when C3 levels are low. Insufficient late complement proteins (C5–C9), on the other hand, may make the person more prone to infections caused by *Neisseria* bacteria, a group that includes the bacteria that cause meningitis and gonorrhea. A complement test does not indicate precisely what condition the patient has; it only indicates that the immune system is involved and narrows down the possible causes. The health-care provider will need to order additional diagnostic tests to determine the underlying disorder.

LYMPHOCYTE TRANSFORMATION TEST

The lymphocyte transformation test (LTT) is performed to assess the function of lymphocytes taken from blood. Lymphocytes are important for fighting infections and diseases. There are two types, B cells and T cells, which work together to protect the body. They recognize and remove harmful invaders such as bacteria and viruses. Lymphocytes are crucial for keeping the body healthy and preventing illnesses. B cells do this by producing antibodies, which attack invasive antigens (foreign substances), while T cells can work in various ways, such as killing invaders directly, sending chemical messages to parts of the immune system, or helping B cells produce antibodies.

When a B lymphocyte makes contact with certain types of antigens, it initiates cell division that forms plasma cells, which then secrete antibodies that bind to specific antigens and label them for destruction, as well as memory cells that recognize the antigen when it is exposed to it again. The LTT uses this principle of antigen-specific initiation of cell division to its advantage. A positive reaction to the test will indicate the presence of antigen-specific memory cells. Based on this, the doctor will then perform further tests to identify and diagnose the underlying condition.

A physician orders an LTT when a patient exhibits symptoms of immune deficiency, such as poor resistance to infections, delay in time taken to recover after an infection, or problems with wound healing. The LTT is primarily used to detect immunodeficiency, pathogens (such as *Chlamydia, Borrelia,* and herpes viruses), and type IV allergy (allergic sensitization to medication, molds, environmental pollutants, or certain foods).

Some other conditions an LTT may help identify are as follows:
- repeated infections in the upper respiratory tract
- bacterial infections
- infections such as those caused by an intestinal virus or *Candida*
- immune deficiency due to protein, vitamin, iron, or zinc deficiency
- immune deficiency as a complication of chronic inflammatory disease

LTT is also performed to assess a person's immunity before and after cancer treatment (surgical, radiation, or chemotherapy) and antiviral treatment for conditions such as HIV infection.

References

ADAM, "Immune Response," MedlinePlus, January 23, 2022. Available online. URL: https://medlineplus.gov/ency/article/000821.htm. Accessed April 21, 2023.

"CBC Blood Test (Complete Blood Count)," OneCare Media, September 28, 2022. Available online. URL: www.testing.com/tests/complete-blood-count-cbc. Accessed April 21, 2023.

"Complement," American Association for Clinical Chemistry (AACC), November 9, 2021. Available online. URL: www.testing.com/tests/complement. Accessed April 21, 2023.

"Complete Blood Count (CBC)," Mayo Foundation for Medical Education and Research (MFMER), January 14, 2023. Available online. URL: www.mayoclinic.org/tests-procedures/complete-blood-count/about/pac-20384919. Accessed April 21, 2023.

"Immune System," BiologyGuide, December 30, 2021. Available online. URL: https://biologyguide.app/notes/immune-system. Accessed April 21, 2023.

"LTT Immune Function Test," Synevo Laboratories, July 11, 2016. Available online. URL: https://synevo.com.tr/en/LTT-Immune-Function-Test. Accessed April 21, 2023.

MacGill, Markus and Rowden, Adam. "What Are the Causes of a Low Platelet Count," Medical News Today, January 12, 2023. Available online. URL: www.medicalnewstoday.com/articles/314123. Accessed April 21, 2023.

Pietrangelo, Ann. "Complement Test," Healthline, May 14, 2018. Available online. URL: www.healthline.com/health/complement. Accessed April 21, 2023.

"What Are the Best Lab Tests for Immune System Function and What They Indicate," Bright Hub, July 13, 2010. Available online. URL: www.brighthub.com/science/medical/articles/77409. Accessed April 21, 2023.

"What Is an Immunoglobulin Test?" WebMD, August 19, 2021. Available online. URL: www.webmd.com/a-to-z-guides/immunoglobulin-test. Accessed April 21, 2023.

Section 56.2 | Antinuclear Antibody Test

WHAT IS AN ANTINUCLEAR ANTIBODY TEST?

An antinuclear antibody (ANA) test is a blood test that looks for antinuclear antibodies in your blood. Antibodies are proteins that your immune system makes to fight foreign substances, such as viruses and bacteria. But an ANA attacks your own healthy cells instead. It is called "antinuclear" because it targets the nucleus (center) of the cells.

It is normal to have a few antinuclear antibodies in your blood. But a large number may be a sign of an autoimmune disorder. If you have an autoimmune disorder, your immune system attacks the cells of your organs and tissues by mistake. These disorders can cause serious health problems. Other names are as follows:

- antinuclear antibody panel
- fluorescent antinuclear antibody
- FANA
- ANA
- ANA reflexive panel

WHAT IS AN ANTINUCLEAR ANTIBODY TEST USED FOR?

An ANA test is used to help diagnose autoimmune disorders such as:

- **Systemic lupus erythematosus (SLE).** SLE is the most common type of lupus, which is a chronic (long-lasting) disease that affects many parts of the body, including the joints, skin, heart, lungs, blood vessels, kidneys, and brain.
- **Rheumatoid arthritis (RA).** RA is a condition that mostly affects joints, causing pain and swelling often in the wrists, hands, and feet.
- **Scleroderma.** This is a rare disease that may affect the skin, blood vessels, and organs.
- **Sjögren syndrome.** This rare disease affects the glands that make tears and saliva (spit) and other parts of the body.
- **Addison disease.** This disease affects your adrenal glands, causing fatigue and weakness.
- **Autoimmune hepatitis.** This disease causes swelling in your liver.

WHY DO YOU NEED AN ANTINUCLEAR ANTIBODY TEST?

Your health-care provider may order an ANA test if you have symptoms of an autoimmune disorder. The symptoms depend on the part of the body that is affected. They may include:

- fever
- rash, blisters, or skin color changes
- fatigue
- joint pain, stiffness, and swelling
- muscle pain

WHAT HAPPENS DURING AN ANTINUCLEAR ANTIBODY TEST?

A health-care professional will take a blood sample from a vein in your arm using a small needle. After the needle is inserted, a small amount of blood will be collected into a test tube or vial. You may feel a little sting when the needle goes in or out. This usually takes less than five minutes.

ARE THERE ANY RISKS IN THE ANTINUCLEAR ANTIBODY TEST?

There is very little risk in having a blood test. You may have slight pain or bruising at the spot where the needle was put in, but most symptoms go away quickly.

WHAT DO THE ANTINUCLEAR ANTIBODY TEST RESULTS MEAN?

Results from an ANA test alone cannot diagnose a specific disease. Your provider will use your ANA test results, along with other tests and information about your health, to make a diagnosis.

- **A negative result on an ANA test**. It means that antinuclear antibodies were not found in your blood, and you are less likely to have an autoimmune disorder. But a negative ANA test does not completely rule out the possibility that you could have an autoimmune disorder.
- **A positive result on an ANA test**. It means that antinuclear antibodies were found in your blood. A positive result may be a sign of:
  - SLE
  - a different type of autoimmune disease
  - a viral infection (antinuclear antibodies from a virus are usually temporary)
  - another health condition that can cause antinuclear antibodies, such as cancer

If your ANA test results are positive, your provider will likely order more tests to make a diagnosis.[1]

---

[1] MedlinePlus, "ANA (Antinuclear Antibody) Test," National Institutes of Health (NIH), August 3, 2022. Available online. URL: https://medlineplus.gov/lab-tests/ana-antinuclear-antibody-test. Accessed May 29, 2023.

Section 56.3 | Rheumatoid Factor Test

WHAT IS A RHEUMATOID FACTOR TEST?

A rheumatoid factor (RF) test looks for RF in a sample of your blood. RFs are proteins made by the immune system. Normally, your immune system makes proteins called "antibodies" to attack germs that could make you sick. But RFs are antibodies that sometimes attack healthy cells and tissues in your body by mistake. When this happens, you have an autoimmune disorder.

Not everyone has RFs in their blood. And some people who have them are healthy. But, if you have certain symptoms and higher levels of RFs, you may have an autoimmune disorder or another health problem related to high RF levels.

RF testing is mostly used with other tests to help diagnose rheumatoid arthritis (RA). RA is a type of autoimmune disorder that damages your joints and causes pain, swelling, and stiffness. It is a chronic (long-lasting) condition that can also affect your organs and cause other symptoms. High levels of RFs may also be a sign of other autoimmune disorders, certain infections, and certain types of cancer.

Another name is RF factor blood test.

WHAT IS A RHEUMATOID FACTOR TEST USED FOR?

An RF test is often used to help diagnose RA and other autoimmune disorders. RF testing may also be used to understand how severe RA may be and whether it is likely to affect organs. An RF test alone cannot diagnose any health problems.

WHY DO YOU NEED A RHEUMATOID FACTOR TEST?

You may need an RF test if you have symptoms of RA. Symptoms often begin in the wrists, hands, and feet. They usually affect the same joints on both sides of the body and tend to come and go. Symptoms of RA may include:
- joint pain
- tenderness, swelling, and warmth of the joint

- joint stiffness that lasts longer than 30 minutes
- fatigue
- occasional low fevers
- loss of appetite
- problems outside of the joints that may include dry eyes or mouth, firm lumps under the skin, or anemia

You may also need an RF test if you are having tests to diagnose another condition that can cause high levels of RF, such as:

- other autoimmune disorders, including:
  - Sjögren syndrome
  - lupus
  - scleroderma
  - juvenile idiopathic arthritis (JIA) in children and teens
- chronic infections, including:
  - hepatitis C (liver)
  - tuberculosis (TB, which mostly affects the lungs)
  - endocarditis (heart)
- certain types of cancer, including leukemia

WHAT HAPPENS DURING A RHEUMATOID FACTOR TEST?

A health-care professional will take a blood sample from a vein in your arm using a small needle. After the needle is inserted, a small amount of blood will be collected into a test tube or vial. You may feel a little sting when the needle goes in or out. This usually takes less than five minutes.

At-home tests for RF are available. The test kit provides everything you need to collect a sample of blood by pricking your finger. You will mail your sample to a lab for testing. If you do a home test, it is important to share your results with your health-care provider.

ARE THERE ANY RISKS IN THE RHEUMATOID FACTOR TEST?

There is very little risk in having a blood test. You may have slight pain or bruising at the spot where the needle was put in, but most symptoms go away quickly.

WHAT DO THE RHEUMATOID FACTOR TEST RESULTS MEAN?

An RF test alone cannot diagnose any conditions. To make a diagnosis, your provider will look at the results of other tests along with your symptoms and medical history:

- **A negative (normal) result**. It means that you have little or no RF in your blood. But that does not rule out RA or another health problem. Many people with RA have little or no RF. If you have symptoms of RA, but your RF test results are normal, your provider may order more tests to make a diagnosis.

- **A positive (abnormal) result**. It means that a higher level of RF was found in your blood. This does not always mean that RFs are causing your symptoms. But the higher your RF test results, the more likely it is that you have a condition linked to RFs. Your provider may do more tests to find out if you have:
  - RA or another autoimmune disease
  - chronic infection
  - certain cancers[2]

[2] MedlinePlus, "Rheumatoid Factor (RF) Test," National Institutes of Health (NIH), September 28, 2022. Available online. URL: https://medlineplus.gov/lab-tests/rheumatoid-factor-rf-test. Accessed May 29, 2023.

Chapter 57 | Inflammatory Markers

Chapter Contents

Section 57.1 | C-Reactive Protein

WHAT IS A C-REACTIVE PROTEIN TEST?

A c-reactive protein (CRP) test measures the level of CRP in a sample of your blood. CRP is a protein that your liver makes. Normally, you have low levels of CRP in your blood. Your liver releases more CRP into your bloodstream if you have inflammation in your body. High levels of CRP may mean you have a serious health condition that causes inflammation.

Inflammation is your body's way of protecting your tissues and helping them heal from an injury, infection, or other disease. Inflammation can be acute (sudden) and temporary. This type of inflammation is usually helpful. For example, if you cut your skin, it may turn red, swell, and hurt for a few days. Those are signs of inflammation. Inflammation can also happen inside your body.

If inflammation lasts too long, it can damage healthy tissues. This is called "chronic (long-term) inflammation." Chronic infections, certain autoimmune disorders, and other diseases can cause harmful chronic inflammation. Chronic inflammation can also happen if your tissues are repeatedly injured or irritated, for example, from smoking or chemicals in the environment. A CRP test can show whether you have inflammation in your body and how much. But the test cannot show what's causing the inflammation or which part of your body is inflamed. Other names are as follows:

- c-reactive protein
- serum

WHAT IS IT USED FOR?

A CRP test may be used to help find or monitor inflammation in acute or chronic conditions, including:

- infections from bacteria or viruses
- inflammatory bowel disease (IBD), disorders of the intestines that include Crohn's disease and ulcerative colitis
- autoimmune disorders, such as lupus, rheumatoid arthritis (RA), and vasculitis
- lung diseases, such as asthma

583

Your health-care provider may use a CRP test to see if treatments for chronic inflammation are working or to make treatment decisions if you have sepsis. Sepsis is your body's extreme response to an infection that spreads to your blood. It is a life-threatening medical emergency.

WHY DO YOU NEED A C-REACTIVE PROTEIN TEST?
You may need this test if you have symptoms of a bacterial infection, such as:
- fever or chills
- rapid heart rate
- rapid breathing
- nausea and vomiting

You may also need a CRP test if your provider thinks you may have a chronic condition that causes inflammation. The symptoms will depend on the condition.

If you have already been diagnosed with an infection or a chronic disease that causes inflammation, you may need this test to monitor your condition and treatment. CRP levels rise and fall depending on how much inflammation is in your body. If your CRP levels fall, it is a sign that your treatment for inflammation is working or you are healing on your own.

WHAT HAPPENS DURING A C-REACTIVE PROTEIN TEST?
A health-care professional will take a blood sample from a vein in your arm using a small needle. After the needle is inserted, a small amount of blood will be collected into a test tube or vial. You may feel a little sting when the needle goes in or out. This process usually takes less than five minutes.

WILL YOU NEED TO DO ANYTHING TO PREPARE FOR THE TEST?
Some medicines may affect your results. So tell your provider about any supplements or medicines that you take, including ibuprofen, aspirin, and other nonsteroidal anti-inflammatory drugs (NSAIDs). Do not stop taking any prescription medicines without talking with your provider first.

ARE THERE ANY RISKS IN THE TEST?

There is very little risk in having a blood test. You may have slight pain or bruising at the spot where the needle was put in, but most symptoms go away quickly.

WHAT DO THE RESULTS MEAN?

Your CRP test results tell you how much inflammation you have in your body. But your test results cannot tell you what is causing the inflammation. To make a diagnosis, your provider will look at your CRP results, along with the results of other tests, your symptoms, and your medical history.

In general, healthy people have very low amounts of CRP in their blood. Any increases above normal mean you have inflammation in your body. But labs measure CRP levels in different ways, and they define "normal" CRP ranges differently, so it is best to ask your provider what your results mean.

IS THERE ANYTHING ELSE YOU NEED TO KNOW ABOUT A C-REACTIVE PROTEIN TEST?

A CRP test is sometimes confused with a high-sensitivity CRP test. They both measure CRP, but they are used for different conditions. A high-sensitivity CRP test measures very tiny increases in your CRP levels. It is used to estimate your risk of heart disease.[1]

Section 57.2 | Erythrocyte Sedimentation Rate

WHAT IS AN ERYTHROCYTE SEDIMENTATION RATE?

An erythrocyte sedimentation rate (ESR) is a blood test that can show if you have inflammation in your body. Inflammation is your immune system's response to injury, infection, and many types of conditions, including immune system disorders, certain cancers, and blood disorders.

[1] MedlinePlus, "C-Reactive Protein (CRP) Test," National Institutes of Health (NIH), September 28, 2022. Available online. URL: https://medlineplus.gov/lab-tests/ana-antinuclear-antibody-test. Accessed May 15, 2023.

Erythrocytes are red blood cells (RBCs). To do an ESR test, a sample of your blood is sent to a lab. A health-care professional places the sample in a tall, thin test tube and measures how quickly the RBCs settle or sink to the bottom of the tube. Normally, RBCs sink slowly. But inflammation makes RBCs stick together in clumps. These clumps of cells are heavier than single cells, so they sink faster.

If an ESR test shows that your RBCs sink faster than normal, it may mean you have a medical condition causing inflammation. The speed of your test result is a sign of how much inflammation you have. Faster ESR rates mean higher levels of inflammation. But an ESR test alone cannot diagnose what condition is causing the inflammation. Other names are as follows:

- ESR
- SED rate sedimentation rate
- Westergren sedimentation rate

WHAT IS IT USED FOR?

An ESR test can be used with other tests to help diagnose conditions that cause inflammation. It can also be used to help monitor these conditions. Many types of conditions cause inflammation, including arthritis, vasculitis, infection, and inflammatory bowel disease (IBD). An ESR may also be used to monitor an existing condition.

WHY DO YOU NEED AN ERYTHROCYTE SEDIMENTATION RATE?

Your health-care provider may order an ESR if you have symptoms of a condition that causes inflammation. Your symptoms will depend on the condition you may have, but they may include:

- anemia
- headaches
- joint stiffness
- loss of appetite
- neck or shoulder pain
- unexplained fever
- weight loss

WHAT HAPPENS DURING AN ERYTHROCYTE SEDIMENTATION RATE?

A health-care professional will take a blood sample from a vein in your arm using a small needle. After the needle is inserted, a small amount of blood will be collected into a test tube or vial. You may feel a little sting when the needle goes in or out. This usually takes less than five minutes.

WILL YOU NEED TO DO ANYTHING TO PREPARE FOR AN ERYTHROCYTE SEDIMENTATION RATE?

You do not need any special preparations for this test. But, if your provider ordered other tests on your blood sample, you may need to fast (not eat or drink) for several hours before the test. Your provider will let you know if there are any special instructions to follow.

ARE THERE ANY RISKS IN THE TEST?

There is very little risk in having an ESR. You may have slight pain or bruising at the spot where the needle was put in, but most symptoms go away quickly.

WHAT DO THE RESULTS MEAN?

Your provider will use the results of your ESR test along with your medical history, symptoms, and other test results to make a diagnosis. An ESR test alone cannot diagnose conditions that cause inflammation.

A high ESR test result may be from a condition that causes inflammation, such as:

- arteritis
- arthritis
- certain cancers
- heart disease
- infection
- IBD

- kidney disease
- polymyalgia rheumatica
- rheumatoid arthritis (RA) and other autoimmune diseases
- systemic vasculitis

A low ESR test result means your RBCs sank more slowly than normal. This may be caused by conditions such as:
- a blood disorder, such as:
  - polycythemia
  - sickle cell disease (SCD)
  - leukocytosis, a very high white blood cell (WBC) count
- heart failure
- certain kidney and liver problems

If your ESR results are not normal, it does not always mean you have a medical condition that needs treatment. Pregnancy, a menstrual cycle, aging, obesity, drinking alcohol regularly, and exercise can affect ESR results. Certain medicines and supplements may also affect your results, so be sure to tell your provider about any medicines or supplements you are taking.

IS THERE ANYTHING ELSE YOU NEED TO KNOW ABOUT AN ERYTHROCYTE SEDIMENTATION RATE?

Because an ESR cannot diagnose a specific disease, your provider may order other tests at the same time. Also, it is possible to have a condition that causes inflammation and still have a normal ESR result. A c-reactive protein (CRP) test is commonly done with an ESR to provide more information.[2]

---

[2] MedlinePlus, "Erythrocyte Sedimentation Rate (ESR)," National Institutes of Health (NIH), November 8, 2022. Available online. URL: https://medlineplus.gov/lab-tests/erythrocyte-sedimentation-rate-esr. Accessed May 15, 2023.

WHAT IS A PROCALCITONIN TEST?

A procalcitonin test (PCT) measures the level of procalcitonin in your blood. Normally, you have very low levels of procalcitonin in your blood. But, if you have a serious bacterial infection, the cells in many parts of your body will release procalcitonin into your bloodstream. A high level of procalcitonin in your blood may be a sign of a serious infection or sepsis.

Sepsis (also called "septicemia") is your immune system's extreme response to an infection, usually from bacteria. Sepsis happens when an infection you already have spread into your bloodstream and triggers a chain reaction throughout your body. It causes inflammation and blood clots. Without quick treatment, sepsis can rapidly lead to tissue damage, organ failure, or even death.

Infections that lead to sepsis most often start in your lungs, urinary tract, skin, or digestive system. A PCT can help your healthcare provider diagnose if you have sepsis from a bacterial infection or if you have a high risk of developing sepsis. This may help you get the right treatment quickly before your condition worsens. Another name is PCT test.

WHAT IS IT USED FOR?

A PCT is mostly used if you are seriously ill and your provider thinks you may have a systemic infection (an infection that affects your entire body). The test helps find out whether bacteria or a virus is causing your infection. For example, a PCT can help tell the difference between bacterial and viral pneumonia. This matters because antibiotics may help bacterial infections but not viral infections. The test may be used to help:
- diagnose or rule out a bacterial infection and/or sepsis
- find out how serious a sepsis infection may be
- make treatment decisions
- monitor how well the treatment is working
- diagnose kidney infections in children with urinary tract infections (UTIs)

This test is usually used in the hospital for very sick people who are in the emergency room (ER) or have already been admitted to the hospital.

WHY DO YOU NEED A PROCALCITONIN TEST?

You may need this test if you have symptoms of sepsis or a serious bacterial infection that could become sepsis. Symptoms of sepsis include:

- clammy or sweaty skin
- confusion
- extreme pain
- fever or chills
- low blood pressure
- rapid heartbeat
- shortness of breath

Sepsis is a medical emergency. If you or your loved one has an infection that is not getting better or is getting worse, get medical help right away.

WHAT HAPPENS DURING A PROCALCITONIN TEST?

A health-care professional will take a blood sample from a vein in your arm using a small needle. After the needle is inserted, a small amount of blood will be collected into a test tube or vial. You may feel a little sting when the needle goes in or out. This usually takes less than five minutes.

WILL YOU NEED TO DO ANYTHING TO PREPARE FOR THE TEST?

You do not need any special preparation for a PCT.

ARE THERE ANY RISKS IN THE TEST?

There is very little risk in having a blood test. You may have slight pain or bruising at the spot where the needle was put in, but most symptoms go away quickly.

WHAT DO THE RESULTS MEAN?

High procalcitonin levels mean that you:

- most likely have sepsis
- may have a high risk of developing severe sepsis and septic shock, a life-threatening condition when your organs do not get enough blood to work properly
- may have a serious systemic bacterial infection that increases your risk for sepsis

The higher your procalcitonin levels, the higher your risk for sepsis and septic shock.

Moderate to mildly high levels of procalcitonin may be a sign of:

- the earlier stages of a systemic bacterial infection
- kidney infection (only in children)
- conditions other than infections, such as tissue damage from trauma, serious burns, recent surgery, and severe heart attack

Slightly high levels of procalcitonin mean that you are unlikely to develop sepsis, but they may be a sign of:

- a local bacterial infection, such as a UTI
- an infection from another cause, such as a virus
- a systemic bacterial infection that is just beginning

If you are being treated for a bacterial infection, decreasing or low procalcitonin levels mean that your treatment is working.

IS THERE ANYTHING ELSE YOU NEED TO KNOW ABOUT A PROCALCITONIN TEST?

A PCT will not show what type of bacteria is causing an infection. To make a full diagnosis, your provider will likely order other tests. But a PCT does give you important information about your risk for sepsis, so you can start treatment sooner, if needed, and avoid more serious illness.[3]

---

[3] MedlinePlus, "Procalcitonin Test," National Institutes of Health (NIH), August 3, 2022. Available online. URL: https://medlineplus.gov/lab-tests/procalcitonin-test. Accessed May 15, 2023.

Part 7 | Drugs and Therapies for Immune Diseases and Disorders

Chapter 58 | Treatments for Allergies and Asthma

Chapter Contents

Section 58.1 | Allergy Immunotherapy

Allergen immunotherapy, often known as "allergy shots," is a treatment that helps minimize how much you react to allergens (such as pollen, pet dander, or dust mites). The treatment is based on receiving small doses of the allergen through injections (shots) over time that helps your body tolerate the allergen, allowing you to respond less strongly to it.

Allergy shots may benefit those with allergies that are difficult to manage with existing medications, those who have difficulty avoiding certain allergens, or those who have severe or year-round chronic symptoms. Patients must be able to follow their health-care provider's treatment plan to receive allergy shots.

An allergist tests for specific allergies and evaluates whether allergy shots are an appropriate therapy choice for the patient. These shots cannot cure an allergy per se, but the symptoms of the allergy can improve.

Allergy shots can be used to control allergies triggered by:
- indoor allergens (e.g., dust, cockroaches, etc.)
- seasonal allergens (e.g., hay fever)
- insect stings (e.g., bee stings)

Allergy shots are recommended when:
- symptoms are severe
- medications do not yield any result or cause adverse side effects
- the cause is unavoidable, such as an allergy due to pollen

HOW DO ALLERGY SHOTS WORK?

Allergy shots make the body accustomed to allergens such as pollen or dust mites. The health-care provider administers a shot containing a trace quantity of the allergen and gradually raises the dose over time. This helps the body gradually build immunity so that when the individual comes in contact with the allergen again, they do not experience as many symptoms. Allergy shots have two phases and must be administered regularly to be effective.

Buildup Phase

During this phase, the person will be given shots containing gradually increasing amounts of allergens one to three times a week for three to six months. This period allows the body to adapt to the allergen and minimizes allergy symptoms.

Maintenance Phase

After reaching an effective dose, the maintenance phase will start. Injections are given every two to four weeks for three to five years or longer throughout this phase. The idea is to keep the body immune to the allergen and avoid allergy symptoms. Maintenance can last up to a few years before an improvement is observed.

HOW EFFECTIVE ARE ALLERGY SHOTS?

Allergy shots can prevent allergies from progressing to chronic conditions such as asthma and stop a person from developing new allergies. The effectiveness of the treatment is determined by the amount of dosage given and the duration of the entire treatment. Even if the shots are no longer being taken, the individual feels better for a long time.

HOW DOES ONE PREPARE BEFORE AN ALLERGY SHOT?

Before administering allergy shots, the health-care provider does a skin or blood test to determine the source of the allergies. The skin test involves applying a small amount of the suspected allergen to the skin and observing whether it causes swelling and redness. It is critical to notify the health-care providers if one feels ill after allergy shots, especially if the individual has asthma. One should avoid vigorous exercise two hours before the shot because it can accelerate the distribution of allergens in the body. Individuals must inform the health-care provider if they have used any vitamins or medications before the shot and if they have experienced any side effects from a previous dose.

WHAT ARE THE RISKS INVOLVED?

Allergy shots can help patients become less allergic to the substances that cause their allergies, but a reaction is possible since they also include the same allergic substances. The reactions might be moderate, such as redness or swelling at the injection site, or severe, such as hives or difficulty in breathing. Anaphylaxis, a potentially fatal reaction, can occur very rarely. However, the chance of a significant reaction can be lowered by following a regular "shot" schedule, being monitored for 30 minutes after each shot, and taking an antihistamine before the shot under the health-care provider's supervision and recommendation. If there is a severe reaction, it is recommended to get immediate medical assistance.

References

"Allergen Immunotherapy," Australasian Society of Clinical Immunology and Allergy (ASCIA), March 2019. Available online. URL: www.allergy.org.au/patients/allergy-treatment/immunotherapy. Accessed April 25, 2023.

"Allergen Immunotherapy," Exton Allergy and Asthma Associates, April 1, 2018. Available online. URL: www.extonallergy.com/allergen-immunotherapy. Accessed April 25, 2023.

"Allergies: Should I Take Allergy Shots?" MyHealth Alberta, April 14, 2022. Available online. URL: https://myhealth.alberta.ca/Health/Pages/conditions.aspx?hwid=aa69795. Accessed April 25, 2023.

"Allergy Immunotherapy (Allergy Shots): What You Should Know," University of Michigan, September 2018. Available online. URL: www.med.umich.edu/1libr/Allergy/AllergyShotsWhatYouShouldKnow.pdf. Accessed April 25, 2023.

"Allergy Shots," Icahn School of Medicine at Mount Sinai, October 30, 2021. Available online. URL: www.mountsinai.org/health-library/discharge-instructions/allergy-shots. Accessed April 25, 2023.

"Allergy Shots," Mayo Foundation for Medical Education and Research (MFMER), January 6, 2022. Available online.

URL: www.mayoclinic.org/tests-procedures/allergy-shots/
about/pac-20392876. Accessed April 25, 2023.

"Allergy Shots (Immunotherapy)," American Academy of
Allergy, Asthma & Immunology (AAAAI), September 28,
2020. Available online. URL: www.aaaai.org/Tools-for-
the-Public/Conditions-Library/Allergies/allergy-shots-
(immunotherapy). Accessed April 25, 2023.

"Immunization Reactions," Seattle Children's Hospital,
December 30, 2022. Available online. URL: www.
seattlechildrens.org/conditions/a-z/immunization-
reactions. Accessed April 25, 2023.

"Immunotherapy," Asthma Allergy Clinic, June 27, 2022.
Available online. URL: https://asthmaallergyclinic.in/
treatment/immunotherapy. Accessed April 25, 2023.

Seymour, Tom. "What to Know about Allergy Shots," Medical
News Today, December 24, 2017. Available online. URL:
www.medicalnewstoday.com/articles/320402. Accessed
April 25, 2023.

Young-Yuen Wu, Adrian. "Immunotherapy–Vaccines for
Allergic Diseases," National Center for Biotechnology
Information (NCBI), April 1, 2012. Available online.
URL: www.ncbi.nlm.nih.gov/pmc/articles/PMC3378232.
Accessed April 25, 2023.

Section 58.2 | Asthma Treatment

HOW IS ASTHMA TREATED?

You can control your asthma and avoid an attack by taking your
medicine exactly as your doctor or other medical professional tells
you to do and by avoiding things that can cause an attack.

Not everyone with asthma takes the same medicine. Some medicines can be inhaled, or breathed in, and some can be taken as a pill.
Asthma medicines come in two types—quick relief and long-term
control. Quick-relief medicines control the symptoms of an asthma
attack. If you need to use your quick-relief medicines more and

more, you should visit your doctor or other medical professional to see if you need a different medicine. Long-term control medicines help you have fewer and milder attacks, but they do not help you if you are having an asthma attack.

Asthma medicines can have side effects, but most side effects are mild and soon go away. Ask your doctor or other medical professional about the side effects of your medicines.

The important thing to remember is that you can control your asthma. With your doctor's or other medical professional's help, make your own asthma action plan (management plan) so that you know what to do based on your own symptoms. Decide who should have a copy of your plan and where she or he should keep it.[1]

QUICK-RELIEF MEDICINES

Quick-relief medicines help prevent or relieve symptoms during an asthma attack. They may be the only medicines needed for mild asthma or asthma that happens only with physical activity.

The types of quick-relief medicines include the following:
- **Inhaled short-acting beta-2 agonists (SABAs)**. They open the airways, so air can flow through them during an asthma attack. Side effects can include tremors and rapid heartbeat.
- **Oral corticosteroids**. They reduce swelling in your airways caused by severe asthma symptoms.
- **Short-acting anticholinergics**. They help open the airways quickly. This medicine may be less effective than SABAs, but it is an option for people who may have side effects from SABAs.

LONG-TERM CONTROL MEDICINES

Your doctor may prescribe medicines, including the following, to take daily to help prevent asthma attacks and control symptoms:
- **Corticosteroids (steroid hormone medicines)**. They reduce inflammation in the body. They may be taken as

[1] "Management and Treatment," Centers for Disease Control and Prevention (CDC), May 4, 2023. Available online. URL: www.cdc.gov/asthma/management.html. Accessed May 25, 2023.

a pill or inhaled. The pill form can have more serious side effects than the inhaled form. Over time, high doses can raise your risk of cataracts (clouding of the eye) or osteoporosis. Osteoporosis makes your bones more likely to break. The common side effects from inhaled corticosteroids include a hoarse voice or a mouth infection called "thrush."

- **Biologic medicines**. They may be prescribed for severe asthma. These include medicines such as benralizumab that are injected into a vein or below the skin.
- **Leukotriene modifiers**. These reduce swelling and keeps your airways open. Your doctor may prescribe these pills alone or with steroid medicine.
- **Inhaled mast cell stabilizers, such as cromolyn**. They help prevent swelling in your airways when you are around allergens or other asthma triggers.
- **Inhaled long-acting bronchodilators, such as long-acting beta-2 agonists (LABAs) or long-acting muscarinic antagonists (LAMAs)**. They may be added to your inhaler to prevent your airways from narrowing.
- **Allergy shots, called "subcutaneous immunotherapy" (SCIT)**. They reduce the body's response to allergens.

BRONCHIAL THERMOPLASTY
Bronchial thermoplasty may help if you have severe asthma and other treatments are not working. In this procedure, your doctor inserts a tube called a "bronchoscope" into your mouth. The bronchoscope has a camera at the end. Your doctor will guide the bronchoscope into your airways to see inside them. Your doctor will then apply heat to the muscles along the airways. This makes them thinner and helps prevent them from narrowing.[2]

[2] "Treatment and Action Plan," National Heart, Lung, and Blood Institute (NHLBI), March 24, 2022. Available online. URL: www.nhlbi.nih.gov/health/asthma/treatment-action-plan. Accessed May 25, 2023.

Chapter 59 | Treatment for Autoimmune Disease

Chapter Contents

WHAT IS PLASMAPHERESIS?

Autoimmune diseases are usually treated with medications that suppress the immune system or reduce inflammation in tissues. However, using these drugs for extended periods or in high amounts can lead to harmful effects on the body. To avoid relying solely on medication, scientists have developed a new approach called "plasmapheresis," which involves mechanically removing autoantibodies from the bloodstream. This process is similar to dialysis and is also known as "plasma exchange," where the liquid part, the plasma, is separated from the blood and is returned to the body, along with fresh plasma or other fluids. This procedure successfully treats some autoimmune diseases, such as multiple sclerosis (MS), Guillain-Barré syndrome (GBS), Miller-Fisher syndrome (MFS), chronic inflammatory demyelinating polyneuropathy (CIDP), Goodpasture syndrome, and Lambert-Eaton syndrome.

The immune system produces antibodies to protect the body from infections, bacteria, viruses, and other invaders, but when the antibodies, which are proteins in blood plasma, attack their own body, they become autoantibodies. Plasma exchange is a process that can help take out harmful proteins called "autoantibodies" from the blood. An alternative treatment for some disorders is to use medication to suppress the immune system. Still, this approach can lead to serious side effects; in some cases, the body may no longer be able to fight infection. So plasmapheresis is often the preferred method of fighting several autoimmune disorders.

PROCEDURE FOR PLASMAPHERESIS

Anesthesia is generally not necessary for the plasmapheresis treatment itself, but it is sometimes used for the placement of the two relatively large needles that must be used. Once the needles are positioned, patients may feel some discomfort, but no pain, for the remainder of the procedure.

Before plasmapheresis, the patient is positioned in a reclining chair or lying down. Two tubes (catheters or needles) are inserted into the body: one in a large vein in the arm and the other in either the opposite arm, foot, groin area, or shoulder. Blood is removed through one of the tubes and passed into an apheresis machine or cell separator. This device separates the plasma from the blood cells by spinning at high speed or passing the blood through a membrane with tiny pores, which allow only the plasma to pass through, but not the blood cells.

The removed plasma is then discarded, along with the autoantibodies it contains. The substitute (replacement) plasma is combined with blood cells and then reintroduced into the body through the other tube. The amount of blood that is outside the body at any given time during the procedure is generally less than the amount a donor would contribute at a blood bank. Plasmapheresis is usually done outpatient, and the procedure can take one to three hours. For an average patient, treatments are repeated 6–10 times over the span of 2–10 weeks. The length and number of treatments depend on the diagnosis and the patient's general condition.

Before the Procedure

Prior to plasmapheresis, the patient will be examined by the physician. The health-care provider will collect a complete medical history and review all medications to decide if the patient needs to stop certain medications before and after treatment.

It is essential to follow the following for a smooth procedure:

- The night before the procedure, it is important to get a good amount of sleep.
- Stay hydrated by drinking fluids during the days leading to the procedure.
- Wear loose-fitting clothes to allow rolling up of sleeves above your elbows.
- Bring something to read or a portable music device with headphones to help pass the time.

After the Procedure

After the procedure, the patient can leave the hospital or medical center after resting briefly. Since many people feel tired or weak after plasmapheresis, the patient will need someone to drive them home. After the procedure, care must be taken to follow the doctor's instructions regarding medication dosages, which may need to be adjusted, and prevent infection. The patient can show improvement within days or, at most, a few weeks, and the positive effects of the course of treatment can be expected to last for several months. But, since plasmapheresis is a temporary treatment, the procedure may have to be repeated on a regular basis.

RISKS AND COMPLICATIONS

Although plasmapheresis is a safe form of treatment, and complications do not occur often, like most medical procedures, it does carry some risks. Awareness of these risks can help the patient be prepared.

A few of the possible risks and complications include:

- bleeding because of the medication given to prevent clotting during the procedure
- low blood pressure, which can be treated by tilting the patient's head downward, raising their legs, and giving them intravenous (IV) fluids
- dizziness, blurred vision, sweating, and abdominal cramps
- allergic reaction resulting in fever, chills, or rashes
- reactions to medication, such as tingling in the mouth or limbs or a metallic taste in the mouth
- swelling, bruises, or rashes where needles or tubes were inserted
- infection
- anaphylaxis, a potentially dangerous reaction to the solutions used in plasma replacement (The procedure needs to be stopped if this complication occurs.)
- fatigue, weakness, or joint pain
- excessive suppression of the immune system during the plasma exchange (However, this generally resolves in a short time as the body produces more antibodies.)
- patients occasionally developing an allergy to the solutions and equipment used in the procedure (If so,

the medical technician or doctor would administer IV medication.)

A health-care provider should be contacted immediately if any of the following serious complications develop:

- seizures
- manifestations of infection, such as chills or fever
- severe bleeding or swelling where the needle or tube was inserted
- persistent itching or rashes
- severe pain
- dizziness, shortness of breath, chest pain, or wheezing

References

"Facts about Plasmapheresis," Muscular Dystrophy Association Inc., July 2011. Available online. URL: www.mda.org/sites/default/files/publications/Facts_ Plasmapheresis_P-206_0.pdf. Accessed April 21, 2023.

Heitz, David. "Plasmapheresis: What to Expect," Healthline, September 3, 2018. Available online. URL: www.healthline. com/health/plasmapheresis. Accessed April 21, 2023.

"Plasma Exchange (Plasmapheresis) for MS," WebMD, May 20, 2021. Available online. URL: www.webmd.com/ multiple-sclerosis/plasma-exchange-ms. Accessed April 21, 2023.

"Plasmapheresis," Northwestern Medicine, August 24, 2017. Available online. URL: www.nm.org/conditions-and-care-areas/treatments/plasmapheresis. Accessed April 21, 2023.

"Plasmapheresis and Plasma Exchange," Cleveland Clinic, September 20, 2022. Available online. URL: https:// my.clevelandclinic.org/health/treatments/24197-plasmapheresis-plasma-exchange. Accessed April 21, 2023.

"Plasmapheresis in the Practice of Autoimmune Diseases Treatment," Manufactura Clinic Medical Center, May 9, 2020. Available online. URL: https://manufacturaclinica.com/en/blog/

plasmapheresis-in-the-practice-of-autoimmune-diseases-
treatment. Accessed April 21, 2023.

Stieglitz, Elliot. "Plasmapheresis Technique," Medscape,
January 25, 2023. Available online. URL: https://
emedicine.medscape.com/article/1895577-
technique?icd=login_success_gg_match_
normisSocialFTC=true. Accessed April 21, 2023.

"Therapeutic Plasma Exchange," The University of Texas
Southwestern Medical Center, March 6, 2018. Available
online. URL: https://utswmed.org/conditions-treatments/
apheresis/therapeutic-plasma-exchange. Accessed
April 21, 2023.

Section 59.2 | Treatment for Rheumatoid Arthritis

Treatment for rheumatoid arthritis (RA) continues to improve, which can give many people relief from symptoms, improving their quality of life (QOL). Doctors may use the following options to treat RA.

MEDICATIONS

Most people who have RA take medications. Studies show that early treatment with combinations of medications, instead of one medication alone, may be more effective in decreasing or preventing joint damage.

Many of the medications that doctors prescribe to treat RA help decrease inflammation and pain and slow or stop joint damage. They may include the following:

- **Anti-inflammatory medications**. These medications provide pain relief and lower inflammation.
- **Corticosteroids**. These can help decrease inflammation, provide some pain relief, and slow joint damage. Because they are potent drugs and have potential side effects, your doctor will prescribe the lowest dose possible to achieve the desired benefit.

- **Disease-modifying antirheumatic drugs (DMARDs).**
  DMARDs can help slow or change the progression of
  the disease.
- **Biologic response modifiers (which are also
  DMARDS).** These drugs are used when your
  disease does not respond to initial therapies. These
  medications target specific immune messages and
  interrupt the signal, helping to decrease or stop
  inflammation.
- **Janus kinase (JAK) inhibitors (which are also
  DMARDs).** These drugs can send messages to specific
  cells to stop inflammation from inside the cell. These
  medications may also be considered if your disease
  does not respond to initial therapies.

PHYSICAL THERAPY AND OCCUPATIONAL THERAPY

Your doctor may recommend physical therapy and occupational
therapy. Physical therapy can help you regain and maintain overall strength and target specific joints that bother you. Occupational
therapy can help develop, recover, improve, and maintain the skills
needed for daily living and working. Sometimes, assistive devices
or braces may be helpful to optimize movement, reduce pain, and
help you maintain the ability to work.

SURGERY

Your doctor may recommend surgery if you have permanent damage or pain that limits your ability to perform day-to-day activities.
Surgery is not for everyone. You and your doctor can discuss the
options and choose what is right for you.

Your doctor will consider the following before recommending
surgery:

- your overall health
- the condition of the affected joint or tendon
- the risks and benefits of the surgery

Types of surgery may include joint repairs and joint replacements.

ROUTINE MONITORING

Regular medical care is important because your doctor can:
- monitor how the disease is progressing
- determine how well the medications are working
- talk to you about any side effects from the medications
- adjust your treatment as needed

Monitoring typically includes regular visits to the doctor. It may also include blood and urine tests, x-rays, or other imaging tests. Having RA increases your risk of developing osteoporosis, particularly if you take corticosteroids. Osteoporosis is a bone disease that causes the bones to weaken and easily break. Talk to your doctor about your risk for the disease and the potential benefits of calcium and vitamin D supplements or other osteoporosis treatments.

Since RA can affect other organs, your doctor may also monitor you for cardiovascular or respiratory health. Many of the medications used to treat RA may increase the risk of infection. Doctors may monitor you for infections. Vaccines may be recommended to lower the risk and severity of infections.

WHO TREATS RHEUMATOID ARTHRITIS?

Diagnosing and treating RA require a team effort involving you and several types of health-care professionals. These may include the following:
- rheumatologists, who specialize in autoimmune diseases, arthritis, and other diseases of the bones, joints, and muscles
- physician assistants, who assist doctors in diagnosing, treating, and monitoring diseases
- primary care providers, such as internists or nurse practitioners, who specialize in the diagnosis and medical treatment of adults
- orthopedists, who specialize in the treatment of and surgery for bone and joint diseases or injuries
- other medical specialty doctors, such as pulmonologists or cardiologists, for people whose RA affects other organs such as the lungs or heart.

- podiatrists, who specialize in the treatment of and surgery for problems in the feet
- physical therapists, who help improve joint function
- occupational therapists, who teach ways to protect joints, minimize pain, perform activities of daily living, and conserve energy
- pharmacists, who dispense medications and help check the dosing and potential for interactions with other medications
- dietitians, who teach ways to eat a good diet to improve health and maintain a healthy weight
- nurse educators, who specialize in helping people understand their overall condition and set up their treatment plans
- mental health professionals and social workers, who help people cope with difficulties in the home and workplace that may result from their medical conditions

LIVING WITH RHEUMATOID ARTHRITIS

Research shows that people who take part in their own care report less pain and make fewer doctor visits. They also enjoy a better QOL.

Self-care can help you play a role in managing your RA and improving your health. You can do the following:

- Learn about RA and its treatments.
- Use exercises and relaxation techniques to reduce your pain and help you stay active.
- Communicate well with your health-care team so that you can have more control over your disease.
- Reach out for support to help cope with the physical, emotional, and mental effects of RA.

Participating in your care can help build confidence in your ability to perform day-to-day activities, allowing you to lead a full, active, and independent life.

Lifestyle Changes

Certain activities can help improve your ability to function on your own and maintain a positive outlook.

- **Rest and exercise.** Balance your rest and exercise, with more rest when your RA is active and more exercise when it is not. Rest helps decrease active joint inflammation, pain, and fatigue. In general, shorter rest breaks every now and then are more helpful than long times spent in bed. Exercise is important for maintaining healthy and strong muscles, preserving joint mobility, and maintaining flexibility. Exercise can help:
  - improve your sleep
  - decrease pain
  - keep a positive attitude
  - maintain a healthy weight

Doctors may sometimes recommend low-impact exercises, such as water exercise programs. Talk to your health-care providers before beginning any exercise program.

- **Joint care.** Some people find wearing a splint for a short time around a painful joint reduces pain and swelling. People use splints mostly on wrists and hands but also on ankles and feet. Talk to your doctor or a physical or occupational therapist before wearing a splint. Other ways you can protect your joints include:
  - using self-help devices, such as items with a large grip, zipper pullers, or long-handled shoehorns
  - using tools or devices that help with activities of daily living, such as an adaptive toothbrush or silverware
  - using devices to help you get on and off chairs, toilet seats, and beds
  - choosing activities that put less stress on your joints, such as limiting the use of the stairs or taking rest periods when walking longer distances

- maintaining a healthy weight to help lower the stress on your joints
- **Monitoring of symptoms**. It is important to monitor your symptoms for any changes or the development of new symptoms. Understanding your symptoms and how they may change can help you and your doctor manage your pain when you have a flare.
- **Stress management**. The emotions you may feel because of RA—fear, anger, and frustration, along with any pain, physical limitations, and the unpredictable nature of flares—can increase your stress level. Stress can make living with the disease more difficult. Stress may also affect the amount of pain you feel. Ways to cope with stress can include:
  - regular rest periods
  - relaxation techniques such as deep breathing, meditating, or listening to quiet sounds or music
  - movement exercise programs, such as yoga and tai chi
- **Mental health management**. Living with RA can be hard and isolating. If you feel alone, anxious, or depressed about having the disease, talk to your doctor, an RA support social worker, or mental health professional. Keep the lines of communication open. Talk to family and friends about your RA to help them understand the disease. You may find it helpful to join an online or community support group.
- **Healthy diet**. A healthy and nutritious diet that includes a balance of calories, proteins, and calcium is important for maintaining overall health. Talk to your doctor about drinking alcoholic beverages because they may interact with the medications you take for RA.

Before making any changes to your diet or activity, talk to your doctor.[1]

---

[1] "Rheumatoid Arthritis," National Institute of Arthritis and Musculoskeletal and Skin Diseases (NIAMS), November 2022. Available online. URL: www.niams.nih.gov/health-topics/rheumatoid-arthritis/diagnosis-treatment-and-steps-to-take. Accessed May 22, 2023.

Chapter 60 | Treatments for Immune Deficiencies

Chapter Contents

Section 60.1 | **Antiretroviral Therapy**

WHAT IS ANTIRETROVIRAL THERAPY?

The treatment for human immunodeficiency virus (HIV) with medicines is called "antiretroviral therapy" (ART). It involves taking a combination of medicines every day. ART is recommended for everyone who has HIV. The medicines do not cure HIV infection but help people with HIV live longer, healthier lives. They also reduce the risk of spreading the virus to others.

HOW DO HUMAN IMMUNODEFICIENCY VIRUS MEDICINES WORK?

Human immunodeficiency virus medicines reduce the amount of HIV (viral load) in your body, which helps by:

- giving your immune system a chance to recover (Even though there is still some HIV in your body, your immune system should be strong enough to fight off infections and certain HIV-related cancers.)
- reducing the risk that you will spread HIV to others

WHAT ARE THE TYPES OF HUMAN IMMUNODEFICIENCY VIRUS MEDICINES?

There are many different types (called "classes") of HIV medicines. Some work by blocking or changing enzymes that HIV needs to make copies of itself. This prevents HIV from copying itself, which reduces the amount of HIV in the body. Several types of medicines do the following:

- **Nucleoside reverse transcriptase inhibitors (NRTIs).** NRTIs block an enzyme called "reverse transcriptase" (RT).
- **Non-nucleoside reverse transcriptase inhibitors (NNRTIs).** NNRTIs bind to and later change RT.
- **Integrase inhibitors.** Also called "integrase strand transfer inhibitors" (INSTIs), these inhibitors block an enzyme called "integrase."
- **Protease inhibitors (PIs).** PIs block an enzyme called "protease."

Some types of HIV medicines interfere with HIV's ability to infect the cluster of differentiation 4 (CD4) immune system cells:

- **Fusion inhibitors.** They block HIV from entering the cells.
- **C-C chemokine receptor type 5 (CCR5) antagonists and post-attachment inhibitors**. They block different molecules on the CD4 cells. To infect a cell, HIV has to bind to two types of molecules on the cell's surface. Blocking either of these molecules prevents HIV from entering the cells.
- **Attachment inhibitors**. They bind to a specific protein on the outer surface of HIV. This prevents HIV from entering the cell.

Pharmacokinetic enhancers are another type of medicine. They are sometimes taken along with certain other HIV medicines. Pharmacokinetic enhancers increase the effectiveness of other medicine. They work by slowing the breakdown of the other medicine. This allows that medicine to stay in the body longer at a higher concentration.

There are also multidrug combinations, which include a combination of two or more different types of HIV medicines.

WHEN DO YOU NEED TO START TAKING HUMAN IMMUNODEFICIENCY VIRUS MEDICINES?

It is important to start taking HIV medicines as soon as possible after your diagnosis, especially if you:

- are pregnant
- have acquired immunodeficiency syndrome (AIDS)
- have certain HIV-related illnesses and infections
- have an early HIV infection (the first six months after infection with HIV)

WHAT ELSE DO YOU NEED TO KNOW ABOUT TAKING HUMAN IMMUNODEFICIENCY VIRUS MEDICINES?

You and your health-care provider will work together to come up with a personal treatment plan.

This plan will be based on many factors, including:
- the possible side effects of HIV medicines
- potential drug interactions with any other medicines you take
- how many medicines you will need to take every day
- any other health problems you may have

It is important to take your medicines every day according to the instructions from your provider. If you miss doses or do not follow a regular schedule, your treatment may not work, and the HIV may become resistant to the medicines.

HIV medicines can cause side effects. Most of these side effects are manageable, but a few can be serious. Tell your provider about any side effects that you are having. Do not stop taking your medicine without first talking to your provider. There may be steps you can take to help manage the side effects. In some cases, your provider may decide to change your medicines.

WHAT ARE HUMAN IMMUNODEFICIENCY VIRUS PRE-EXPOSURE AND POST-EXPOSURE PROPHYLAXIS MEDICINES?

Human immunodeficiency virus medicines are not just used for treatment. Some people take them to prevent HIV. Pre-exposure prophylaxis (PrEP) is for people who do not already have HIV but are at a very high risk of getting it. Post-exposure prophylaxis (PEP) is for people who have possibly been exposed to HIV.[1]

Section 60.2 | Immune Globulin Intravenous Injection

Immune globulin intravenous (IGIV) injection is a sterilized, highly purified medication made from human plasma that contains antibodies to help fight infections and other diseases. Its principal use is

---

[1] MedlinePlus, "HIV Medicines," National Institutes of Health (NIH), February 14, 2023. Available online. URL: https://medlineplus.gov/hivmedicines.html. Accessed May 22, 2023.

in the treatment of primary immunodeficiency (PI), a group of hundreds of mostly genetic disorders in which the body's immune system is unable to produce enough antibodies on its own, as well as some secondary immunodeficiencies, those caused by other conditions.

PI disorders include:
- X-linked agammaglobulinemia
- common variable immunodeficiency
- Wiskott-Aldrich syndrome
- DiGeorge syndrome
- chronic mucocutaneous candidiasis
- chronic granulomatous disease
- C2 deficiency

Secondary immunodeficiencies, also known as "acquired immunodeficiencies," include disorders such as:
- human immunodeficiency virus (HIV)
- lymphocytic leukemia
- severe malnutrition
- chronic diseases, such as diabetes

It can also be caused by certain immunosuppressive medications or by chemotherapy.

In addition, IGIV injection may be used to increase the platelet count in individuals with blood disorders, such as idiopathic thrombocytopenia purpura, blood vessel diseases, such as Kawasaki syndrome, and nerve disorders, such as chronic inflammatory demyelinating polyneuropathy (CIDP).

HOW IT IS MADE

Immune globulin intravenous injection is made from plasma collected from large numbers of donors who have been carefully screened to ensure that they are healthy, are free of disease, have not traveled to high-risk areas, and have not engaged in behaviors that might increase their risk of contracting an infectious disease.

The plasma from many donors is pooled together, purified to remove any viruses or other pathogens, and treated to extract the immune globulins. Depending on the particular type of IGIV injection being prepared, sugars, amino acids, or other substances may be added to help preserve the solution for storage and transportation. The product is then packaged, stored, and finally shipped to health-care providers.

ADMINISTERING IMMUNE GLOBULIN INTRAVENOUS INJECTION

Immune globulin intravenous injection is known as a "replacement therapy" because it replenishes substances (such as antibodies) that the body is incapable of producing—or produces in insufficient quantities—on its own. It does not prompt the immune system to begin producing antibodies. Instead, it provides the necessary antibodies from an outside source. Since the supply of antibodies constantly gets depleted, IGIV injection is a temporary treatment that must be repeated on a regular basis.

IGIV treatments are usually given by infusion but in some cases may also be administered by intramuscular or subcutaneous injection. With infusion, the medication is introduced directly into a vein through a needle or catheter over a two- to four-hour period in sessions that are repeated approximately every three to four weeks. Prior to the introduction of infusion therapy, intramuscular injections were the norm, but this method fell out of favor because it is less effective and causes pain in many patients. A better alternative for some types of immunoglobulins is subcutaneous (under the skin) injection, which is more convenient but may need to be repeated more often, depending on the condition.

IGIV injection can be administered at a medical facility or at home. If self-administered, it is important that the patient fully understands the proper storage method of the medication, the exact dosages required, and the cleaning, usage, and disposal of needles and other equipment. Some types of IGIV injection need to be kept in a refrigerator, while others may be stored at room temperature. Medication that has changed color or contains foreign particles is unsafe to use. The prescribing health-care provider will explain the proper storage and use of the IGIV injection to the patient, and the instructions must be followed carefully to ensure the safe and effective use of the medication.

RISKS ASSOCIATED WITH IMMUNE GLOBULIN INTRAVENOUS INJECTION

Although multiple precautions are taken in screening donors, treating fluids, and testing the product, because the IGIV injection is made from human plasma, there is a very slight chance that the medication could transmit viruses or other diseases. But, with modern screening and processing methods, this risk is so low that the benefits of treatment far outweigh this risk.

In an unlikely event where transmission of infection via IGIV injection is suspected, it is important to consult a physician as soon as possible. The signs of infection include the following:

- high fever
- flu symptoms
- mouth sores
- severe headache
- neck stiffness
- increased sensitivity to light
- nausea and vomiting

IGIV injection has been associated with kidney failure and other severe renal disorders. The physician must be informed if the patient has ever had kidney disease, diabetes, sepsis, plasma cell disease, paraproteinemia, or fluid volume depletion. Many other drugs, including over-the-counter (OTC) medications, can increase the chance of kidney disease. So patients taking medicines such as antivirals, chemotherapy, certain antibiotics, or drugs for pain, osteoporosis, and bowel disorders or to prevent rejection of organ transplants may be at even greater risk when undergoing IGIV treatment.

Most IGIV solutions contain additives such as amino acids or sugars, which help preserve them and also reduce the incidence of side effects. These substances are harmless for most patients; however, some of them may cause adverse reactions in a small percentage of individuals. The administering physician monitors the responses and recommends a different type of IGIV injection if necessary.

SIDE EFFECTS

Immune globulin intravenous injection is a well-established form of treatment that has proven safe and effective for most patients. However, as with any medication, some individuals may experience side effects, which commonly include the following:

- chills
- diarrhea
- dizziness
- fatigue
- headache
- low-grade fever
- muscle cramps
- muscle or back pain
- skin irritation and redness
- uneasiness, inflammation, or discoloration at the injection site
- vomiting

Some reactions to the IGIV injection require the immediate attention of a medical professional. These uncommon but more serious side effects may include the following:

- aseptic meningitis
- blood clots
- chest pain
- difficulty breathing
- fainting
- hives
- kidney problems (indicated by rapid weight gain, swelling, or low urine output)
- liver problems (characterized by jaundice or dark urine)
- pulmonary embolism
- severe allergic reactions
- severe headaches
- signs of infection (including fever, neck stiffness, or flu-like symptoms)

- slurred speech
- sudden cough

In preparation for receiving the IGIV treatment, it is crucial for the patient to ensure they are well hydrated and to inform their health-care provider of their medical history, any allergies, current medications, and pregnancy status and plans.

References

"How to Use Immune Globulin Solution, Reconstituted (Recon Soln)," WebMD, August 26, 2015. Available online. URL: www.webmd.com/drugs/2/drug-22523/immune-globulin-intravenous/details. Accessed April 24, 2023.

"Immune Globulin (Human) (IgG) Solution—Uses, Side Effects, and More," WebMD, August 27, 2014. Available online. URL: www.webmd.com/drugs/2/drug-20642/immune-globulin-human-igg-intravenous/details. Accessed April 24, 2023.

"Immune Globulin Injection," Cleveland Clinic, October 28, 2018. Available online. URL: https://my.clevelandclinic.org/health/drugs/20705-immune-globulin-injection. Accessed April 24, 2023.

"The Immune System and Primary Immunodeficiency," Immune Deficiency Foundation, June 25, 2013. Available online. URL: https://primaryimmune.org/immune-system-and-primary-immunodeficiency. Accessed April 24, 2023.

"Immunoglobulin (Ig) Replacement Therapy," Immune Deficiency Foundation, March 27, 2020. Available online. URL: https://primaryimmune.org/immunoglobulin-replacement-therapy. Accessed April 24, 2023.

Katz, Jessica. "Intravenous Immunoglobulin," Medscape, April 21, 2023. Available online. URL: https://emedicine.medscape.com/article/210367-overview. Accessed April 24, 2023.

Chapter 61 | **Cancer Immunotherapy**

Cancer treatment vaccines are a type of immunotherapy that treats cancer by strengthening the body's natural defenses against the cancer. Unlike cancer prevention vaccines, cancer treatment vaccines are designed to be used in people who already have cancer—they work against cancer cells, not against something that causes cancer.

The idea behind treatment vaccines is that cancer cells contain substances, called "tumor-associated antigens," that are not present in normal cells or, if present, are at lower levels. Treatment vaccines can help the immune system learn to recognize and react to these antigens and destroy cancer cells that contain them.

Cancer treatment vaccines may be made in three main ways:

- They can be made from your own tumor cells. This means they are custom-made so that they cause an immune response against features that are unique to your cancer.
- They may be made from tumor-associated antigens that are found on cancer cells of many people with a specific type of cancer. Such a vaccine can cause an immune response in any patient whose cancer produces that antigen. This type of vaccine is still experimental.
- They may be made from your own dendritic cells, which are a type of immune cell. Dendritic cell vaccines stimulate your immune system to respond to an antigen on tumor cells. One dendritic cell vaccine has been approved, sipuleucel-T, which is used to treat some men with advanced prostate cancer.

A different type of cancer treatment, called "oncolytic virus therapy," is sometimes described as a type of cancer treatment vaccine. It uses an oncolytic virus, which is a virus that infects and breaks down cancer cells but does not harm normal cells.

The first oncolytic virus therapy approved by the U.S. Food and Drug Administration (FDA) is talimogene laherparepvec (T-VEC, or Imlygic®). It is based on herpes simplex virus type 1. Although this virus can infect both cancer and normal cells, normal cells are able to kill the virus while cancer cells cannot.

T-VEC is injected directly into a tumor. As the virus makes more and more copies of itself, it causes cancer cells to burst and die. The dying cells release new viruses and other substances that can cause an immune response against cancer cells throughout the body.

WHICH CANCERS ARE TREATED WITH CANCER TREATMENT VACCINES?

Sipuleucel-T is used to treat people with prostate cancer:
- that has spread to other parts of the body
- who have few or no symptoms
- whose cancer does not respond to hormone treatment

T-VEC is used to treat some people with melanoma that returns after surgery and cannot be removed with more surgery.

WHAT ARE THE SIDE EFFECTS OF CANCER TREATMENT VACCINES?

Cancer treatment vaccines can cause side effects, which affect people in different ways. The side effects you may have and how they make you feel will depend on how healthy you are before treatment, your type of cancer, how advanced it is, the type of treatment vaccine you are getting, and the dose.

Doctors and nurses cannot know for sure when or if side effects will occur or how serious they will be. Therefore, it is important to know which signs to look for and what to do if you start to have problems.

Cancer treatment vaccines can cause flu-like symptoms, which include:
- chills
- dizziness
- fatigue
- fever
- headache
- low or high blood pressure
- muscle or joint aches
- nausea or vomiting
- trouble breathing
- weakness

You may have a severe allergic reaction. Sipuleucel-T can cause a stroke.

T-VEC can cause tumor lysis syndrome. In this syndrome, the tumor cells die and break apart in the blood. This changes certain chemicals in the blood, which may cause damage to organs such as the kidneys, heart, and liver.

Since T-VEC is made from the herpesvirus, it can sometimes cause a herpesvirus infection that can lead to:
- pain, burning, or tingling in a blister around the mouth, genitals, fingers, or ears
- eye pain, sensitivity, discharge from the eyes, and blurry vision
- weakness in the arms and legs
- extreme fatigue and drowsiness
- confusion[1]

---

[1] "Cancer Treatment Vaccines," National Cancer Institute (NCI), September 24, 2019. Available online. URL: www.cancer.gov/about-cancer/treatment/types/immunotherapy/cancer-treatment-vaccines. Accessed May 22, 2023.

Chapter 62 | Gene Therapy

WHAT IS GENE THERAPY?

Gene therapy is a medical approach that treats or prevents disease by correcting the underlying genetic problem. Gene therapy techniques allow doctors to treat a disorder by altering a person's genetic makeup instead of using drugs or surgery.

Gene therapies are being used to treat a small number of diseases, including an eye disorder called "Leber congenital amaurosis" (LCA) and a muscle disorder called "spinal muscular atrophy" (SMA). Many more gene therapies are undergoing research to make sure that they will be safe and effective. Genome editing is a promising technique also under study that doctors hope to use soon to treat disorders in people.

HOW DOES GENE THERAPY WORK?

Gene therapy works by altering the genetic code to recover the functions of critical proteins. Proteins are the workhorses of the cell and the structural basis of the body's tissues. The instructions for making proteins are carried in a person's genetic code, and variants (or mutations) in this code can impact the production or function of proteins that may be critical to how the body works. Fixing or compensating for disease-causing genetic changes may recover the role of these important proteins and allow the body to function as expected.

Gene therapy can compensate for genetic alterations in a couple different ways:

- Gene transfer therapy introduces new genetic material into cells. If an altered gene causes a necessary protein to be faulty or missing, gene transfer therapy can introduce a normal copy of the gene to recover the function of the protein. Alternatively, the therapy can introduce a different gene that provides instructions for a protein that helps the cell function normally, despite the genetic alteration.

- Genome editing is a newer technique that may potentially be used for gene therapy. Instead of adding new genetic material, genome editing introduces gene editing tools that can change the existing deoxyribonucleic acid (DNA) in the cell. Genome editing technologies allow genetic material to be added, removed, or altered at precise locations in the genome. Clustered regularly interspaced palindromic repeats (CRISPR) associated protein 9 (Cas9) is a well-known type of genome editing.

Genetic material or gene editing tools that are inserted directly into a cell usually do not function. Instead, a carrier called a "vector" is genetically engineered to carry and deliver the material. Certain viruses are used as vectors because they can deliver the material by infecting the cell. The viruses are modified so that they cannot cause disease when used in people. Some types of viruses, such as retroviruses, integrate their genetic material (including the new gene) into a chromosome in the human cell. Other viruses, such as adenoviruses, introduce their DNA into the nucleus of the cell, but the DNA is not integrated into a chromosome. Viruses can also deliver the gene editing tools to the nucleus of the cell.

The vector can be injected or given intravenously (IV) directly into a specific tissue in the body, where it is taken up by individual cells. Alternatively, a sample of the patient's cells can be removed and exposed to the vector in a laboratory setting. The cells containing the vector are then returned to the patient. If the treatment is successful, the new gene delivered by the vector will make a functioning protein, or the editing molecules will correct a DNA error and restore protein function.

Gene therapy with viral vectors has been successful, but it does carry some risks. Sometimes, the virus triggers a dangerous immune response. In addition, vectors that integrate the genetic material into a chromosome can cause errors that lead to cancer. Researchers are developing newer technologies that can deliver genetic material or gene editing tools without using viruses. One such technique uses special structures called "nanoparticles" as vectors to deliver the genetic material or gene editing components into cells. Nanoparticles are incredibly small structures that have been developed for many uses. For gene therapy, these tiny particles are designed with specific characteristics to target them to particular cell types. Nanoparticles are less likely to cause immune reactions than viral vectors, and they are easier to design and modify for specific purposes.

Researchers continue to work to overcome the many technical challenges of gene therapy. For example, scientists are finding better ways to deliver genes or gene editing tools and target them to particular cells. They are also working to more precisely control when the treatment is functional in the body.

IS GENE THERAPY SAFE?

The first gene therapy trial was run more than 30 years ago. The earliest studies showed that gene therapy could have very serious health risks, such as toxicity, inflammation, and cancer. Since then, researchers have studied the mechanisms and developed improved techniques that are less likely to cause dangerous immune reactions or cancer. Because gene therapy techniques are relatively new, some risks may be unpredictable; however, medical researchers, institutions, and regulatory agencies are working to ensure that gene therapy research, clinical trials, and approved treatments are as safe as possible.

Comprehensive federal laws, regulations, and guidelines help protect people who participate in research studies (called "clinical trials"). The U.S. Food and Drug Administration (FDA) regulates all gene therapy products in the United States and oversees research in this area. Researchers who wish to test an approach in a clinical trial must first obtain permission from the FDA. The FDA has the authority to reject or suspend clinical trials that are suspected of being unsafe for participants.

The National Institutes of Health (NIH) also plays an important role in ensuring the safety of gene therapy research. The NIH provides guidelines for investigators and institutions (such as universities and hospitals) to follow when conducting clinical trials with gene therapy. These guidelines state that clinical trials at institutions receiving NIH funding for this type of research must be registered with the NIH Office of Biotechnology Activities. The protocol, or plan, for each clinical trial is then reviewed by the NIH Recombinant DNA Advisory Committee (RAC) to determine whether it raises medical, ethical, or safety issues that warrant further discussion at an RAC public meeting.

An Institutional Review Board (IRB) and an Institutional Biosafety Committee (IBC) must approve each gene therapy clinical trial before it can be carried out. An IRB is a committee of scientific and medical advisors and consumers that reviews all research within an institution. An IBC is a group that reviews and approves an institution's potentially hazardous research studies. Multiple levels of evaluation and oversight ensure that safety concerns are a top priority in the planning and carrying out of gene therapy research.

The clinical trial process occurs in three phases. Phase I studies determine if a treatment is safe for people and identify its side effects. Phase II studies determine if the treatment is effective, meaning whether it works. Phase III studies compare the new treatment to the current treatments available. Doctors want to know whether the new treatment works better or has fewer side effects than the standard treatment. The FDA reviews the results of the clinical trial. If it determines that the benefits of the new treatment outweigh the side effects, it approves the therapy, and doctors can use it to treat a disorder.

Successful clinical trials have led to the approval of a small number of gene therapies, including therapies to treat inherited disorders such as SMA and LCA.

WHAT ARE THE ETHICAL ISSUES SURROUNDING GENE THERAPY?

Because gene therapy involves making changes to the body's basic building blocks (DNA), it raises many unique ethical concerns. The ethical questions surrounding gene therapy and genome editing include the following:

- How can "good" and "bad" uses of these technologies be distinguished?

- Who decides which traits are normal and which constitute a disability or disorder?
- Will the high costs of gene therapy make it available only to the wealthy?
- Could the widespread use of gene therapy make society less accepting of people who are different?
- Should people be allowed to use gene therapy to enhance basic human traits such as height, intelligence, or athletic ability?

Current research on gene therapy treatment has focused on targeting body (somatic) cells such as bone marrow or blood cells. This type of genetic alteration cannot be passed to a person's children. Gene therapy could be targeted to egg and sperm cells (germ cells), however, which would allow the genetic changes to be passed to future generations. This approach is known as "germline gene therapy."

The idea of these germline alterations is controversial. While it could spare future generations in a family from having a particular genetic disorder, it might affect the development of a fetus in unexpected ways or have long-term side effects that are not yet known. Because people who would be affected by germline gene therapy are not yet born, they cannot choose whether to have the treatment. Because of these ethical concerns, the U.S. government does not allow federal funds to be used for research on germline gene therapy in people.

IS GENE THERAPY AVAILABLE TO TREAT YOUR DISORDER?

Gene therapy is currently available primarily in a research setting. The FDA has approved only a small number of gene therapy products for sale in the United States. For example, FDA-approved gene therapies are available for conditions that include a rare eye disorder called "LCA," a form of skin cancer known as "melanoma," and a genetic muscle condition called "SMA." Other genetic therapies have been approved for blood cell cancers such as lymphoma and multiple myeloma. Gene therapies to treat additional conditions have been approved in other countries.

Hundreds of research studies (clinical trials) are underway to test gene therapy as a treatment for genetic conditions, cancer, and human immunodeficiency virus (HIV)/acquired immuno-deficiency syndrome (AIDS). If you are interested in participating in a clinical trial, talk with your doctor or a genetics professional about how to participate.

WHAT ARE CHIMERIC ANTIGEN RECEPTOR T-CELL THERAPY, RIBONUCLEIC ACID THERAPY, AND OTHER GENETIC THERAPIES?

Several treatments have been developed that involve genetic material but are typically not considered gene therapy. Some of these methods alter DNA for a slightly different use than gene therapy. Others do not alter genes themselves, but they change whether or how a gene's instructions are carried out to make proteins.

Cell-Based Gene Therapy

Chimeric antigen receptor T-cell therapy (CAR T-cell therapy) is an example of cell-based gene therapy. This type of treatment combines the technologies of gene therapy and cell therapy. Cell therapy introduces cells to the body that have a particular function to help treat a disease. In cell-based gene therapy, the cells have been genetically altered to give them the special function. CAR T-cell therapy introduces a gene to a person's T cells, which are a type of immune cell. This gene provides instructions for making a protein, called the "chimeric antigen receptor" (CAR), that attaches to cancer cells. The modified immune cells can specifically attack cancer cells.

Ribonucleic Acid Therapy

Several techniques, called "ribonucleic acid (RNA) therapies," use pieces of RNA, which is a type of genetic material similar to DNA, to help treat a disorder. In many of these techniques, the pieces of RNA interact with a molecule called "messenger RNA" (mRNA). In cells, mRNA uses the information in genes to create a blueprint for making proteins. By interacting with mRNA, these therapies influence how much protein is produced from a gene, which can compensate for the effects of a genetic alteration. Examples of these RNA therapies include antisense oligonucleotide (ASO), small interfering RNA (siRNA), and microRNA (miRNA) therapies. An RNA therapy, called "RNA aptamer therapy," introduces small pieces of RNA that attach directly to proteins to alter their function.

Epigenetic Therapy

Another gene-related therapy, called "epigenetic therapy," affects epigenetic changes in cells. Epigenetic changes are specific modifications (often called "tags") attached to DNA that control whether genes are turned on or off. Abnormal patterns of epigenetic modifications alter gene activity and, subsequently, protein production. Epigenetic therapies are used to correct epigenetic errors that underlie genetic disorders.

WHAT ARE MRNA VACCINES, AND HOW DO THEY WORK?

Vaccines help prevent infection by preparing the body to fight foreign invaders (such as bacteria, viruses, or other pathogens). All vaccines introduce into the body a harmless piece of a particular bacterium or virus, triggering an immune response. Most vaccines contain a weakened or dead bacterium or virus. However, scientists have developed a new type of vaccine that uses a molecule called "mRNA" rather than part of an actual bacterium or virus. mRNA is a type of RNA that is necessary for protein production. Once cells finish making a protein, they quickly break down the mRNA. mRNA from vaccines does not enter the nucleus and does not alter DNA.

mRNA vaccines work by introducing a piece of mRNA that corresponds to a viral protein, usually a small piece of a protein found on the virus's outer membrane. (Individuals who get an mRNA vaccine are not exposed to the virus, nor can they become infected with the virus by the vaccine.) By using this mRNA, cells can produce the viral protein. As part of a normal immune response, the immune system recognizes that the protein is foreign and produces specialized proteins called "antibodies." Antibodies help protect the body against infection by recognizing individual viruses or other pathogens, attaching to them, and marking the pathogens for destruction. Once produced, antibodies remain in the body, even after the body has rid itself of the pathogen so that the immune system can quickly respond if exposed again. If a person is exposed to a virus after receiving mRNA vaccination for it, antibodies can quickly recognize it, attach to it, and mark it for destruction before it can cause serious illness.

Like all vaccines in the United States, mRNA vaccines require authorization or approval from the FDA before they can be used. Currently, vaccines for coronavirus disease of 2019 (COVID-19), the disease caused by the severe acute respiratory syndrome coronavirus 2 (SARS-CoV-2), are the only authorized or approved mRNA vaccines. These vaccines use mRNA that directs cells to produce copies of a protein on the outside of the coronavirus known as the "spike protein." Researchers are studying how mRNA might be used to develop vaccines for additional diseases.[1]

THERAPY REPAIRS THE RAVAGED IMMUNE SYSTEM

Gene therapy can safely restore immune function in children with severe combined immunodeficiency (SCID) and allow some to stop taking painful weekly injections. The finding, from a small clinical trial, offers hope for children born with this deadly condition.

Children with SCID cannot produce healthy microbe-fighting white blood cells (WBCs) called "lymphocytes." As a result, these children are susceptible to a wide range of infections. Most die by the age of two if untreated.

One type of SCID arises from a faulty gene for the enzyme adenosine deaminase (ADA). Without this enzyme, toxic compounds build up in the body and inhibit the production of lymphocytes. Once- or twice-weekly injections of ADA can partly restore immune function. But this therapy is expensive and must continue for a lifetime.

---

[1] MedlinePlus, "What Is Gene Therapy?" National Institutes of Health (NIH), February 28, 2022. Available online. URL: https://medlineplus.gov/genetics/understanding/therapy/genetherapy. Accessed May 25, 2023.

For two decades, researchers have been exploring an alternative approach that uses gene therapy to replace the damaged *ADA* gene in the blood-forming stem cells found in the bone marrow. But they have had trouble developing a method that effectively raises ADA levels and leads to lasting improvements in immune function.

An 11-year effort to test two different gene therapy regimens was led by Dr. Donald B. Kohn of the University of California, Los Angeles, and Dr. Fabio Candotti of the NIH's National Human Genome Research Institute (NHGRI). The research was supported in part by several NIH components, including the National Heart, Lung, and Blood Institute (NHLBI). The results appeared on September 11, 2012, in the online edition of *Blood*.

Ten patients with ADA-deficient SCID were treated at either the NIH Clinical Center or the Children's Hospital Los Angeles. Blood-forming stem cells were isolated from their bone marrow. The cells were treated with retroviral vectors, which delivered healthy *ADA* genes. The corrected cells were then infused back into the patients' bloodstream.

The first four patients remained on ADA replacement therapy throughout the gene therapy procedure and follow-up. Although the gene therapy had no negative effect, it did not improve ADA function. The scientists suspect that ongoing enzyme replacement therapy might have diluted the number of corrected lymphocytes in the patients' immune systems. As a result, the corrected cells could not establish themselves.

For the six additional patients, the doctors modified the treatment. Enzyme replacement therapy was stopped before the procedure, and patients received low-dose chemotherapy, which depletes bone marrow stem cells. "This step proved to be important," says Dr. Candotti. "By adjusting the chemotherapy dosage, we found its optimal level for enhancing the efficacy of the corrected stem cells."

Three children who received the refined procedure have had improved health for up to five years and have not needed enzyme replacement injections. The other three patients did not have lasting improvements from the procedure. Now that the scientists have identified a regimen that can be effective, eight children have been added to a second phase of the study.

"We are encouraged by the outcome of our gene therapy trial," Dr. Candotti says. "We will continue to follow the progress of our patients and to enroll those who can benefit from this promising gene therapy strategy."[2]

[2] "Therapy Repairs Ravaged Immune System," National Institutes of Health (NIH), October 1, 2012. Available online. URL: www.nih.gov/news-events/nih-research-matters/therapy-repairs-ravaged-immune-system. Accessed May 25, 2023.

Chapter 63 | **Stem Cell Transplantation**

The body's main line of defense against invasion by infectious organisms is the immune system. To succeed, an immune system must distinguish the many cellular components of its own body (self) from the cells or components of invading organisms (nonself). "Nonself" should be attacked while "self" should not. Therefore, two general types of errors can be made by the immune system. If the immune system fails to quickly detect and destroy an invading organism, an infection will result. However, if the immune system fails to recognize self cells or components and mistakenly attacks them, the result is known as an "autoimmune disease."

HOW DOES THE IMMUNE SYSTEM NORMALLY KEEP YOU HEALTHY?

The "soldiers" of the immune system are white blood cells (WBCs), including T and B lymphocytes, which originate in the bone marrow from hematopoietic stem cells. Every day the body comes into contact with many organisms such as bacteria, viruses, and parasites. Unopposed, these organisms have the potential to cause serious infections, such as pneumonia or acquired immunodeficiency syndrome (AIDS). When a healthy individual is infected, the body responds by activating a variety of immune cells. Initially, invading bacteria or viruses are engulfed by an antigen-presenting cell (APC), and their component proteins (antigens) are cut into pieces and displayed on the cell's surface.

Pieces of the foreign protein (antigen) bind to the major histocompatibility complex (MHC) proteins, also known as "human leukocyte antigen" (HLA) molecules, on the surface of the APCs.

This complex, formed by a foreign protein and an MHC protein, then binds to a T-cell receptor (TCR) on the surface of another type of immune cell, the CD4 helper T-cell. They are so named because they "help" immune responses proceed and have a protein called "CD4" on their surface. This complex enables these T cells to focus the immune response to a specific invading organism.

The antigen-specific CD4 helper T cells divide and multiply while secreting substances called "cytokines," which cause inflammation and help activate other immune cells. The particular cytokines secreted by the CD4 helper T cells act on cells known as the "CD8 cytotoxic T cells" (because they can kill the cells that are infected by the invading organism and have the CD8 protein on their surface). The helper T cells can also activate antigen-specific B cells to produce antibodies, which can neutralize and help eliminate bacteria and viruses from the body. Some of the antigen-specific T and B cells that are activated to rid the body of infectious organisms become long-lived "memory" cells. Memory cells have the capacity to act quickly when confronted with the same infectious organism at later times. It is the memory cells that cause us to become "immune" from later reinfections with the same organism.

HOW DO THE IMMUNE CELLS OF THE BODY KNOW WHAT TO ATTACK AND WHAT NOT TO?

All immune and blood cells develop from multipotent hematopoietic stem cells that originate in the bone marrow. Upon their departure from the bone marrow, immature T cells undergo a final maturation process in the thymus, a small organ located in the upper chest, before being dispersed to the body with the rest of the immune cells (e.g., B cells). Within the thymus, T cells undergo an important process that "educates" them to distinguish between self (the proteins of their own body) and nonself (the invading organism's) antigens. Here, the T cells are selected for their ability to bind to the particular MHC proteins expressed by the individual. The particular array of MHCs varies slightly between individuals, and this variation is the basis of the immune response when a transplanted organ is rejected. MHCs and other less easily characterized molecules called "minor histocompatibility antigens (MiHAs)" are genetically determined, and this is the reason why donor organs from relatives of the recipient are preferred over unrelated donors.

In the bone marrow, a highly diverse and random array of T cells is produced. Collectively, these T cells are capable of recognizing an almost unlimited number of antigens. Because the process of generating a T cell's antigen specificity is a random one, many immature T cells have the potential to react with the body's own (self) proteins. To avoid this potential disaster, the thymus provides an environment where T cells that recognize self-antigens (autoreactive or self-reactive T cells) are deleted or inactivated in a process called "tolerance induction."

Tolerance usually ensures that T cells do not attack the "auto-antigens" (self-proteins) of the body. Given the importance of this task, it is not surprising that there are multiple checkpoints for destroying or inactivating T cells that might react to auto-antigens.

Autoimmune diseases arise when this intricate system for the induction and maintenance of immune tolerance fails. These diseases result in cell and tissue destruction by antigen-specific CD8 cytotoxic T cells or autoantibodies (antibodies to self-proteins) and the accompanying inflammatory process. These mechanisms can lead to the destruction of the joints in RA, the destruction of the insulin-producing beta cells of the pancreas in type 1 diabetes, or damage to the kidneys in lupus. The reasons for the failure to induce or maintain tolerance are enigmatic. However, genetic factors, along with environmental and hormonal influences and certain infections, may contribute to tolerance and the development of autoimmune disease.

HEMATOPOIETIC STEM CELL THERAPY FOR AUTOIMMUNE DISEASES

The current treatments for many autoimmune diseases include the systemic use of anti-inflammatory drugs and potent immunosuppressive and immunomodulatory agents (i.e., steroids and inhibitor proteins that block the action of inflammatory cytokines). However, despite their profound effect on immune responses, these therapies are unable to induce clinically significant remissions in certain patients. In years, researchers have contemplated the use of stem cells to treat autoimmune disorders. Discussed here are some of the rationales for this approach, with a focus on experimental stem cell therapies for lupus, RA, and type 1 diabetes.

The immune-mediated injury in autoimmune diseases can be organ-specific, such as type 1 diabetes, which is the consequence of the destruction of the pancreatic beta islet cells, or MS, which results from the breakdown of the myelin covering of nerves. These autoimmune diseases are amenable to treatments involving the repair or replacement of damaged or destroyed cells or tissue. In contrast, nonorgan-specific autoimmune diseases, such as lupus, are characterized by widespread injury due to immune reactions against many different organs and tissues.

One approach is being evaluated in early clinical trials of patients with poorly responsive, life-threatening lupus. This is a severe disease affecting multiple organs in the body including muscles, skin, joints, and kidneys as well as the brain and nerves. Over 239,000 Americans, of which more than 90 percent are women, suffer from lupus. In addition, lupus disproportionately afflicts African American and Hispanic women. A major obstacle in the treatment of nonorgan-specific autoimmune diseases such as lupus is the lack of a single specific target for the application of therapy.

The objective of hematopoietic stem cell therapy for lupus is to destroy the mature, long-lived, and autoreactive immune cells and to generate a new, properly functioning immune system. In most of these trials, the patient's own stem cells have been used in a procedure known as "autologous (from "one's self") hematopoietic stem cell transplantation." First, patients receive injections of a growth factor, which coaxes large numbers of hematopoietic stem cells to be released from the bone marrow into the bloodstream. These cells are harvested from the blood, purified away from mature immune cells, and stored. After sufficient quantities of these cells are obtained, the patient undergoes a regimen of cytotoxic (cell-killing) drug and/or radiation therapy, which eliminates the mature immune cells. Then, the hematopoietic stem cells are returned to the patient via a blood transfusion into the circulation where they migrate to the bone marrow and begin to differentiate to become mature immune cells. The body's immune system is then restored. Nonetheless, the recovery phase, until the immune system is reconstituted, represents a period of dramatically increased susceptibility to bacterial, fungal, and viral infection, making this a high-risk therapy.

Reports suggest that this replacement therapy may fundamentally alter the patient's immune system. Richard Burt and his colleagues conducted a long-term follow-up (one to three years) of seven lupus patients who underwent this procedure and found that they remained free from active lupus and improved continuously after transplantation, without the need for immunosuppressive medications. One of the hallmarks of lupus is that during the natural progression of the disease, the normally diverse repertoire of T cells becomes limited in the number of different antigens they recognize, suggesting that an increasing proportion of the patient's T cells are autoreactive. Burt and colleagues found that following hematopoietic stem cell transplantation, levels of T-cell diversity were restored to those of healthy individuals. This finding provides evidence that stem cell replacement may be beneficial in reestablishing tolerance in T cells, thereby decreasing the likelihood of disease reoccurrence.

DEVELOPMENT OF HEMATOPOIETIC STEM CELL LINES FOR TRANSPLANTATION

The ability to generate and propagate unlimited numbers of hematopoietic stem cells outside the body—whether from adult, umbilical cord blood, fetal, or embryonic sources—would have a major impact on the safety, cost, and availability of stem cells for transplantation. The current approach of isolating hematopoietic stem cells from a patient's own peripheral blood places the patient at risk for a flare-up of their autoimmune disease. This is a potential consequence of repeated administration of the stem cell growth factors needed to mobilize hematopoietic stem cells from the bone marrow to the bloodstream in numbers sufficient for transplantation. In addition, contamination of the purified hematopoietic stem cells with the patient's mature autoreactive T and B cells could affect the success of the treatment in some patients. Propagation of pure cell lines in the laboratory would avoid these potential drawbacks and increase the number of stem cells available to each patient, thus shortening the at-risk interval before full immune reconstitution.

Whether embryonic stem cells will provide advantages over stem cells derived from cord blood or adult bone marrow hematopoietic stem cells remains to be determined. However, hematopoietic stem cells, whether from umbilical cord blood or bone marrow, have a more limited potential for self-renewal than pluripotent embryonic stem cells. Although information will be needed to direct the differentiation of embryonic stem cells into hematopoietic stem cells, hematopoietic cells are present in differentiated cultures from human embryonic stem cells and from human-fetal-derived embryonic germ stem cells.

One potential advantage of using hematopoietic stem cell lines for transplantation in patients with autoimmune diseases is that these cells could be generated from unaffected individuals or, as predisposing genetic factors are defined, from embryonic stem cells lacking these genetic influences. In addition, the use of genetically selected or genetically engineered cell types may further limit the possibility of disease progression or reemergence.

One risk of using nonself hematopoietic stem cells is the immune rejection of the transplanted cells. Immune rejection is caused by MHC protein differences between the donor and the patient (recipient). In this scenario, the transplanted hematopoietic stem cells and their progeny are rejected by the patient's own T cells, which are originating from the patient's surviving bone marrow hematopoietic stem cells. In this regard, embryonic stem-cell-derived hematopoietic stem cells may offer distinct advantages over cord blood and bone marrow hematopoietic stem cell lines in avoiding rejection of the transplant. Theoretically, banks of embryonic stem cells expressing various combinations of the three most critical MHC proteins could be generated to allow close matching to the recipient's MHC composition.

Additionally, there is evidence that embryonic stem cells are considerably more receptive to genetic manipulation than hematopoietic stem cells.

This characteristic means that embryonic stem cells could be useful in strategies that could prevent their recognition by the patient's surviving immune cells. For example, it may be possible to introduce the recipient's MHC proteins into embryonic stem cells through targeted gene transfer. Alternatively, it is theoretically possible to generate a universal donor embryonic stem cell line by genetic alteration or removal of the MHC proteins. Researchers have accomplished this by genetically altering a mouse so that it has little or no surface expression of MHC molecules on any of the cells or tissues. There is no rejection of pancreatic beta islet cells from these genetically altered mice when the cells are transplanted into completely MHC-mismatched mice. Additional research will be needed to determine the feasibility of these alternative strategies for the prevention of graft rejection in humans.

Jon Odorico, M.D., Faculty, UW School of Medicine and Public Health, and colleagues have shown that the expression of MHC proteins on mouse embryonic stem cells and differentiated embryonic stem cell progeny is either absent or greatly decreased compared with MHC expression on adult cells. These preliminary findings raise the intriguing possibility that lines derived from embryonic stem cells may be inherently less susceptible to rejection by the recipient's immune system than lines derived from adult cells. This could have important implications for the transplantation of cells other than hematopoietic stem cells.

Another potential advantage of using pure populations of donor hematopoietic stem cells achieved through stem cell technologies would be a lower incidence and severity of graft versus host disease, a potentially fatal complication of bone marrow transplantation. Graft versus host disease results from the immune-mediated injury to recipient tissues that occurs when mature organ-donor T cells remain within the organ at the time of transplant. Such mature donor alloreactive T cells would be absent from pure populations of multipotent hematopoietic stem cells, and under ideal conditions of immune tolerance induction in the recipient's thymus, the donor-derived mature T-cell population would be tolerant to the host.

GENE THERAPY AND STEM CELL APPROACHES FOR THE TREATMENT OF AUTOIMMUNE DISEASES

Gene therapy is the genetic modification of cells to produce a therapeutic effect. In most investigational protocols, DNA containing the therapeutic gene is transferred into cultured cells, and these cells are subsequently administered to the animal or patient. DNA can also be injected directly, entering cells at the site of the injection or in the circulation. Under ideal conditions, cells take up the DNA and produce the therapeutic protein encoded by the gene.

Currently, there is an extensive amount of gene therapy research being conducted in animal models of autoimmune diseases. The goal is to modify the aberrant, inflammatory immune response that is characteristic of autoimmune diseases. Researchers most often use one of two general strategies to modulate the immune system. The first strategy is to block the actions of an inflammatory cytokine (secreted by certain activated immune cells and inflamed tissues) by transferring a gene into cells that encodes a "decoy" receptor for that cytokine. Alternatively, a gene is transferred that encodes an anti-inflammatory cytokine, redirecting the auto-inflammatory immune response to a more "tolerant" state. In many animal studies, promising results have been achieved by using these approaches, and the studies have an advanced understanding of the disease processes and the particular inflammatory cytokines involved in disease progression.

Serious obstacles to the development of effective gene therapies for humans remain, however. Foremost among these are the difficulty of reliably transferring genetic material into adult and slowly dividing cells (including hematopoietic stem cells) and of producing long-lasting expression of the intended protein at levels that can be tightly controlled in response to disease activity. Importantly, embryonic stem cells are substantially more permissive to gene transfer than adult cells, and embryonic cells sustain protein expression during extensive self-renewal. Whether adult-derived stem cells, other than hematopoietic stem cells, are similarly amenable to gene transfer has not yet been determined.

Ultimately, stem cell gene therapy should allow the development of novel methods for immune modulation in autoimmune diseases. One example is the genetic modification of hematopoietic stem cells or differentiated tissue cells with a "decoy" receptor for the inflammatory cytokine interferon gamma to treat lupus.

Researchers are exploring similar genetic approaches to prevent progressive joint destruction and loss of cartilage and to repair damaged joints in animal models of RA. RA is a debilitating auto-immune disease characterized by acute and chronic inflammation, in which the immune system primarily attacks the joints of the body. In a study, investigators genetically transferred an anti-inflammatory cytokine, interleukin-4 (IL-4), into a specialized, highly efficient APC, called a "dendritic cell," and then injected these IL-4-secreting cells into mice that can be induced to develop a form of arthritis similar to RA in humans. These IL-4-secreting dendritic cells are presumed to act on the CD4 helper T cells to reintroduce tolerance to self-proteins. Treated mice showed complete suppression of their disease, and, in addition to its immune-modulatory properties, IL-4 blocked bone resorption (a serious complication of RA), making it a particularly attractive cytokine for this therapy. However, one obstacle to this approach is that human dendritic cells are difficult to isolate in large numbers.

Investigators have also directed the differentiation of dendritic cells from mouse embryonic stem cells, indicating that a stem-cell-based approach might work in patients with RA. Longer-term follow-up and further characterization will be needed in animal models before researchers proceed with the development of such an approach in humans. In similar studies, using other inhibitors of inflammatory cytokines, such as a decoy receptor for tumor necrosis factor-A (a prominent inflammatory cytokine in inflamed joints), an inhibitor of nuclear factor-κB (a protein within cells that turns on the production of many inflammatory cytokines), and interleukin-13 (an anti-inflammatory cytokine), researchers have shown promising results in animal models of RA. Because of the complexity and redundancy of immune system signaling networks, it is likely that a multifaceted approach involving inhibitors of several different inflammatory cytokines will be successful, whereas approaches targeting single cytokines might fail or produce only short-lived responses. In addition, other cell types may prove to be even better vehicles for the delivery of gene therapy in this disease.

Chondrocytes, cells that build cartilage in joints, may provide another avenue for stem-cell-based treatment of RA. These cells have been derived from human bone marrow stromal stem cells. Little is known about the intermediate cells that ultimately differentiate into chondrocytes. In addition to the adult bone marrow as a source for stromal stem cells, human embryonic stem cells can differentiate into precursor cells believed to lead ultimately to the stromal stem cells. However, extensive research is needed to reliably achieve the directed derivation of the stromal stem cells from embryonic stem cells and, subsequently, the differentiation of chondrocytes from these stromal stem cells.

The ideal cell for optimum cartilage repair may be a more primitive cell than the chondrocyte, such as the stromal cell, or an intermediate cell in the pathway (e.g., a connective tissue precursor) leading to the chondrocyte. Stromal stem cells can generate new chondrocytes and facilitate cartilage repair in a rabbit model. Such cells may also prove to be ideal targets for the delivery of immune-modulatory gene therapy. As hematopoietic stem cells, stromal stem cells have been used in animal models for the delivery of gene therapy. For example, a study demonstrated that genetically engineered chondrocytes, expressing a growth factor, can enhance the function of transplanted chondrocytes.

Two obstacles to the use of adult stromal stem cells or chondrocytes are the limited numbers of these cells that can be harvested and the difficulties in propagating them in the laboratory. Embryonic stem cells, genetically modified and expanded before directed differentiation to a connective tissue stem cell, may be an attractive alternative.

Collectively, these results illustrate the tremendous potential these cells may offer for the treatment of RA and other autoimmune diseases.[1]

[1] Stem Cell Information, "Autoimmune Diseases and the Promise of Stem Cell-Based," National Institutes of Health (NIH), June 17, 2001. Available online. URL: https://stemcells.nih.gov/info/2001report/chapter6.htm. Accessed May 29, 2023.

Part 8 | Coping with Immune Diseases

Chapter 64 | **Coping with Autoimmune and Immune Disorders**

Autoimmune disorders occur when the immune system misidentifies the body's healthy cells and tissues as foreign invaders (viruses and bacteria) and releases autoantibodies to target healthy cells. An immune disease is distinguished by common inflammatory pathways that lead to inflammation resulting in the dysregulation of the normal immune response. On the one hand, statistics from 2018 by American Autoimmune Related Disorders Association (AARDA) show that around 50 million Americans have a chronic autoimmune condition, but on the other hand, studies say it takes several years to diagnose these conditions.

However, with appropriate medical support and effective changes in one's lifestyle, environment, and working conditions, one is able to cope with these disorders and live a successful, fulfilling, and productive life. Though there are different ways to cope with these disorders, the two most essential steps are to learn to accept one's sense of self and invest in patience within relationships, as disorders like these are lifelong conditions. An individual will benefit much from speaking about the condition with the nearest of kin who could, in turn, support in coping with the illness.

EXPLAIN YOUR ILLNESS
It is very important for your family and friends to know what you are going through, and it is essential that you understand your disease.

Therefore, a good start upon diagnosis is to read about the illness and be informed about what may or may not happen. This knowledge will empower you enough to explain to your family exactly what happens to your body due to this illness—which, in turn, will help your family and friends support you however they can.

TALK WITH YOUR CHILDREN

Make sure you prepare your family well so that they can adjust to this change. Most importantly, if you have children, talk to them about your illness and explain how it may affect life at home.

LIFE AFTER DIAGNOSIS

It may happen that you live in denial for a long time and ignore that you have been diagnosed with a condition that will alter the course of your life. You may go about your routine as usual. But these responses—or the lack thereof—may worsen your condition. Therefore, it is important to acknowledge the diagnosis and get on with your life, which does not necessarily mean giving in to the disease. Fight the disease, but do not ignore you are having it.

KICK-START YOURSELF

Although it is critical to learn as much as you can about the condition of your health, paradoxically, it is also necessary that you divert your focus from the disease. Even though many changes in your lifestyle may be required after you are diagnosed with an autoimmune or immune disease, it is necessary that you take time for yourself and do what you have always enjoyed doing. This will help you transition to a "new normal" while remaining connected with the "old you."

TAKE THE DRUGS AS PRESCRIBED

In some cases, the only way to keep the disease under check is by taking prescribed doses of medications. This reality may not suit everyone's lifestyle, and you may experience adverse side effects.

Hence, before taking your medications, know and understand the risks and possible side effects, which may help you avoid any adverse effects.

IDENTIFY WORK-AROUNDS

Many people can continue to work or go to school after being diagnosed with an autoimmune or immune disorder. Depending on the disease and its symptoms, you may continue with the job at hand or look for a change. In some scenarios, quitting your job or school altogether might be the best decision for your health.

- **Disability benefits**. Seek information about benefits for people with disabilities from your company's human resources office or the Social Security Administration (SSA). Also, there is a policy concerning benefits in the Americans with Disabilities Act (ADA), which the employer should offer to help a person meet the requirements for his or her job.
- **Relax your child's routine**. Analyses have shown that even children afflicted with autoimmune and immune disorders succeed in school. For children to do well in school, besides keeping a check on their health, make sure you:
  - do not overload their schedule
  - leave time for relaxation
  - communicate with the school about the medical condition of the child
  - learn about financial assistance opportunities—your child might be eligible for federal financial aid and several scholarship programs

FIND THE SUPPORT YOU NEED

It is always recommended to be socially connected if you have any autoimmune or immune disorders. Social networks and forums will help you understand your condition better and act as support systems.

The following are other ways you can find reinforcement:
- **Individual therapy**. This therapy can help you deal with anxiety and depression related to your illness.
- **Couples therapy**. This therapy can help you find support for yourself and your partner to cope with the diagnosis.
- **Online support group**. This type of group can help you connect with other people affected by the same disorder as yours.

Life with an autoimmune or immune disease might be challenging; however, it does not mean you have to stop doing things that matter to you. Like any other average person, you, too, can balance your health and life.

References

"Coping with Lupus: A Guide," Lupus Foundation of America, January 12, 2018. Available online. URL: www. lupus.org/resources/coping-with-lupus-guide. Accessed April 19, 2023.

Tucker, Miriam E. "Closing the Care Gap in Autoimmune Disease," The Autoimmune Association, October 5, 2018. Available online. URL: https://autoimmune.org/closing-care-gap-autoimmune-disease. Accessed April 19, 2023.

Watson, Stephanie. "Autoimmune Diseases: Types, Symptoms, Causes, and More," Healthline, July 15, 2022. Available online. URL: www.healthline.com/health/autoimmune-disorders. Accessed April 19, 2023.

"Who Am I Now? Living with an Autoimmune Disease," Hospital for Special Surgery (HSS), August 23, 2012. Available online. URL: www.hss.edu/conditions_who-am-i-now-living-with-autoimmune-disease.asp. Accessed April 19, 2023.

Chapter 65 | **Autoimmune Community**

Individuals and families affected by rare medical conditions might look to nonprofit support and advocacy groups for different reasons. Some may want to find other people who understand how having the condition affects their lives. Others are searching for medical information, treatment options, the latest research, or financial-aid resources. This guide will help you learn more about the different types of information and services offered by nonprofit support and advocacy groups. The information about how to connect with others is also included when your specific condition does not have a support and advocacy group.

Nonprofit support and advocacy groups may be referred to as "nonprofits," "patient support groups," "condition-specific organizations," "advocacy groups," "public charities," or "registered charities." These terms tend to be used interchangeably rather than being specific to the focus of the group. It is best to look beyond the label to find out what the group offers. In the remainder of this chapter, these groups will be referred to as "nonprofit advocacy groups."

WHAT ARE THE DIFFERENT TYPES OF NONPROFIT ADVOCACY GROUPS?
- **Condition-specific groups**. Many nonprofit advocacy groups focus on one rare or genetic condition or a group of closely related conditions. Condition-specific groups often vary in their mission or focus. For example, some groups may focus on providing support or driving research, while other groups will offer a range of services,

such as helping you find a doctor, organizing conferences, or working to gain the support of local, state, or federal legislators.

- **Umbrella groups or alliances**. Nonprofit advocacy groups may join together to tackle larger issues, such as advocating for legislation to help or protect all individuals with rare and genetic conditions. Umbrella groups include the National Organization for Rare Disorders (NORD), Genetic Alliance, Global Genes, and European Rare Disease Organisation (EURORDIS). Examples of their accomplishments include the passage of the Orphan Drug Act, the Genetic and Information Nondiscrimination Act (GINA), and the European Union Regulation on Orphan Medicinal Products. These groups may also provide information and resources for specific medical conditions, but their activities and resources tend to be focused more on helping the rare disease community at large.
- **General support groups**. Some nonprofit advocacy groups focus on a symptom that may have many different causes, such as vision loss or developmental disabilities. Other groups may focus on a part of the body or a body system, such as the liver or the immune system. These groups tend to offer general information and resources that may help anyone dealing with challenges addressed by the group. For example, the Center for Parent Information and Resources (www.parentcenterhub.org) offers services to any family who has a child with disabilities.

WHAT DO NONPROFIT ADVOCACY GROUPS DO?

Nonprofit advocacy groups typically offer the following types of services. Individual groups may not provide all of these services, so it is important to check each group's website or contact them to learn more about what they offer.

- **Support**. Most nonprofit advocacy groups help people connect with each other. Ways to connect online may include Facebook, blogs, Listservs, Yahoo groups, and Twitter chats. Groups may provide opportunities to meet in person at yearly conferences, summer camps, or local meetings. Whether in person or online, support from others can empower you to take charge of your health.

- **Medical information**. Most nonprofit advocacy groups provide medical information in easy-to-understand terms to help you learn more about your medical condition, available treatment options, and current research. Information is often on the group's website but may also be available by mail, phone, or email. If you do call and leave a voice mail or send an email, keep in mind that many groups have a very small staff, so it may take a few days to get a reply.

- **Resources**. Nonprofit advocacy groups often have a list of helpful resources, such as related nonprofit advocacy groups, financial assistance resources, and sources for special medical equipment. They may also be able to give advice on dealing with school or health insurance issues.

- **List of doctors or clinics**. Many nonprofit advocacy groups have a list of medical-care professionals and clinics to help you find specialists with experience in diagnosing or treating a rare medical condition. Groups may work closely with clinical centers, sometimes called "Centers of Excellence," or be involved in the training of specialists. Other nonprofit advocacy groups may have a list of doctors recommended by their members. Many groups also have a medical advisory board made up of experts in the field. If you cannot find this information on the group's website, call or email the group to see if they can provide you with a list of doctors or clinics.

- **Registry**. A registry is a collection of information about individuals, usually focused on a specific diagnosis or medical condition. Many rare disease registries are maintained by nonprofit advocacy groups to help advance medical research for a particular medical condition. If the group does not have its own disease registry, it may know of an appropriate registry for your medical condition.

- **Research and clinical trials**. Clinical trials are medical research studies in which people participate as volunteers. These studies may be evaluating new treatments or medications, searching for the cause(s) of a medical condition, or researching how the symptoms of the condition change over a person's lifetime. Whether you are interested in enrolling in a clinical trial or aim to stay aware of potential new treatments and advances, you may want to find a nonprofit advocacy group that provides information about the latest medical research. Some groups raise money to offer grants to medical researchers or pharmaceutical companies who are developing new treatments. Often, these groups will keep information on their website about the progress of supported research.
- **Advocacy**. Advocacy for a rare medical condition may involve educating the public or the medical community about the condition. A group may also take issues to local, state, and federal governments in an effort to pass legislation that will improve the lives of those affected by rare and genetic conditions.

WHAT SHOULD YOU LOOK FOR IN A SUPPORT AND ADVOCACY GROUP?

Evaluating a group is not always easy. When you are looking for a nonprofit advocacy group, you want to make certain that the group offers helpful and up-to-date information. The mission statement of the group can help you understand the focus of the group's activities. Also, look at who is involved in running the group. The group's staff members may have the medical condition themselves or have an affected family member. Other staff members may have a degree in a related field, such as social work, public health, education, communication, or medicine.

Learn about the group's funding sources and how they spend donations. The activities of 501(c)(3) groups are strictly regulated, which makes certain that the donations and grants are used properly. A similar status in many European countries is registered charity. Some groups have a membership fee, have corporate sponsors, or use website advertisements. If you cannot afford the membership fee, contact the group to see if it can be waived.

WHAT IF YOU CANNOT FIND A NONPROFIT ADVOCACY GROUP?

In some cases, a condition does not have a specific nonprofit advocacy group. The following online resources can help you search for other people with your diagnosis:

- **Social media sites**. These sites can be a great way to connect with others, especially if a medical condition is very rare. You can try searching for the condition name on Facebook to find a group. Other social media tools, such as Twitter, may also be options for rare and genetic conditions. Medical information that is suggested by others on social media is usually not reviewed by medical professionals, so it is suggested to discuss any medical recommendations with your doctor or another trusted medical-care professional.
- **GenomeConnect**. This is an online tool (www. clinicalgenome.org/genomeconnect/for-patients-genomeconnect) people can use to share their genetic test results and health information with researchers and health-care providers. You can also connect with other individuals who have a similar diagnosis or related symptoms.
- **MyGene²**. This is an online tool (www.mygene2. org/MyGene2) that families, who are interested in sharing their health and genetic information, can use to connect with other families, clinicians, and researchers.
- **RareConnect**. This platform (www.rareconnect. org/en/communities) has online communities for patients and families with rare medical conditions so they can connect with others and share their

experiences. The project is a joint collaboration between EURORDIS and NORD.

- **RareShare**. This online social hub (rareshare. org) is dedicated to patients, families, and health-care professionals who are affected by rare medical disorders.
- **DNAandU.org**. This is a website and has a blog page that collects firsthand stories from people making tough decisions about using genomic (deoxyribonucleic acid (DNA)) information in their own health-care choices.[1]

---

[1] Genetic and Rare Diseases Information Center (GARD), "Support for Patients and Families," National Center for Advancing Translational Sciences (NCATS), August 11, 2016. Available online. URL: https://rarediseases.info. nih.gov/guides/pages/120/support-for-patients-and-families. Accessed May 29, 2023.

Chapter 66 | **Immunization Recommendations for People with a Weakened Immune System**

Getting vaccinated is one of the safest ways for you to protect your health. Vaccines help prevent the getting and spreading of serious diseases that could result in poor health, missed work, medical bills, and not being able to care for the family.

ASPLENIA
Vaccines You Need
Vaccines are especially critical for people with chronic health conditions such as asplenia (without a functioning spleen) to protect them from vaccine-preventable diseases. In addition to vaccines recommended for all adults (coronavirus disease 2019 (COVID-19), influenza (flu), and tetanus, diphtheria, and pertussis (Tdap) or tetanus and diphtheria (Td) vaccines), make sure you are up-to-date on the following vaccines:
- *Haemophilus influenzae* type b (Hib) vaccine
- meningococcal vaccines—both MenACWY and MenB
- pneumococcal vaccine

You May Need Other Vaccines, Too

You may need other vaccines based on your age or other factors, too. Talk with your doctor to find out which vaccines are recommended for you. These may include the following:

- **Chickenpox vaccine (varicella)**. It is recommended for all adults born in 1980 or later.
- **Hepatitis B virus (HBV) vaccine**. It is recommended for all adults up to 59 years of age and for some adults aged 60 and over with known risk factors.
- **Human papillomavirus (HPV) vaccine**. It is recommended for all adults up to 26 years of age and for some adults aged 27–45.
- **Measles, mumps, and rubella (MMR) vaccine**. It is recommended for all adults born in 1957 or later.
- **Shingles vaccine (zoster)**. It is recommended for all adults aged 50 and over.

DIABETES, TYPE 1 AND TYPE 2
Vaccines You Need

People with diabetes (both type 1 and type 2) are at higher risk of serious problems, including hospitalization or death, from certain vaccine-preventable diseases. Vaccines are one of the safest ways for you to protect your health, even if you are taking prescription medications. In addition to vaccines recommended for all adults (COVID-19, flu, and Tdap or Td), make sure you are up-to-date on the pneumococcal vaccine.

You May Need Other Vaccines, Too

You may need other vaccines based on your age or other factors, too. Talk with your doctor to find out which vaccines are recommended for you. These may include the following:

- **Chickenpox vaccine (varicella)**. It is recommended for all adults born in 1980 or later.

- **HBV vaccine**. It is recommended for all adults up to 59 years of age and for some adults aged 60 and over with known risk factors.
- **HPV vaccine**. It is recommended for all adults up to 26 years of age and for some adults aged 27–45.
- **MMR vaccine**. It is recommended for all adults born in 1957 or later.
- **Shingles vaccine (zoster)**. It is recommended for all adults aged 50 and over.

HEART DISEASE, STROKE, OR OTHER CARDIOVASCULAR DISEASES
Vaccines You Need

People with heart disease and those who have suffered stroke are at higher risk of serious problems or complications from certain vaccine-preventable diseases. Other vaccine-preventable diseases, such as the flu, can even increase the risk of another heart attack. In addition to vaccines recommended for all adults (COVID-19, flu, and Tdap or Td), make sure you are up-to-date on the pneumococcal vaccine.

You May Need Other Vaccines, Too

You may need other vaccines based on your age or other factors, too. Talk with your cardiologist or primary care doctor to find out which vaccines are recommended for you. These may include the following:
- **Chickenpox vaccine (varicella)**. It is recommended for all adults born in 1980 or later.
- **HBV vaccine**. It is recommended for all adults up to 59 years of age and for some adults aged 60 and over with known risk factors.
- **HPV vaccine**. It is recommended for all adults up to 26 years of age and for some adults aged 27–45.
- **MMR vaccine**. It is recommended for all adults born in 1957 or later.
- **Shingles vaccine (zoster)**. It is recommended for all adults aged 50 and over.

HUMAN IMMUNODEFICIENCY VIRUS INFECTION
Vaccines You Need
Vaccines are especially critical for people with chronic health conditions such as human immunodeficiency virus (HIV) infection. Vaccine recommendations may differ based on CD4 count. In addition to vaccines recommended for all adults (COVID-19, flu, and Tdap or Td), make sure you are up-to-date on the following vaccines:
- hepatitis A vaccine
- HBV vaccine
- meningococcal conjugate vaccine (MenACWY)
- pneumococcal vaccine
- shingles vaccine (zoster)

If Your CD4 Count Is 200 (or 15%) or Greater
In addition to the vaccines listed above, you may need the following vaccines:
- **Chickenpox vaccine (varicella).** It is recommended for all adults born in 1980 or later.
- **MMR vaccine.** It is recommended for all adults born in 1957 or later.

You May Need Other Vaccines, Too
You may need other vaccines based on your age or other factors, too. Talk with your doctor to find out which vaccines are recommended for you. This may include the following:
- **HPV vaccine.** It is recommended for all adults up to 26 years of age and for some adults aged 27–45.

LIVER DISEASE
Vaccines You Need
Vaccines are especially critical for people with health conditions such as liver disease. Getting vaccinated is one of the safest ways for you to protect your health, even if you are taking prescription medications for liver disease. In addition to vaccines recommended

for all adults (COVID-19, flu, and Tdap or Td), make sure you are up-to-date on the following vaccines:
- hepatitis A vaccine
- HBV vaccine
- pneumococcal vaccine

You May Need Other Vaccines, Too

You may need other vaccines based on your age or other factors, too. Talk with your doctor to find out which vaccines are recommended for you. These may include the following:
- **Chickenpox vaccine (varicella).** It is recommended for all adults born in 1980 or later.
- **HPV vaccine.** It is recommended for all adults up to 26 years of age and for some adults aged 27–45.
- **MMR vaccine.** It is recommended for all adults born in 1957 or later.
- **Shingles vaccine (zoster).** It is recommended for all adults aged 50 and over.

LUNG DISEASE (INCLUDING ASTHMA OR CHRONIC OBSTRUCTIVE PULMONARY DISEASE)
Vaccines You Need

People with lung disease (including asthma or chronic obstructive pulmonary disease (COPD)) are at higher risk of serious problems, including hospitalization or death, from certain vaccine-preventable diseases. Getting vaccinated is one of the safest ways for you to protect your health, even if you are taking prescription medications for your condition. In addition to vaccines recommended for all adults (COVID-19, flu, and Tdap or Td), make sure you are up-to-date on the pneumococcal vaccine.

You May Need Other Vaccines, Too

You may need other vaccines based on your age or other factors, too. Talk with your doctor to find out which vaccines are recommended for you.

These may include the following:

- **Chickenpox vaccine (varicella).** It is recommended for all adults born in 1980 or later.
- **HBV vaccine.** It is recommended for all adults up to 59 years of age and for some adults aged 60 and over with known risk factors.
- **HPV vaccine.** It is recommended for all adults up to 26 years of age and for some adults aged 27–45.
- **MMR vaccine.** It is recommended for all adults born in 1957 or later.
- **Shingles vaccine (zoster).** It is recommended for all adults aged 50 and over.

END-STAGE RENAL (KIDNEY) DISEASE
Vaccines You Need

Getting vaccinated is one of the safest ways for you to protect your health, even if you are taking prescription medications for end-stage renal (kidney) disease or are on hemodialysis. In addition to vaccines recommended for all adults (COVID-19, flu, and Tdap or Td), make sure you are up-to-date on the following vaccines:

- HBV vaccine
- pneumococcal vaccine

You May Need Other Vaccines, Too

You may need other vaccines based on your age or other factors, too. Talk with your doctor to find out which vaccines are recommended for you. These may include the following:

- **Chickenpox vaccine (varicella).** It is recommended for all adults born in 1980 or later.
- **HPV vaccine.** It is recommended for all adults up to 26 years of age and for some adults aged 27–45.
- **MMR vaccine.** It is recommended for all adults born in 1957 or later.
- **Shingles vaccine (zoster).** It is recommended for all adults aged 50 and over.

WEAKENED IMMUNE SYSTEM (EXCLUDING HIV INFECTION)
Vaccines You Need

Vaccines are especially critical for people with a weakened immune system from diseases such as cancer or patients taking immuno-suppressive drugs. Having a weakened immune system means that it is more difficult to fight off infections or diseases in the body. In addition to vaccines recommended for all adults (COVID-19, flu, and Tdap or Td), adults with weakened immune systems caused by immunocompromising conditions such as cancer should make sure they are up-to-date on the following vaccines:

- Hib vaccine (recommended for adults with complement deficiency, which is a specific type of immune deficiency, and for adults who have received a hematopoietic stem cell transplant (hematopoietic stem cell transplantation, or HSCT, or a bone marrow transplant))
- pneumococcal vaccines (PCV15 or PCV20 and PPSV23)
- meningococcal vaccines (MenACWY and MenB; recommended for adults with complement deficiency, which is a specific type of immune deficiency)
- shingles vaccine (zoster)

You May Need Other Vaccines, Too

You may need other vaccines based on your age or other factors, too. Talk with your doctor to find out which vaccines are recommended for you. These may include the following:

- **HBV vaccine.** It is recommended for all adults up to 59 years of age and for some adults aged 60 and over with known risk factors.
- **HPV vaccine.** It is recommended for all adults up to 26 years of age and for some adults aged 27–45.[1]

---

[1] "What Vaccines Are Recommended for You," Centers for Disease Control and Prevention (CDC), May 19, 2023. Available online. URL: www.cdc.gov/vaccines/adults/rec-vac/index.html. Accessed May 31, 2023.

Chapter 67 |
Recommendations for Travelers with Immune System Disorders

Many chronic illnesses, underlying health conditions, and medicines can weaken a person's immune system, which is called being "immunocompromised." If you are immunocompromised and are planning a trip, take steps to prepare for a safe and healthy trip.

BEFORE YOU START YOUR TRIP
- **Make an appointment with your health-care provider or a travel health specialist**. This should be done at least one month before you leave. They can help you get destination-specific vaccines, medicines, and information. Discussing your health concerns, itinerary, and planned activities with your provider allows them to give more specific advice and recommendations.
- **Make sure you are up-to-date on all of your routine vaccines**. Routine vaccinations protect you from infectious diseases such as measles that can spread quickly in groups of unvaccinated people. Many diseases prevented by routine vaccination are not common in the United States but are still common in other countries.
  - If you are immunocompromised, you can safely get most vaccines recommended for travelers. However,

vaccines may be less effective in people who are immunocompromised.

- Vaccines made from live viruses, such as measles, mumps, and rubella (MMR) and varicella, may not be safe for people who are immunocompromised. Talk to your health-care provider about your options for protecting yourself against these diseases.
- Yellow fever vaccine is a vaccine made from a live virus. People whose immune systems are very weak, such as people with low T cell counts due to human immunodeficiency virus (HIV) infection or people receiving cancer chemotherapy, should not receive the yellow fever vaccine. If there is a risk of yellow fever at your destination, the Centers for Disease Control and Prevention (CDC) recommends delaying your trip until your immune system is healthy enough for you to receive the vaccine. Some countries may require the vaccine, even if there is no risk of yellow fever. If that is the case, ask your health-care provider about a medical waiver for the vaccine.

- **Take recommended medicines as directed**. If your doctor prescribes medicine for you, take the medicine as directed before, during, and after travel. Counterfeit drugs are common in some countries, so only take the medicine that you bring from home and make sure to pack enough for the duration of your trip, plus extra in case of travel delays.
- **Take medicine that prevents malaria**. All travelers should take malaria medication when it is recommended for their destination. However, depending on your condition and the medications you are taking, you may need to avoid some medications that prevent malaria. All travelers should take steps to avoid bugbites.
- **Get travel insurance**. Find out if your health insurance covers medical care abroad. Travelers are usually responsible for paying hospital and other medical

expenses out of pocket at most destinations. Make sure you have a plan to get care overseas in case you need it. Consider buying additional insurance that covers health care and emergency evacuation, especially if you will be traveling to remote areas.

- **Prepare a travel health kit with items you may need**. It is important that the travel kit includes items that may be difficult to find at your destination. Include your prescriptions and over-the-counter (OTC) medicines in your travel health kit and take enough to last your entire trip, plus extra in case of travel delays. Depending on your destination, you may also want to pack a mask, insect repellent, sunscreen (SPF15 or higher), aloe, alcohol-based hand sanitizer, water disinfection tablets, and your health insurance card.

DURING TRAVEL

- **Wash your hands**. Regular handwashing is one of the best ways to remove germs, avoid getting sick, and prevent the spread of germs to others. Wash your hands with soap and water. If soap and water are not available, use a hand sanitizer containing at least 60 percent alcohol.
- **Choose safe food and drink**. Contaminated food or drinks can cause traveler's diarrhea and other diseases and disrupt your travel. Travelers to low- or middle-income destinations are especially at risk. Generally, foods served hot and dry and packaged foods are usually safe to eat. Bottled, canned, and hot drinks are usually safe to drink.
- **Protect yourself from the sun**. Apply sunscreen with SPF15 or higher when traveling. Protecting yourself from the sun is not just for tropical beaches—you can get sunburn even if it is cloudy or cold. You are at the highest risk of ultraviolet (UV) exposure when you are traveling during summer months, near the equator, at high altitudes, or between 10 a.m. and 4 p.m.

AFTER TRAVEL

If you traveled and feel sick, particularly if you have a fever, talk to a health-care provider and tell them about your travel.[1]

HEALTH-CARE RESOURCES FOR TRAVELERS

The following list of resources may help international travelers identify health-care providers and facilities around the world. The CDC does not endorse any particular provider or medical insurance company, and accreditation does not ensure a good outcome.

- The nearest U.S. embassy or consulate can help travelers locate medical services and notify their friends, family, or employer of an emergency. They are available for emergencies 24 hours a day, seven days a week, overseas and in Washington, DC (888-407-4747 or 202-501-4444).
- The U.S. Department of State maintains a list of travel medical and evacuation insurance providers.
- The International Society of Travel Medicine maintains a directory of health-care professionals with expertise in travel medicine in more than 80 countries.
- The International Association for Medical Assistance to Travelers maintains a network of physicians, hospitals, and clinics that have agreed to provide care to members.
- Travel agencies, hotels, and credit card companies may also provide information on local health-care resources.[2]

[1] "Travelers with Weakened Immune Systems," Centers for Disease Control and Prevention (CDC), August 18, 2022. Available online. URL: wwwnc.cdc.gov/travel/page/weakened-immune-systems. Accessed May 25, 2023.
[2] "Getting Health Care during Travel," Centers for Disease Control and Prevention (CDC), October 31, 2022. Available online. URL: wwwnc.cdc.gov/travel/page/health-care-during-travel. Accessed May 25, 2023.

Chapter 68 | **Students with Chronic Illnesses: Guidance for Families, Schools, and Students**

Chronic illnesses affect at least 10–15 percent of American children. Responding to the needs of students with chronic conditions, such as asthma, allergies, diabetes, and epilepsy (also known as "seizure disorders"), in the school setting requires a comprehensive, coordinated, and systematic approach. Students with chronic health conditions can function to their maximum potential if their needs are met. The benefits to students can include better attendance, improved alertness and physical stamina, fewer symptoms, fewer restrictions on participation in physical activities and special activities such as field trips, and fewer medical emergencies. Schools can work together with parents, students, health-care providers, and the community to provide a safe and supportive educational environment for students with chronic illnesses and to ensure that students with chronic illnesses have the same educational opportunities as other students.

FAMILY'S RESPONSIBILITIES
- Notify the school of the student's health management needs and diagnosis when appropriate. Notify schools as early as possible and whenever the student's health needs change.

673

- Provide a written description of the student's health needs at school, including authorizations for medication administration and emergency treatment, signed by the student's health-care provider.
- Participate in the development of a school plan to implement the student's health needs:
  - Meet with the school team to develop a plan to accommodate the student's needs in all school settings.
  - Authorize appropriate exchange of information between school health program staff and the student's personal health-care providers.
  - Communicate significant changes in the student's needs or health status promptly to the appropriate school staff.
- Provide an adequate supply of the student's medication in pharmacy-labeled containers and other supplies to the designated school staff and replace medications and supplies as needed. This supply should remain at school.
- Provide the school with a means of contacting you or another responsible person at all times in case of an emergency or medical problem.
- Educate the student to develop age-appropriate self-care skills.
- Promote good general health, personal care, nutrition, and physical activity.

SCHOOL'S RESPONSIBILITIES

- Identify students with chronic conditions and review their health records as submitted by families and health-care providers.
- Arrange a meeting to discuss health accommodations and educational aids and services that a student may need and to develop a 504 Plan, individualized education program (IEP), or other school plans, as appropriate. The participants should include the family, student (if appropriate), school health staff, 504/IEP coordinator (as applicable), individuals trained to assist the student, and

the teacher who has primary responsibility for the student. Health-care provider input may be provided in person or in writing.

- Provide nondiscriminatory opportunities to students with disabilities. Be knowledgeable about and ensure compliance with applicable federal laws, including the Americans with Disabilities Act (ADA), Individuals with Disabilities Education Act (IDEA), Section 504, and Family Educational Rights and Privacy Act of 1974 (FERPA). Be knowledgeable about any state or local laws or district policies that affect the implementation of students' rights under federal law.
- Clarify the roles and obligations of specific school staff and provide the education and communication systems necessary to ensure that students' health and educational needs are met in a safe and coordinated manner.
- Implement strategies that reduce disruption in the student's school activities, including physical education, recess, offsite events, extracurricular activities, and field trips.
- Communicate with families regularly and, as authorized, with the student's health-care providers.
- Ensure that the student receives prescribed medications in a safe, reliable, and effective manner and has access to needed medication at all times during the school day and at school-related activities.
- Be prepared to handle health needs and emergencies and to ensure that there is a staff member available who is properly trained to administer medications or other immediate care during the school day and at all school-related activities, regardless of time or location.
- Ensure that all staff who interact with the student on a regular basis receive appropriate guidance and training on routine needs, precautions, and emergency actions.
- Provide appropriate health education to students and staff.
- Provide a safe and healthy school environment.
- Ensure that case management is provided as needed.

- Ensure proper recordkeeping, including appropriate measures to both protect confidentiality and share information.
- Promote a supportive learning environment that views students with chronic illnesses the same as other students except to respond to health needs.
- Promote good general health, personal care, nutrition, and physical activity.

STUDENT'S RESPONSIBILITIES

- Notify an adult about concerns and needs in managing his or her symptoms or the school environment.
- Participate in the care and management of his or her health as appropriate to his or her developmental level.[1]

---

[1] "Students with Chronic Illnesses: Guidance for Families, Schools, and Students," National Heart, Lung, and Blood Institute (NHLBI), February 28, 2003. Available online. URL: www.nhlbi.nih.gov/files/docs/public/lung/guidfam.pdf. Accessed May 30, 2023.

Part 9 | Additional Help and Information

Chapter 69 | **Glossary of Terms Related to Immunology**

acquired immunodeficiency syndrome (AIDS): A medical condition where the immune system cannot function properly and protect the body from disease. As a result, the body cannot defend itself against infections (such as pneumonia).

adaptive immune response: Second line of the immune response that is specific to a given foreign molecule or pathogen and leads to an "immuno-logical memory" after the first response to the molecule or pathogen.

Addison disease: A condition that occurs when the adrenal glands (a pair of glands situated on top of the kidneys) fail to secrete enough corticosteroid hormones.

adjuvant: A substance added to a vaccine to enhance the immune response to the antigen, improving the vaccine's effectiveness.

adrenal gland: Gland located on each kidney that secretes hormones regulating metabolism, sexual function, water balance, and stress.

agammaglobulinemia: Congenital or acquired absence of, or extremely low levels of, gamma globulins in the blood.

antigen-presenting cell (APC): Cells, such as dendritic cells, macrophages, and B cells, that process and present antigens to T cells, initiating immune responses.

antigen: A molecule or substance that triggers an immune response by binding to specific receptors on immune cells.

This glossary contains terms excerpted from documents produced by several sources deemed reliable.

antinuclear antibody (ANA): A type of antibody directed against the nuclei of the body's cells. Because these antibodies can be found in the blood of children with lupus and some other rheumatic disorders, testing for them can be useful in diagnosis.

arthritis: A group of diseases affecting the joints. Common symptoms include pain, swelling, and reduced range of motion in the affected joints. Treatment options may include physical therapy or medications to alleviate symptoms.

autoimmune disease: A condition in which the immune system mistakenly attacks and damages healthy tissues in the body, leading to chronic inflammation and various symptoms.

B cells: Also known as "B lymphocytes," these white blood cells play a key role in the adaptive immune response by producing antibodies.

B lymphocyte: A type of lymphocyte. B lymphocytes (B cells) produce antibodies to help the body fight infection.

bacteria: Microscopic organisms composed of a single cell. Some cause disease.

Behçet disease: A condition characterized by sores in the mouth and on the genitals and by inflammation in parts of the eye. In some people, the disease also results in inflammation of the joints, digestive tract, brain, and spinal cord.

bone marrow: Bone marrow transplants are often used to treat blood cancers. Bone marrow is a spongy tissue found inside bones. For a bone marrow transplant, cells are taken from the bone marrow of a donor and put inside a patient to make new blood cells.

C-reactive protein: A protein produced by the body during the process of inflammation. A positive blood test for the protein indicates the presence of inflammation in the body.

celiac disease: A digestive disease that damages the small intestine and interferes with the absorption of nutrients from food. When people with celiac disease eat foods containing gluten, their immune system responds by damaging the small intestine.

cell-mediated immunity: The branch of adaptive immunity involving T cells, which targets intracellular pathogens, infected cells, and abnormal cells.

Glossary of Terms Related to Immunology

complement system: A group of proteins in the blood that enhances the immune response by assisting antibodies in destroying pathogens and promoting inflammation.

Crohn's disease: A chronic medical condition characterized by inflammation of the bowel.

cytokines: Small proteins released by immune cells that regulate the immune response by signaling between cells.

dendritic cells: Specialized antigen-presenting cells that capture, process, and present antigens to T cells, playing a critical role in initiating immune responses.

deoxyribonucleic acid (DNA): The molecule containing the genetic information necessary for cells to divide and produce proteins. DNA carries the code for every inherited characteristic of an organism; see gene.

enzyme: A protein that speeds up chemical reactions in the body.

erythrocyte sedimentation rate (ESR): A blood test that signals the presence of inflammatory disease by measuring the speed at which red blood cells (RBCs) settle to the bottom of a test tube.

fungi: Members of a class of relatively primitive vegetable organisms. They include mushrooms, yeasts, rusts, molds, and smuts.

gene: A hereditary unit that is composed of a sequence of deoxyribonucleic acid (DNA) and occupies a specific position or locus.

granulocyte: A type of white blood cell characterized by the presence of granules in the cytoplasm, including neutrophils, eosinophils, and basophils, involved in immune defense against various pathogens.

Graves disease: An autoimmune disease of the thyroid gland that results in the overproduction of thyroid hormone. This causes such symptoms as nervousness, heat intolerance, heart palpitations, and unexplained weight loss.

Guillain-Barré syndrome (GBS): A rare neurological disease characterized by loss of reflexes and temporary paralysis. Muscle paralysis starts in the feet and legs and moves upward to the arms and hands. Sometimes, paralysis can result in the respiratory muscles causing breathing difficulties.

human leukocyte antigen (HLA): A group of genes that encode proteins responsible for presenting antigens to T cells, contributing to the recognition of self and nonself.

immune evasion: Strategies employed by pathogens or cancer cells to evade or subvert the immune system's detection and elimination mechanisms.

immune response: The coordinated set of cellular and molecular events triggered by the immune system to eliminate pathogens or foreign substances.

immune system: The complex network of cells, tissues, and organs that work together to defend the body against pathogens and foreign substances.

immune tolerance: The ability of the immune system to recognize and tolerate the body's own cells and tissues, preventing autoimmune reactions.

immunity: Protection against disease caused by infectious microorganisms or by other foreign substances. Immunity can be acquired through vaccination, by contracting the disease, or by transfer of antibodies produced by another person or animal.

immunoglobulin A (IgA): A class of immunoglobulin that is the second most common immunoglobulin in blood. It is the main immunoglobulin found in secretions, such as tears, saliva, colostrum, mucous membranes of the intestine, and respiratory and reproductive tracts. IgA provides a local defense against microorganisms as they try to infect mucous membranes.

immunosuppression: The intentional or unintentional suppression of the immune system, often through medication or disease, which can increase susceptibility to infections and other diseases.

immunotherapy: Therapeutic approaches that harness or manipulate the immune system to treat diseases, including cancer, autoimmune disorders, and allergies.

inflammation: A localized immune response characterized by redness, swelling, heat, and pain. Inflammation is an essential part of the immune response but can also contribute to tissue damage.

inflammatory bowel disease (IBD): A general term for any disease characterized by inflammation of the bowel. Examples include colitis and Crohn's disease. Symptoms include abdominal pain, diarrhea, fever, loss of appetite, and weight loss.

keratoconus: A degenerative condition characterized by conical protrusion of the cornea and irregular astigmatism.

lichen planus: A chronic inflammatory condition affecting the skin and mucosal surfaces.

lymphocyte: A type of white blood cell involved in adaptive immune responses, including B cells, T cells, and natural killer (NK) cells.

major histocompatibility complex (MHC): A group of genes that encode proteins on the surface of cells, which are responsible for presenting antigens to T cells and initiating an immune response.

myasthenia gravis: A disease in which the immune system attacks the nerves and muscles in the neck, causing weakness and problems with seeing, chewing, and/or talking.

myocarditis: Inflamed and degenerating muscle tissue of the heart that can cause chest pain and shortness of breath. This can lead to congestive heart failure.

natural killer (NK) cells: White blood cells that can recognize and kill infected or abnormal cells without prior exposure or activation.

opsonization: The process of coating pathogens or other foreign substances with antibodies or complement proteins, facilitating their recognition and engulfment by phagocytes.

pathogen: Any disease-causing microorganism, such as a bacterium or virus.

phagocytes: Cells, such as macrophages and neutrophils, that engulf and destroy pathogens or debris through a process called "phagocytosis."

psoriasis: A chronic skin disease that occurs when cells in the outer layer of the skin reproduce faster than normal and pile up on the skin's surface. This results in scaling and inflammation. An estimated 10–30 percent of people with psoriasis develop an associated arthritis called "psoriatic arthritis."

rheumatoid factor (RF): An antibody that is eventually present in the blood of most people with rheumatoid arthritis. Not all people with rheumatoid arthritis test positive for rheumatoid factor, and some people test positive for rheumatoid factor yet never develop the disease.

sarcoidosis: A disease characterized by granulomas (small growths of blood vessels, cells, and connective tissue) that can lead to problems in the skin, lungs, eyes, joints, and muscles.

scleroderma: An autoimmune disease characterized by abnormal growth of connective tissue in the skin and blood vessels. In more severe forms, connective tissue can build up in the kidneys, lungs, heart, and gastrointestinal tract, leading, in some cases, to organ failure.

severe combined immunodeficiency (SCID): Included in a group of rare, life-threatening disorders caused by at least 15 different single gene defects that result in profound deficiencies in T- and B-lymphocyte function.

Sjögren syndrome: A condition in which the body's immune system attacks the moisture-producing glands, resulting in uncomfortable and sometimes damaging dryness of tissues, particularly those of the eyes and mouth.

spleen: The organ that cleans the blood and makes white blood cells. White blood cells attack bacteria and other foreign cells.

stem cells: Cells made by the bone marrow that can differentiate into different kinds of blood cells as needed by the body.

T cells: T lymphocytes are white blood cells that are crucial for cell-mediated immune responses. They recognize and eliminate infected or abnormal cells directly.

thymus: A gland located in the chest, essential for T cell development and maturation.

type 1 diabetes: A condition in which the immune system destroys insulin-producing cells of the pancreas, resulting in the body's inability to use glucose (blood sugar) for energy. Type 1 diabetes usually occurs in children and young adults.

ulcerative colitis: A disease that causes ulcers in the top layers of the lining of the large intestine. This leads to abdominal pain and diarrhea.

virus: Microorganisms composed of a piece of genetic material—ribonucleic acid (RNA) or deoxyribonucleic acid (DNA)—surrounded by a protein coat. Viruses can reproduce only in living cells.

vitiligo: A disorder in which the immune system destroys pigment-making cells called "melanocytes." This results in white patches of skin on different parts of the body.

x-ray: A type of high-energy radiation. In low doses, x-rays are used to diagnose diseases by making pictures of the inside of the body.

Chapter 70 | **Directory of Organizations Related to Immune Disorders**

GOVERNMENT ORGANIZATIONS THAT PROVIDE INFORMATION ABOUT IMMUNE SYSTEM DISORDERS

Centers for Disease Control and Prevention (CDC)
1600 Clifton Rd.
Atlanta, GA 30329-4027
Toll-Free: 800-232-4636
(800-CDC-INFO)
TTY: 888-232-6348
Website: www.cdc.gov
Email: cdcinfo@cdc.gov

Clinical Center (CC)
10 Center Dr.
Bethesda, MD 20892
Phone: 301-496-4000
Website: clinicalcenter.nih.gov

ClinicalInfo
5601 Fishers Ln., Bldg. 5601 Fl.,
Rm. 2F02
MSC 9840
Rockville, MD 20892
Toll-Free: 800-448-0440
(800-HIV-0440)
Website: https://clinicalinfo.hiv.gov
Email: HIVinfo@NIH.gov

Genetic and Rare Diseases Information Center (GARD)
P.O. Box 8126
Gaithersburg, MD 20898-8126
Toll-Free: 888-205-2311
Website: https://rarediseases.info.nih.gov

About This Chapter: Resources in this chapter were compiled from several sources deemed reliable; all contact information was verified and updated in June 2023.

MedlinePlus

8600 Rockville Pike
Bethesda, MD 20894
Website: https://medlineplus.gov

National Cancer Institute (NCI)

9609 Medical Center Dr.
Rockville, MD 20850
Toll-Free: 800-422-6237
(800-4-CANCER)
Website: www.cancer.gov
Email: NCIinfo@nih.gov

National Center for Complementary and Integrative Health (NCCIH)

9000 Rockville Pike
Bethesda, MD 20892
Toll-Free: 888-644-6226
Website: www.nccih.nih.gov
Email: info@nccih.nih.gov

National Eye Institute (NEI)

31 Center Dr.
MSC 2510
Bethesda, MD 20892
Phone: 301-496-5248
Website: www.nei.nih.gov
Email: 2020@nei.nih.gov

National Heart, Lung, and Blood Institute (NHLBI)

31 Center Dr., Bldg. 31
Bethesda, MD 20892
Toll-Free: 877-645-2448
(877-NHLBI4U)
Website: www.nhlbi.nih.gov
Email: nhlbiinfo@nhlbi.nih.gov

National Human Genome Research Institute (NHGRI)

9000 Rockville Pike, 31 Center Dr.,
Bldg. 31, Rm. 4B09
MSC 2152
Bethesda, MD 20892
Phone: 301-402-0911
Fax: 301-402-2218
Website: www.genome.gov

National Institute of Allergy and Infectious Diseases (NIAID)

5601 Fishers Ln.
MSC 9806
Bethesda, MD 20892
Toll-Free: 866-284-4107
Phone: 301-496-5717
TDD: 800-877-8339
Fax: 301-402-3573
Website: www.niaid.nih.gov
Email: ocpostoffice@niaid.nih.gov

National Institute of Arthritis and Musculoskeletal and Skin Diseases (NIAMS)

1 AMS Cir.
Bethesda, MD 20892-3675
Toll-Free: 877-226-4267
(877-22-NIAMS)
Phone: 301-495-4484
Fax: 301-718-6366
Website: www.niams.nih.gov
Email: NIAMSinfo@mail.nih.gov

National Institute of Diabetes, Digestive, and Kidney Diseases (NIDDK)

9000 Rockville Pike
Bethesda, MD 20892
Toll-Free: 800-860-8747
Website: www.niddk.nih.gov
Email: healthinfo@niddk.nih.gov

National Institute of Environmental Health Sciences (NIEHS)

P.O. Box 12233
MD K3-16
Research Triangle Park, NC 27709
Phone: 919-541-3345
Fax: 919-541-4395
Website: www.niehs.nih.gov
Email: webcenter@niehs.nih.gov

National Institute of General Medical Sciences (NIGMS)

45 Center Dr.
MSC 6200
Bethesda, MD 20892
Phone: 301-496-7301
Website: www.nigms.nih.gov

National Institute of Mental Health (NIMH)

6001 Executive Blvd., Rm. 6200
MSC 9663
Bethesda, MD 20892
Toll-Free: 866-615-6464
Website: www.nimh.nih.gov
Email: nimhinfo@nih.gov

National Institute of Neurological Disorders and Stroke (NINDS)

P.O. Box 5801
Bethesda, MD 20824
Toll-Free: 800-352-9424
Website: www.ninds.nih.gov
Email: braininfo@ninds.nih.gov

National Institutes of Health (NIH)

9000 Rockville Pike
Bethesda, MD 20892
Phone: 301-496-4000
TTY: 301-402-9612
Website: www.nih.gov
Email: olib@od.nih.gov

Office on Women's Health (OWH)

1101 Wootton Pkwy.
Rockville, MD 20852
Toll-Free: 800-994-9662
Phone: 202-690-7650
Fax: 202-205-2631
Website: www.womenshealth.gov

U.S. Department of Health and Human Services (HHS)

200 Independence Ave., S.W.
Washington, DC 20201
Toll-Free: 877-696-6775
Website: www.hhs.gov

U.S. Food and Drug Administration (FDA)

10903 New Hampshire Ave.
Silver Spring, MD 20993-0002
Toll-Free: 888-463-6332
(888-INFO-FDA)
Website: www.fda.gov

PRIVATE ORGANIZATIONS THAT PROVIDE INFORMATION ABOUT IMMUNE SYSTEM DISORDERS

American Academy of Dermatology (AAD)
P.O. Box 1968
Des Plaines, IL 60017
Toll-Free: 888-462-3376
(888-462-DERM)
Phone: 847-240-1280
Fax: 847-240-1859
Website: www.aad.org
Email: mrc@aad.org

Arthritis Foundation
1355 Peachtree St., N.E., Ste. 600
Atlanta, GA 30309
Toll-Free: 800-283-7800
Website: www.arthritis.org
Email: corporate@arthritis.org

Celiac Disease Foundation
20350 Ventura Blvd., Ste. 240
Woodland Hills, CA 91364
Phone: 818-716-1513
Website: https://celiac.org
Email: info@celiac.org

Cleveland Clinic
9500 Euclid Ave.
Cleveland, OH 44195
Toll-Free: 800-223-2273
Phone: 216-444-2200
Website: my.clevelandclinic.org

Crohn's & Colitis Foundation
733 Third Ave., Ste. 510
New York, NY 10017
Toll-Free: 800-932-2423
Website: www.crohnscolitisfoundation.org
Email: info@crohnscolitisfoundation.org

Graves' Disease and Thyroid Foundation
P.O. Box 2793
Rancho Santa Fe, CA 92067
Toll-Free: 877-643-3123
Fax: 877-643-3123
Website: https://gdatf.org
Email: info@gdatf.org

Immune Deficiency Foundation
7550 Teague Rd., Ste. 220
Hanover, MD 21076
Phone: 410-321-6647
Fax: 410-321-9165
Website: https://primaryimmune.org

Lupus Foundation of America, Inc.
2121 K St., N.W., Ste. 200
Washington, DC 20037
Phone: 202-349-1155
Fax: 202-349-1156
Website: www.lupus.org
Email: info@lupus.org

Multiple Sclerosis Foundation (MSF)

6520 N. Andrews Ave.
Fort Lauderdale, FL 33309-2132
Toll-Free: 888-673-6287
(888-MSFOCUS)
Phone: 954-776-6805
Fax: 954-351-0630
Website: https://msfocus.org
Email: support@msfocus.org

Muscular Dystrophy Association (MDA)

161 N. Clark St., Ste. 3550
Chicago, IL 60601
Toll-Free: 800-572-1717
Website: www.mda.org
Email: ResourceCenter@mdausa.org

Myocarditis Foundation

800 Rockmead Dr., Ste. 155
Kingwood, TX 77339
Phone: 281-713-2962
Website: www.myocarditisfoundation.org
Email: info@myocarditisfoundation.org

National Alopecia Areata Foundation (NAAF)

65 Mitchell Blvd., Ste. 200-B
San Rafael, CA 94903
Phone: 415-472-3780
Website: www.naaf.org
Email: info@naaf.org

National Celiac Association (NCA)

20 Pickering St.
Needham, MA 02492
Toll-Free: 888-423-5422
(888-4-CELIAC)
Phone: 617-262-5422
Website: https://nationalceliac.org
Email: info@nationalceliac.org

National Organization for Rare Disorders (NORD)

1900 Crown Colony Dr., Ste. 310
Quincy, MA 02169
Phone: 617-249-7300
Website: www.rarediseases.org

National Psoriasis Foundation® (NPF)

1800 Diagonal Rd., Ste. 360
Alexandria, VA 22314
Toll-Free: 800-723-9166
Phone: 503-244-7404
Fax: 703-842-8105
Website: www.psoriasis.org
Email: getinfo@psoriasis.org

National Scleroderma Foundation

300 Rosewood Dr., Ste. 105
Danvers, MA 01923
Toll-Free: 800-722-4673
(800-722-HOPE)
Phone: 978-463-5843
Fax: 978-777-1313
Website: https://scleroderma.org
Email: info@scleroderma.org

Pfizer Inc.
235 E. 42nd St.
New York, NY 10017
Toll-Free: 800-879-3477
Website: www.pfizer.com

Scleroderma Research Foundation (SRF)
220 Montgomery St., Ste. 484
San Francisco, CA 94104
Toll-Free: 800-441-2873
(800-441-CURE)
Phone: 415-834-9444
Website: https://srfcure.org
Email: info@srfcure.org

Sepsis Alliance
3180 University Ave., Ste. 310
San Diego, CA 92104
Phone: 619-232-0300
Website: www.sepsis.org
Email: info@sepsis.org

Sjögren's Foundation
10701 Parkridge Blvd., Ste. 170
Reston, VA 20191
Phone: 301-530-4420
Fax: 301-530-4415
Website: https://sjogrens.org
Email: info@sjogrens.org

INDEX

INDEX

Page numbers followed by "n" refer to citation information; by "t" indicate tables; and by "f" indicate figures.

Index

Index

H

I

Index

Index